Public health: building innovative practice

Edited by Linda Jones and Jenny Douglas

The Open University

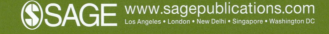
SAGE www.sagepublications.com
Los Angeles • London • New Delhi • Singapore • Washington DC

Published by

SAGE Publications
1 Oliver's Yard
55 City Road
London EC1Y 1SP

in association with

The Open University
Walton Hall
Milton Keynes
MK7 6AA
United Kingdom

First published 2012

Edited, designed and typeset by The Open University.

Printed in the United Kingdom by Bell & Bain Ltd, Glasgow.

A catalogue record for this book is available from the British Library.

Library of Congress Control Number: 2011923905.

ISBN 978-1-4462-0773-4 (hardback)

ISBN 978-1-4462-0774-1 (paperback)

ISBN 978-1-4462-5280-2 (ebook)

1.1

Contents

About the authors

Philippa Bird has conducted public health research in low/middle and high income country contexts. She is currently at the University of York, where her research focuses on the relationship between income inequality and health.

Ian Bowns is a medically qualified public health specialist with over 20 years experience in the NHS, academia and public sector consultancy. He currently runs his own independent consultancy across a range of public health practice and interventions.

Alan Cribb is Director of the Centre for Public Policy Research, King's College London. His work links applied philosophy, sociology and practitioner concerns in health and education. He has published extensively on applied ethics and public health.

Mark Dooris is Director of the Healthy Settings Unit and Reader in Health and Sustainable Development at the University of Central Lancashire. He is currently engaged in coordinating the UK Healthy Cities Network and the English Network of Healthy Universities.

Jenny Douglas is a Senior Lecturer in Health Promotion in the Faculty of Health & Social Care at the Open University. Her research interests include inequalities in health and 'race', gender, ethnicity and health.

Peter Duncan works on the Postgraduate Programmes in Health Promotion and Health and Society, Centre for Public Policy Research, King's College London. His publications include *Critical Perspectives on Health* (2007) and *Values, Ethics and Health Care* (2010).

Linda Finlay is an occupational therapist and integrative psychotherapist. She teaches psychology and is involved in course production with The Open University. She also offers training on the use of qualitative methodology in healthcare research.

Jackie Green is Emeritus Professor of Health Promotion at Leeds Metropolitan University and a former President of the Institute of Health Promotion and Education. Her particular interests include the planning and evaluation of health promotion.

Jenny Griffiths is a moderator with the UK Public Health Register and a Non-Executive Director with the National Institute of Health and Clinical Excellence. After a career in NHS general management, she is now an independent health consultant.

Linda Jones is Professor of Health at The Open University, with research and teaching interests in public health policy and professional development. She has contributed to OU courses in public health, nursing and social care.

Cathy Lloyd is a Senior Lecturer in Health & Social Care at The Open University. She has a particular interest in epidemiology, health care delivery and the impact of long-term conditions.

Angela Scriven has been teaching and researching in the field of health promotion for over 25 years and is currently a Reader in Health Promotion at Brunel University. She has published widely, including nine books.

Moyra Sidell, formerly Senior Lecturer at The Open University, has published in the fields of women's and older people's health and researched end of life care for the Department of Health.

Jane Springett is Professor and Director of the Centre for Health Promotion Studies, University of Alberta, Canada. Previously based in Liverpool, she is known internationally for her participatory evaluation work and co-leads the International Collaboration on Participatory Health Research.

Margaret Whitehead is WH Duncan Professor of Public Health at the University of Liverpool, where she is also Head of the World Health Organization Collaborating Centre for Policy Research on Social Determinants of Health.

Jane Wills is Professor of Health Promotion at London South Bank University. She has written extensively on health promotion and been influential in its development as a field of activity over the past 20 years.

Foreword

As you read this book, we face an array of challenges to public health: from disease, the threat of climate change, and health inequalities within and between nations. The state of our health reflects our physical, social, economic and emotional circumstances. Health is created or destroyed in the places where people live out their everyday lives. Effective public health action is essential if we are to promote and protect health today, and secure that of generations to come.

Public health: building innovative practice responds to these challenges. It takes the reader on a journey, embracing the key knowledge and skills needed to design and build a healthier future. It investigates the two arms of public health – disease prevention and health promotion – recognising the need to support individuals to achieve their maximum potential for health. It acknowledges that health is everybody's business, with all sectors having a part to play as policy makers, suppliers, employers, neighbours, family or friends. Ethical considerations, the public health research base and public health planning are explored.

But theory in the absence of competent practice is not enough. National policy without local action will have limited impact. We have more than sufficient evidence to take effective action on the fundamental determinants of health. Every neighbourhood, district and region has assets and resources on which public health can build. This book recognises that, above all else, public health is about people. People themselves must play a prominent role in the design and delivery of all we do in their name.

The future is not a destination we just travel to; it is something we need to build: a construct born out of evidence-based policy and effective action. At the end of the journey through this book you will have a better understanding of public health. The prospects for a healthier society will be one step closer.

Professor Richard Parish,

Chief Executive of the Royal Society for Public Health and Chair of the National Pharmacy and Public Health Forum

Introduction

Linda Jones and Jenny Douglas

This book is aimed at public health practitioners and at the increasingly large 'wider workforce' in public health, which includes groups ranging from teachers, nurses and housing officers to informal carers and parents. It provides key insights into all the major areas of public health work, including issues that have been relatively neglected in public health until recently, such as ethics, reflective practice and managing change. It is aimed largely at a UK audience and the divergence of national systems is noted. However, it also includes discussion of global trends, challenges and policy responses.

Public health is becoming a multi-professional, multi-sectoral activity that embraces health improvement, prevention, health protection and health promotion. In all UK nations and elsewhere in Europe, steps have been taken to integrate parts of the public health function, so that health improvement and health protection become more effective. This has happened partly through restructuring, for example in the creation of national agencies for health protection or food standards. The latest examples of restructuring in the UK have been the creation of national public health agencies in Wales, Northern Ireland and England and the consolidation of public health within NHS Scotland. There have also been initiatives in all four countries to facilitate joint planning and action between local authorities, public health, primary care, social care and other local stakeholders.

Amid such upheaval, there has been increasing recognition of the challenges that public health practitioners face in working in these new ways. Engaging with communities, building partnerships and planning health action across organisations and localities is difficult work, especially when practitioners are more used to hands-on work with defined groups or discrete interventions to respond to a health 'problem' or government initiative. Yet within both the core and wider workforce, public health practice needs to become more strategic. People working for public health will need negotiating, influencing, boundary-spanning and effective social learning skills to persuade other agencies, businesses and sectors (including the NHS) to give population health and wellbeing a higher priority.

In the UK, there is wide agreement on the core skills, knowledge and understanding needed for public health work. This is evidenced by the

UK Public Health Skills and Careers Framework (2008) and by the 12 standards developed under the auspices of the UK Public Health Register (UKPHR, 2011) for public health practitioners. However, these standards also have much wider relevance because they define key public health competencies for the wider public health workforce. The 2008 Framework indicates that people can be working for public health at a whole range of levels. Even if the wider workforce is focused on only part of the public health function, or bound by other professional standards, understanding how their work fits into the 'bigger picture' of public health can help to build a sense of common purpose and shared identity.

This book also aims to foster a sense of shared identity and common purpose, hence the title: 'Public health: building innovative practice'. It seeks to become part of the solution, enabling anyone with an interest in public health to develop knowledge and gain insights into skills for evidence-based practice. It investigates the wider determinants of health and underlying health inequalities, explores work with communities and alliances with other agencies and sectors, and builds understanding of how to plan, implement and evaluate interventions and influence public health policy. But beyond this, it highlights some core skills: to lead and be part of a team, become a reflective practitioner, engage positively with change, communicate effectively, work ethically and make effective use of theories and ideas.

The 15 chapters that make up this book take the reader on a journey of discovery through contemporary public health. Chapters 1 and 2 explore the scope and nature of public health and of the health challenges facing it. Chapter 1 reviews the changing focus and priorities of public health within the context of approaches to health itself. After all, how we view health and wellbeing will influence what type of public health service is created for us and what priorities are set. Chapter 2 highlights UK and international trends in health and disease. It identifies key global and UK health challenges, including the pervasiveness of social gradients in health. Peeling back the layers, it explores the wider social determinants of health and the generation of inequality. It concludes by identifying priorities for public health action to tackle and reduce health inequalities.

Chapters 3 and 4 build some core skills for public health, skills often assumed to be in place but with which practitioners sometimes struggle. Chapter 3 looks at team building, leading and learning, which are important skills given that much public health work takes place across organisational and sector boundaries. In addition, since restructuring is a continuing feature of public health work, it shares some insights which can help practitioners to 'surf the waves' of change. Chapter 4 focuses on reflective practice. This has recently become a required feature for public health (see Standard 4 of the UKPHR Standards, 2011) but few techniques are taught to help practitioners reflect productively and devise strategies to become more effective.

Chapter 5 encourages the reader to stand back from everyday practice and reflect on the ethics of public health. Some key debates, for example about the proper balance between individual and collective responsibility for health, are, at root, ethical debates sustained by conflicts of value. This chapter engages readers in working through how to address such dilemmas and manage conflict in practice. Chapter 6 also encourages greater reflexivity about practice by exploring key theories in public health and health promotion. It notes their role in conceptualising these fields and the socio-cultural and personal values that underpin them. It considers the role that theories and models can play in enhancing practice.

Chapters 7, 8 and 9 focus on building skills for evidence-based practice. Chapter 7 takes the reader through techniques in statistics and epidemiology that will enable them to understand and manage data with more confidence. Such grounding is vital if the health needs of their service users, communities and populations are to be understood. Chapter 8 focuses on the uses and value of qualitative approaches, noting the importance of reflexivity and triangulation. It investigates the scope for using mixed methodologies in the field of public health to capture its complexity, including techniques such as Health Impact Assessment. Chapter 9 explores the theory and practice of public health planning and evaluation, drawing on research approaches and techniques. It considers how to assess needs, set priorities and determine effective strategies. The chapter introduces a range of tools that can be used for the practical evaluation of health interventions, noting their increasing use in public health and considering their relevance and utility.

Chapter 10 is the first of three chapters exploring aspects of public health practice at the local level. It reassesses the contribution of health education and unpacks some of the key skills that it offers. These include effective communication and influencing skills to engage individuals and communities and support health literacy and empowerment. Communication and social marketing techniques are investigated and evaluated. Chapter 11 focuses on working in localities and community settings, exploring why so much local-level work is 'targeted at' rather than 'working with' communities. It provides examples of new ways of working that combine action with research and enable local people to be full participants in action for their health. Chapter 12 investigates one of the most enduring legacies of the global health promotion movement: the settings approach. From the launch of Healthy Cities in the 1980s, settings have formed a spine of work to enhance health. The chapter provides advice on developing, managing and evaluating a settings-based intervention through a range of case studies.

Chapter 13 analyses partnership at several levels. Partnerships and alliances are seen as an unqualified good in public health but this chapter focuses on unpacking the rhetoric and investigating what lies underneath. It considers what drives partnership work, how far and in what circumstances it can work and what are its limitations. Chapter 14 investigates how policy is conceptualised, made and changed, aiming to educate and energise readers to influence policy development, especially at organisational and local level. It then uses the case study of food policy to explore influences on policymaking and the contested nature of public health policy. Finally, Chapter 15 investigates new challenges for public health, such as climate change and globalisation. It assesses progress, potential and pitfalls in global, regional and national public health development. It reflects on the 'toolbox' of contemporary public health, considers how this needs expanding and sketches out alternative public health futures.

References

Public Health Resource Unit and Skills for Health (2008) *Public Health Skills and Career Framework*, London, Public Health Resource Unit. Available at: www.sph.nhs.uk/sph-files/PHSkills-CareerFramework_Launchdoc_April08.pdf (accessed 27 August 2011).

United Kingdom Public Health Register (UKPHR) (2011) *Public Health Practitioner Assessment and Regulation*, London, UKPHR. Available at: www.publichealthregister.org.uk/ (accessed 31 August 2011).

Chapter 1: Public health in context

Linda Jones

Introduction

Public health is a complex area of activity marked by changing ideals and shifting realities. It is an area of intense debate, not least because it involves political and value judgements about whether, when and how to intervene and limit people's freedom. It is a growing focus of interest not just for professionals but also for the general public, who are encouraged to think of it as 'everybody's business'. It is becoming our business to make 'healthy choices' and to change to 'healthier lifestyles' and it is becoming the business of central and local governments to create social environments in which health can flourish. The public health workforce has a key role to play in both endeavours. But is any of this achievable and, just as important, is it appropriate?

This chapter explores the scope and focus of public health, unpacking its various dimensions and considering the shifting relationships between health, healthcare and public health. It suggests that there are important connections between people's views about health and the types of public health action they are prepared to tolerate. Some important debates are outlined, in particular about the level and focus of public health work and the degree to which it should be concerned with a social change agenda.

1.1 What is public health?

Unravelling 'public health' is not a simple task, yet in its essentials it is clear. A good starting point is Donald Acheson's description of public health as the:

> science and art of preventing disease, prolonging life and promoting health through the organised efforts of society.
>
> (Acheson, 1998, p. 4)

The breadth of Acheson's definition is surprising, encompassing action at all levels and across all sectors. It appeared in his influential report on inequalities in health (1998) and is reflected in subsequent statements by public health bodies such as the Faculty of Public Health, which views public health as encompassing health improvement, health protection and health services quality (Griffiths and Dark, 2006; Faculty of Public Health, 2011). So why has the National Health Service (NHS), which spends 95 per cent of its budget on treating disease and very little on prevention or health promotion, dominated public health for so long? Why has there been so much emphasis on 'prolonging life' rather than focusing on the other aspects that Acheson identifies: 'preventing disease' and 'promoting health'?

With these questions we begin to move into more complex territory, since public health has had a chequered history. It has been bitterly contested: fought over by reformers and traditionalists; claimed by various parts of the health sector as their own; discovered and rediscovered several times; and generally been situated as a marginal player in society. Public health is not just practical, as Acheson makes it sound; it is also charged with ideology, shaped by competing politics and infused with conflicting values. In Section 1.3, we unpick a little of its history in order to understand the dynamics of contemporary public health and its multidisciplinary character. First, however, it is worth considering the scope of activity that Acheson's definition includes.

Before you move on, compare Acheson's definition of public health with your own. What similarities and differences can you see?

Preventing disease

'Preventing disease' embraces active measures to protect populations from infectious diseases, environmental hazards and so on, using legislation, public health regulation and emergency planning procedures. It relies on statistical surveillance at a population level, as do all aspects of public health, to understand disease patterns and potential threats to health and to counter these where possible. It also merges into primary prevention, which involves preventing the onset of disease in a population.

Immunisation is a good example of an intervention that both protects the population and prevents disease at a primary stage. Not everyone who was immunised with the 'swine flu' vaccine would have caught H1N1 influenza in the pandemic which swept through the UK between April and December 2009, but widespread vaccination of at-risk groups probably created a high enough level of immunity to help prevent a more prolonged outbreak (Box 1.1). Note the use of the word 'probably'. We do not always know whether action has been justified because we do not know what might have happened had the action not been taken. Acheson acknowledges this in his characterisation of public health as 'art and science', relying on evidence, experience and judgement.

> **Box 1.1 The 2009 H1N1 'swine flu' pandemic**
>
> H1N1/09 'swine flu' reached the UK in late April 2009 and affected well over half a million people by the end of the year, 360 of whom died. It was declared a pandemic by the World Health Organization (WHO) in June 2009. There were two peaks in the UK: July/August, after which governments approved mass vaccination of at-risk population groups (including pregnant women, frontline health workers and under 5s) and October/ November, after which it subsided. Mass vaccination in England and Wales reached around 40 per cent of an estimated nine million people in at-risk categories, but nearly 60 per cent elsewhere in the UK. The Health Protection Agency coordinated responses using its 2007 Pandemic Plan, monitoring trends, using specialist virus laboratories for diagnosis, building stocks of vaccine and anti-viral drugs and issuing guidance to the NHS and general public.
>
> (Health Protection Agency, 2010)

Prolonging life

The second dimension of Acheson's definition is 'prolonging life'. This focuses on secondary and tertiary prevention (see Table 1.1, page 8), which involves detecting and curing disease at an early stage or slowing down/reversing the effects of an established disease. For example, bowel and cervical cancer screening are well established examples of secondary prevention. Although screening does not prevent disease, it aims to detect disease and treat it at an early stage. However, health services are mainly focused on tertiary prevention in sick people, such as bypass surgery, transplants, hip replacement, medications or interventions to help people manage longer-term conditions like diabetes, stroke or mental health problems. Tertiary prevention, or medical treatment as we should call it, is the most expensive and usually the least efficient form of public health. Increasing quality and efficiency by using guidance on clinical effectiveness produced by the National Institute for Health and Clinical Excellence (NICE), for example, is therefore very important.

Table 1.1 Primary, secondary and tertiary prevention

	Primary prevention	**Secondary prevention**	**Tertiary prevention**
Aim	To prevent the onset of disease	To detect and cure a disease at an early stage before it causes irreversible problems	To minimise the effects, reduce or slow the progress of an already established irreversible disease
Examples	Immunisation No-smoking areas	Cervical cancer screening Stress management	Hip replacement surgery False teeth

Promoting health

'Promoting health' is the third dimension of Acheson's definition and it refers to efforts at an individual, community and population level to improve and enhance people's health and wellbeing. It is the most challenging and problematic part of public health and focuses on improving health by tackling health inequalities and supporting community development and healthy lifestyles. It requires action on the wider determinants of health by improving socioeconomic infrastructure and the health-promoting potential of public policies. It cannot be achieved by public health alone and relies on a coalition of agencies and services.

The boundaries between 'promoting health' and 'preventing disease' are unclear. In the cause of disease prevention, for example, considerable legislation has been passed which regulates air quality, food hygiene and the wearing of seat belts. These can also be viewed as healthy public policy making initiatives. In a similar blurring of boundaries, population surveillance has uncovered deep-rooted health inequalities between social groups and this has led to an increasing emphasis on health improvement as one way of preventing avoidable disease. Thus the agendas of prevention and promotion are brought closer together.

Perhaps the distinguishing feature of 'promoting health' is its commitment to comprehensive intervention to enhance health as a progressive programme. The WHO Ottawa Charter for Health Promotion (1986) embodied this approach with its emphasis on five different dimensions of activity (see Box 1.2).

Box 1.2 Focus of the WHO Ottawa Charter for Health Promotion (1986)

- Build healthy public policy – putting health on the agenda of policy makers in all sectors and at all levels, directing them to be aware of the health consequences of their actions and to accept their responsibilities for health.

- Create supportive environments – systematic assessment of the health impact of a rapidly changing environment … protection of the natural and built environment and the conservation of natural resources.

- Strengthen community action – concrete and effective community action in setting priorities, making decisions, planning strategies and implementing them to achieve better health. At the heart of this process is the empowerment of communities.

- Develop personal skills – health promotion supports personal and social development through providing information, education for health and enhancing life skills.

- Reorient health services – the role of the health sector must move increasingly in a health promotion direction, beyond its responsibility for providing clinical and curative services.

(WHO, 1986)

The Charter situated health promotion as an overtly political and radical area of action, committed to changing priorities in health services, putting health higher on the public policy agenda, creating stronger communities and more healthful environments for people.

It required cooperation with other sectors that influence health – such as housing, transport, planning and retail – and framing policies to protect and enhance people's health. It situated developing 'personal skills', which is often the main focus for governments which want to reduce costs by persuading people into more healthy habits (eating more fruit, taking more exercise, stopping smoking), as one aspect of an agenda that aims for societal change, not as the whole picture. It demanded a focus on the wider influences on people's health – what we term the 'social determinants of health' – rather than just on individual behaviour change. These social determinants, which are explored in

Chapter 2, have been described as 'the causes of the causes' of ill health (Marmot, 2010), encompassing:

> the range of interacting factors that shape health and well-being. These include: material circumstances, the social environment, psychosocial factors, behaviours, and biological factors. In turn, these factors are influenced by social position, itself shaped by education, occupation, income, gender, ethnicity and race. All these influences are affected by the socio-political and cultural and social context in which they sit.
>
> (Marmot, 2010, p. 16)

A shifting focus

In this way, a deceptively simple definition from Acheson uncovers a rich and contested territory that is in continual flux. Table 1.2 indicates the current 'view from the top' as seen by Faculty of Public Health specialists. The headings and ranking of various action areas have changed over time (e.g. inequalities have risen higher) and will probably do so again in the future.

Table 1.2 Domains of public health, 2011

Health protection	Improving services	Health improvement
Infectious diseases	Clinical effectiveness	Inequalities/exclusion
Chemicals and poisons	Efficiency	Education
Radiation	Service planning	Housing
Emergency response	Audit and evaluation	Employment
Environmental health hazards	Clinical governance	Family/community
	Equity	Lifestyle advice Surveillance and monitoring of specific diseases and risk factors

(Source: Faculty of Public Health, 2011)

1.2 Interconnections: health, healthcare and public health

At the core of contemporary public health practice is the view that people have health needs which should be met and the right to a reasonable standard of health. An influential report for the WHO argued that:

> Action on the social determinants of health must involve the whole of government, civil society and local communities, business, global fora and international agencies.
>
> (WHO, 2008, p. 20)

In the UK there is a recognition that, in spite of a national health service, there is still a significant gap between high and low income groups in terms of life expectancy, likelihood of ill health and disability, and experiencing long-term sickness (Figure 1.1, page 12). Interventions to reduce these inequalities in health are now a significant aspect of the work of the public health workforce (see Chapter 2). In parts of the UK, such as Scotland, where there has been a move to enshrine patient rights in legislation (albeit in very general terms), we might anticipate future challenges if inequalities are not reduced (Scottish Government, 2011).

Health as absence of disease and death

This focus on the right to health and the notion of 'health' as a positive state to which we should aspire is of recent origin. In the West, health has been defined and measured much more often in terms of disease and death (Jones, 2000a). The Registrar General began to systematically collect and publish the UK mortality statistics in the 1840s. The statistics revealed huge differences in life expectancy and rates of ill health between professional and manual workers, and between people (especially children) living in inner-city slum housing and those in outer suburbs.

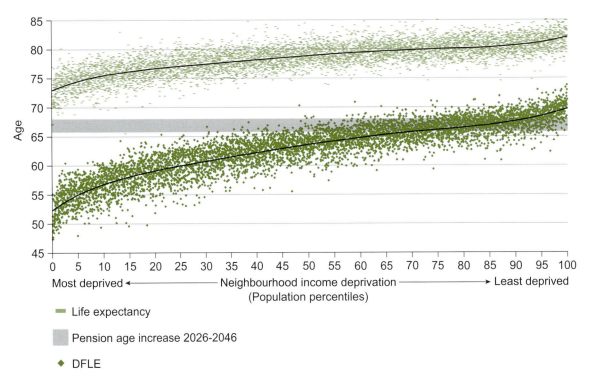

Figure 1.1 Life expectancy and disability-free life expectancy (DFLE) at birth, persons by neighbourhood income level, England, 1999–2003

(Source: Marmot, 2010, p. 17)

While such evidence had a significant impact on public health policy and provided support for the arguments of public health reformers for environmental cleansing of inner cities, the conceptualisation of health as 'not dead' and 'not sick' remained strong. This was reinforced by the growing power of the medical profession, which focused on treating (mainly physical) disease in individual patients. In a classic analysis, Friedson (1975) charted the rise of clinical pathology and the scientific investigation of disease and definition of normality by a growing body of specialist doctors and researchers. Health work emerged as a formal, professionalised area of expertise, in which patients were conceptualised as largely inactive recipients of expert knowledge and intervention. Some key features of what is termed 'the medical' (or 'biomedical') model can be seen in Table 1.3.

Table 1.3 The medical and social models of health compared

Dimension	Medical model	Social model
Definition of health	Predominantly as absence of disease and functional fitness	A 'resource for living' embodying positive health and wellbeing
Primary focus of intervention	Treatment of sick people and those with disabilities in mainly institutional settings: a 'sickness service'	Individual and community capacity; creation of social, economic and physical environment in which ill health is minimised, health is protected and wellbeing is advanced: a 'health service'
Key workforce	Specialist medical and health services	Health practitioners, politicians, organisations, local authorities, communities
Goals	Alleviate suffering or cure people and return them to productive labour	Treat disease and create/sustain health for the whole population through socially just policies; reduce inequalities in health
Explanation of disease and sickness	Biological reductionist framework that emphasises the physical nature of disease	Interrelationship of social structures, culture, social environment, health behaviour, psychological factors and genes; emphasising social nature and social determinants of disease
Focus and methods	Pathogenic, emphasising risk factors, establishing normality and abnormality	Health-ease–dis-ease continuum emphasising whole person, adaptation and 'health despite disease'
Research approach	Scientific method (hypothetico-deductive) emphasising quantitative methods and epidemiology	Scientific method encompassing quantitative and qualitative methods and the inclusion of a 'lay perspective'

Health as a resource for living

A more positive concept of health emerged formally after World War II, when the WHO declared in its constitution that 'health is not merely the absence of disease, but a state of complete physical, mental and social well-being' (WHO, 1946). This idealistic statement conceptualises health as a positive state rather than a state of 'absence of disease' or not being sick. People are viewed not only in physical terms but also in psychological and social terms and all-round health is seen as including wellbeing, a much more slippery and elusive concept.

The WHO had recast health as a goal to be worked towards on a community, national and global level. However, there was recognition that a more focused and detailed definition was required and in 1984 a WHO working group report on health promotion defined health more guardedly as:

> … the extent to which an individual or group is able, on the one hand, to realize aspirations and satisfy needs and on the other hand, to change or cope with the environment. Health is therefore seen as a resource for everyday life, not the objective of living: it is a positive concept emphasizing social and personal resources as well as physical capabilities.
>
> (WHO, 1984, p. 23)

This definition emphasises that health is embedded in the processes and actions of people's everyday lives. It relates health to the ability to cope and adapt within a particular environment. Health is not an object of life but 'a resource for living' and it might be understood in different ways by different individuals and groups. This directs attention to the embedded nature of health as part of the dynamic interaction between individuals and their environment. Above all, it reminds us of the potential contribution to health not just of individual biology and medical services but also of wider determinants in the natural, social, economic, cultural and political environment.

Today, a much wider range of statistics is collected by each UK nation to enable detailed analysis of life expectancy, morbidity and mortality patterns and help guide interventions to prevent or treat disease and improve health. Health economists have developed more positive measures of health (see Box 1.3), such as potential years of life lost (PYLL) and quality-adjusted life years (QALY), which measure people's quality of life in terms of relative freedom from disability and distress as well as years of life added (Bowling, 1991). These measures are explored in Chapter 9.

Box 1.3 **Positive measures of health**

Potential years of life lost (PYLL) – estimates average years someone would have lived if they had not died prematurely.

Disability adjusted life years (DALY) – combines calculation of years of life lost (YLL) with years of good health lost through disability (YLD) to calculate total years lost due to morbidity or premature death. Adopted by the WHO as a measure in 2000.

Quality adjusted life years (QALY) – cost–benefit analysis of the value of an intervention based on the extra number of years of life it is likely to deliver for an individual set against the cost of the procedure.

Disability-free life expectancy (DFLE) – calculates length of time that people in different income groups are likely to live free of disability, thus measuring an aspect of inequality in health.

The Marmot Report, *Fair Society: Healthy Lives* (2010), used a DFLE measure to assess how long people in different income groups could expect to live free of disability. One startling conclusion, as Figure 1.1 shows, is that three-quarters of the population in England 'do not have disability-free lives as long as 68 … the pensionable age to which England is moving' (Marmot, 2010, p. 38).

Lay concepts of health

How far are these definitions and concepts of health shared by ordinary, non-specialist 'lay' people? When people are asked about their health through in-depth studies, as opposed to on-the-spot questionnaires, some of this complex picture of health does emerge (Cox et al., 1987; Stainton-Rogers, 1991; Popay et al., 2003; Blaxter, 2004; Hughner and Klein, 2004). People define health in various ways: as absence of disease, functional capacity, physical fitness, strength and energy. They relate it to healthy habits, ability to cope, psychological wellbeing and taking care of oneself. They attribute health (and disease) to moral standing, religious faith, luck, genetics, government policy and lifestyle. However, in a classic and comprehensive study of the health and lifestyles of 9000 adults in the late 1980s, 37 per cent of all respondents described someone they thought of as healthy in purely negative terms as 'never ill, no disease, never see a doctor', suggesting that absence of disease may retain its power as an image of health (Cox et al., 1987). Interestingly, when the same study asked about people's own health, 54 per cent described it as 'feeling psychologically fit, good, happy, able to cope'.

 How would you define health? Does your definition align with one or more than one of the research findings summarised above?

It seems likely that many of us hold several potentially conflicting views about health, with variation across our life span and by circumstances. Indeed, researchers note considerable differences between people's concepts of health depending on their state of health, age, gender, ethnicity and socioeconomic circumstances (Blaxter, 2004). Views about health and illness are also influenced by cultural change. For example, a survey of women's mental health by Platform 51 (2011) suggested that (scaling up from the study sample) over half of all women in the UK had some type of mental health problem. These findings were influenced by the redefinition of 'mental ill health' to include 'low self-esteem' and 'lack of confidence'. It may be that such findings, in their turn, will begin to redefine people's concepts of 'mental health'.

Discourses about health and their critics

Accounts of health 'weave stories' not only about beliefs but also about practices (Jones, 2000a). In the eighteenth and nineteenth centuries, as scientific medical knowledge developed and challenged older ways of thinking about health, medical power also grew (Foucault, 1973). Doctors exerted increasing control over the human body, creating a whole regulatory framework of observation, diagnosis, categorisation, treatment and segregation. Healthy people became those with 'normal' functioning, as measured within a medically defined range and with no evident pathology. By the early twentieth century, medicine had consolidated its power base within the health field and was able to influence the training of other health professionals, so that medical concepts and practices became generalised and normalised. Foucault (1973) termed this a 'discourse'; that is, a comprehensive way of conceptualising (seeing) and practising (doing) health work.

The medical model in Table 1.3 is still the most powerful discourse about health and one which has defined health quite narrowly, largely as 'absence of disease'. In some ways its approach is quite helpful in everyday life, enabling us to suffer minor complaints – aching feet, a cold, back ache – and still see ourselves as healthy. But it has also led to people with acute and long-term conditions being labelled in terms of their disease, even if they are otherwise healthy. While this has slowly changed, public health and even health promotion (which has long positioned itself as a force for change) are still influenced significantly by the medical model. They attach a high value to research methods drawn from medical science, using medical risk factors such as obesity and targeting 'at risk' groups.

The medical discourse of health has been challenged in several ways, each of which has reconceptualised and 'reframed' health and disease and gradually shifted the focus towards positive health and resilience. For example, research by Antonovsky focused for almost the first time on what kept people healthy. Studying concentration camp survivors, among other groups, he developed the theory of 'salutogenesis'; that is, the origins (genesis) of health (salus) rather than the causes of disease. Antonovsky argued that stress and disruption were unavoidable aspects of life and that most people move back and forth along a health-ease–dis-ease continuum. But ability to cope successfully depended on individuals having acquired what he called 'behavioural immunology'. By this he meant that if, by early adulthood, individuals felt confident that the world had meaning for them and was predictable, that they could cope with challenge and adversity, and that it was worthwhile to respond positively to challenges, then they had gained a certain level of immunity against disruption and despair (Box 1.4).

> **Box 1.4 Components of the 'sense of coherence'**
>
> **'Sense of coherence'** is defined as an orientation in which people feel a sense of:
>
> **Comprehensibility** – the world has meaning for them and is predictable
>
> **Manageability** – the challenge and adversity they face can be managed
>
> **Meaningfulness** – they view it as worthwhile to respond to the challenge and adversity they face
>
> (Antonovsky, 1979)

These three components – comprehensibility, manageability and meaningfulness – together created what Antonovsky called a 'sense of coherence' (1979, 1987, 1993). Even under extreme pressure, this sense of coherence could enable individuals to survive. Ensuring that young adults gained such behavioural immunology could enable them to flourish despite adversity. Helping people and communities to gain a greater sense of coherence could enhance their health.

> The sense of coherence is a global orientation that expresses the extent to which one had a pervasive, enduring though dynamic feeling of confidence that one's internal and external environments are predictable and that there is a high probability that things will work out as well as can reasonably be expected.
>
> (Antonovsky, 1979, p. 123)

More recent studies have explored the theory of salutogenesis and its relevance to various situations and population groups (Eriksson and Lindstrom, 2005; Sidell, 2007). Sidell suggests that it makes a useful framework for exploring older people's health and that thinking about their health in terms of a health-ease–dis-ease continuum is much more meaningful in older age than the binary health/disease divide. She also comments that sense of coherence links strongly to promoting health in communities and groups, as Antonovsky himself claimed.

Antonovsky's measurement scale, which uses a series of questions to assess an individual's 'sense of coherence', has been tested and found valid and reliable in a range of settings and across cultures (Eriksson and Lindstrom, 2005), and its relevance for positive mental health has been indicated. In a contribution to debates about health promotion theory (Eriksson and Lindstrom, 2008), the authors also argue that salutogenesis could provide a theoretical basis for the field of health promotion. They offer a salutogenic interpretation of the Ottawa Charter, highlighting its concern with creating supportive environments, building community action and developing personal skills.

The health-ease–dis-ease continuum has been incorporated into healthcare practice (for example, nursing theory) together with a focus on a 'holistic' approach that treats body, mind and spirit. Healthcare has shifted towards a better appreciation of the complexities of health and illness. Sense of coherence has also been influential and, indeed, has much in common with the concept of 'resilience', which is an emerging area for study in child welfare and health. As Box 1.5 highlights, 'resilience' has been identified as ability to cope in adversity and is linked to protective factors in childhood such as good health, sufficient resources and coping with challenges (Luthar et al., 2000). Taken together, these approaches move us on towards a more complex 'social model of health'.

Box 1.5 The concept of resilience

'Resilience' is defined as a set of protective factors or qualities that:

- enable 'positive adaption' within the context of significant adversity or in spite of serious threats to adaptation or development
- include the 'ability to cope' with uncertainty and recover more successfully from traumatic events or episodes
- may include: good health, lack of vulnerability (e.g. of mental health problems), exposure to some degree of risk in childhood and 'adequate resources'.

(Ungar, 2008; Luthar et al., 2000)

The social model of health

Much has been written about the 'social' (or 'bio-psycho-social') model of health (The Open University, 1992; Jones, 2000a) and it has been developed explicitly and implicitly through the strategic thinking of the WHO (1986, 1997, 2005) and the practical impact of health-promoting initiatives and community projects. It is closely associated with the rise of health promotion and attempts to reorient health services and act on the social causes of ill health through policy, community and environmental action, as Ottawa analysed them (WHO, 1986). In various ways, national and international reports over the last two decades have increasingly adopted the language (if not the imperatives) of the social model of health, viewing health as being influenced by political, social, economic, psychological, cultural and environmental as well as biological factors.

As noted in Section 1.1, these diverse material–structural and behavioural–cultural influences on health have been characterised collectively as social determinants of health (Dahlgren and Whitehead, 1991). In the social model they are not only a key tenet of belief but also an imperative for action. The implication is that many causes of ill health, such as diabetes or heart disease, arise through a set of complex interactions between individuals and their environment. Just looking at one dimension – be it genetic inheritance, behaviour, income, culture or social structure – will not explain health and disease. All of the interactions and causes, immediate and underlying, need to be acted on (Marmot, 2010).

Table 1.3 sets out other major features, including the significance of modern medicine. The social model does not reject but incorporates modern medicine, setting it in a larger landscape populated by other approaches to protecting and improving health. These encompass reducing health inequalities, creating equity in access to health, valuing and including lay people and communities in decision making (Jones, 2000a).

The social model has not survived unchallenged and three distinct sets of criticism have been made about it. First, that it is confused and confusing, used variously to describe a 'philosophical approach', a 'set of guiding principles' and a 'set of practice objectives'. Even in practice it is 'an umbrella concept underneath which several different sets of priorities have sheltered, variously emphasising large-scale statutory intervention, small-scale self-help, lay power and shared lay and professional leadership' (Jones, 2000a, p. 34).

Second, while it purports to be new, replacing the epistemology (ways of seeing and knowing) of the medical model, it is actually a similar expert discourse about the social causes of disease that is analogous to the medical model's concern with biological causes. Instead of blaming viruses or germs, social structures are blamed.

> In the medical model the pathogens are microbes, viruses or malfunctioning cellular reproduction. In the social model they are poor housing, poverty, unemployment and powerlessness. The discourse may be different but the epistemology is the same. The social model is not, in our view, an alternative to the discredited medical model. It is a partner in crime.
>
> (Kelly and Charlton, 1995, p. 82)

Third, the social model of health is characterised by some sociologists as imperialistic, gradually encompassing and regulating the whole of our lives and intruding into private and social life in the name of 'wellness' (Lupton, 1995; O'Brien, 1995).

In addition, it might be criticised for lack of delivery. It has proved much more difficult than health promoters in the 1980s expected to reorient health services, redirect resources to tackle the social determinants of health and systematise policy change and action at community level. This is partly for political reasons: health is not just about health but about politics. But it is also because the tasks themselves are very difficult.

Even when large-scale programmes have been implemented it has proved very difficult to deliver health improvement. The stop–start and short-term character of many community-level interventions and lack of funding for evaluation have also made it difficult to demonstrate what community action can deliver. Governments have been reluctant in many cases to regulate advertising or develop cross-governmental approaches that enable health to be considered in all policies. Instead, significant levels of resource have been directed at persuading individuals to change their behaviour. Consequently, private life has been targeted as O'Brien argued and, in rhetorical terms, health has been equated with healthy behaviours and burgeoning 'wellness' messages from food and leisure industries. For devotees, the main criticism of the social model of health is that they are still waiting for its analysis to be matched by effective action.

1.3 Public health: back to the future?

After a brief ascendency in the later nineteenth and early twentieth centuries, the public health movement and its sanitary reform approach were downgraded in importance by the triumphant march of clinical medicine (see Table 1.4, page 22). This was not because public health had failed; quite the contrary. It had been spectacularly successful in helping to bring down rates of infectious disease, clear away noxious slums, and press for clean water, unadulterated food supplies, adequate drainage and sewage treatment. But it was assumed that public health had delivered most of what it could in terms of health improvement. Any further gains in human health would be made either through continued regulation of housing and environmental hazards (a routine job for local councils and environmental health officers) or through clinical medicine.

Table 1.4 Major phases in the development of UK public health

Phase	Main focus	Characteristic action	Other relevant action
Sanitary reform – early nineteenth to early twentieth century	Populations and infectious diseases: typhoid, cholera, etc. Cleaning up physical environment – belief in 'miasma' (foul air) as cause of disease. Sanitary engineering; quarantine; medical officer (Ministry of Health) role.	1842 Sanitary Report sets out link between environment and health. 1848–1875 Public Health Acts pushed local authorities into cleaning up towns and cities. 1853 Compulsory vaccination for smallpox.	Factory and Mines Acts 1833, 1842, limited female/child labour. Poor Laws and workhouses. Temperance movement. 1866–1869 Contagious Diseases Acts.
Preventive medicine – twentieth century	Personal health and hygiene. Germ theory/medical laboratory science. Surveillance and epidemiology. Ministry of Health remit grew but rivalry with GPs.	1908 Children's Act – medical inspection. 1919 Ministry of Health created. Growing influence of clinical medicine. 1948 NHS established GP primary care role.	1929 Local Government Act; Local health committees lead public health and ex-poor law provision. Welfare legislation, 1940s welfare state.
Community medicine – mid to late twentieth century	Prevention. Behaviour change. Specialist public health advice to NHS and local authorities.	1974 Ministry of Health shift to 'community physician' role in NHS; status reduced. Commissioning for health gain; targets.	1956 Clean Air Act. 1974 Local authorities retain community health services. 1980s Internal market, GP fund-holding.
'New Public Health' (1980s) **Integrated public health? – late twentieth century to present**	Health improvement, protection and healthcare quality. Making healthy choices; tackling inequalities; social determinants. Multidisciplinary teams; Acheson and Wanless Reports recommend stronger public health function. Intersectoral focus.	From late 1980s – national health strategies. 2000s Public health strategies and targets. 1990s Public Health Minister post emerges. 1999 Health Protection Agency. 2009–2012 Dedicated public health agencies in UK nations.	Increasing linkage of social care, healthcare and public health services. 1999 Sure Start. Minimum wage. NHS restructurings. 2013 Local authorities regain responsibility for public health in England.

Public health medicine

Until the 1970s, public health in the UK was led from local authorities (see Table 1.4). Public health physicians focused much attention on re-creating themselves as a specialism to rival other medical specialisms. This defensive approach, although understandable, saw public health recast as 'preventive' and then 'community' medicine, increasingly divorced from its progressive and campaigning roots. After 1974, when public health medicine moved into the NHS, health surveillance and secondary and tertiary prevention became the main focus of activity. Health education – both in its narrow sense of persuading people to change their behaviour and in its broader, more radical approach of working with individuals, groups and communities to enable them to take control over their lives and live in a more healthy way – was increasingly promoted outside public health medicine. Agencies involved included the Health Education Council, the Health Education Authority and the Health Development Agency. They variously fell out of favour with government as they developed more innovative approaches to health education, incorporated health promotion and community change approaches and, in doing so, highlighted the underlying structural causes of unhealthy behaviour.

There are several landmarks in the refocusing of public health medicine into contemporary 'multidisciplinary public health', with its broader vision of public health goals, greater inclusiveness (it opened the register to non-medical public health specialists in 2002) and potential for achieving integration. The publication of *The Black Report on Inequalities in Health* in 1980 was a key moment in raising the consciousness of health professionals and the general public. Over 30 years after the foundation of the NHS, health inequalities were shown to be still marked and widespread across the UK (Townsend and Davidson, 1982).

In the 1980s, the work of WHO and its health promotion teams was also influential in reframing health and health work through the Ottawa Charter and developing initiatives such as Healthy Cities and intersectoral public policy making for health. It helped to prompt the emergence of the New Public Health movement, an alliance of public health practitioners, health promotion specialists, innovative local authorities, activists and climate change scientists (Ashton and Seymour, 1988). New Public Health linked together health and sustainability agendas (as they were being linked at the WHO and on other global stages), emphasising environmental interventions and the social determinants of health. In the late 1990s, having been off the government agenda for nearly two decades, reducing health inequalities re-emerged as a major plank of public health policy in all the UK nations.

 How far does the broad vision of public health emerging here agree with your views about the role of public health in today's society?

Myth and ideology have both played a part in the creation of twenty-first-century multidisciplinary public health: myth, through the discovery of supposed continuity between nineteenth-century public health reformers and the late twentieth-century New Public Health Movement (Sram and Ashton, 2010); ideology, through the (largely unacknowledged) incorporation and adaptation of health promotion analysis, approaches and strategies into aspects of public health practice (Ashton and Seymour, 1988; Wills, 2010). Wills regards this as the squeezing out of health promotion by a more cautious, mainstream and influential public health. It could also be argued that, in some ways, health promotion has at last moved centre stage in public health.

A positive balance sheet?

There is some evidence in all four UK nations that a broader, more progressive vision of public health is emerging. If we use an Ottawa Charter test and consider progress in its five domains – public policy, supportive environments, community action, personal skills and health services – the record looks encouraging. Personal skills remain a strong focus in all four countries, with emerging behaviour change techniques, such as the use of personal trainers, 'motivational interviewing' and 'nudge theory' being deployed to varying degrees alongside more established health-education approaches (Boyce and Robertson, 2008).

The reorientation of health services could be viewed as a 'work in progress' as all UK nations attempt to create a more primary-care-led NHS, focusing on assessing and responding to the needs of local populations. There have been continued efforts to encourage general practitioners to focus more on prevention and health promotion, for example by rewarding them through the 'Quality and Outcomes Framework' from 2004 onwards (Boyce et al., 2010). Since the late 1990s, systematic work on tackling health inequalities across the UK has yielded some positive outcomes, including a fall in the numbers of children living in poverty between 1997 and 2005 (Marmot, 2010).

Public policy has been deployed in the cause of health to create more supportive environments in some areas. There has been some further use of health regulation, notably the bans on smoking in public places, led by Scotland but now effective across the UK. Interdepartmental committees at UK and national levels have made efforts to consider health impacts in policy areas other than health. A range of health promotion inspired initiatives, such as the Healthy Cities and Healthy Schools movements of the last two decades, has delivered tangible health benefits to localities and population groups (see Chapter 12).

Restructuring of public health, most recently in England (Department of Health [DoH], 2010, 2011), is creating stronger links between health, social services and other local authority functions (see Box 1.6, page 26). Scotland has created community health partnerships for joint health and social care planning and commissioning and Wales has linked together the activities of its health boards and local authorities. Northern Ireland already had combined health and social care services.

Greater integration of public health should follow, facilitating joint commissioning of services, pooling of resources, more joined-up delivery and, through these changes, more effective local public health services that create supportive environments. For example, if an urban built environment becomes more safe, convenient and pleasant for walking and cycling, those means of transport may gain in popularity and, in doing so, increase physical activity levels and benefit health. If children's services are better integrated, fewer children will 'slip through the net' and fail to receive the support they need to thrive. Community action should be enhanced by closer working between local authorities and health services, building on existing successful practice funded from statutory and voluntary sectors. The Big Lottery, for example, has funded a wide range of health projects and there is evidence of wide take-up of such activities, although evaluation is not always well funded.

Box 1.6 Organisational arrangements for public health in the UK

Northern Ireland Public Health Agency, established in 2009, is responsible for health and social wellbeing improvement, health protection, public health support to commissioning and policy development and research. It is headed by a chief executive officer, with three directors responsible for broad areas of work and assistant directors managing work streams such as screening and health improvement.

Public Health Wales, established in 2009 as an NHS trust, has four functions: managing services for public health; health protection and health improvement; research, information and communication with the public; population health research and screening. It has a chief executive officer, board and executive directors and provides support to the seven local health boards in Wales.

NHS Health Scotland has a chief executive officer and four directorates: public health sciences focused on information and research programme; design and delivery, focused on topics, sectors/settings and lifestyles work; quality, people and performance, which includes health inequalities work; resource management. Health protection is managed through a separate body: the **Scotland Health Protection Agency**.

Public Health England is planned to take over full responsibilities as an executive agency from 2013, incorporating regional and strategic public health staff, plus bodies such as the Health Protection Agency and specialist Public Health Observatories. It will research, commission, fund and oversee health improvement, provide policy advice and deliver health protection services. Directors of public health and public health services will move into local authorities, which will become responsible for local health improvement and service integration, managed through local health and wellbeing boards.

All national public health bodies are responsible to their national government's minister for health.

Or 'could do much better'?

As yet, much of the evidence of impact remains to be gathered and evaluated. The vision has certainly shifted but the realities of priorities and delivery have changed rather less. The Wanless Report (2004) commented on the history of public health policy in the UK as follows:

> So much is written often covering similar ground ... but rigorous implementation of identified solutions has often been sadly lacking ... There is limited assessment of long-term impact on population health of key policies such as agriculture or the built environment.
>
> (Wanless, 2004, p. 3)

The findings and recommendations of the Marmot Report (2010) bear this out. Focusing largely on England, but with many findings relevant for the UK as a whole, its conclusions are depressingly similar to those of the Black Report. While average life expectancy between 1979 and 2010 increased, inequalities in health remained stubbornly resistant and social class gradients in health were almost as evident in 2010 as they had been in 1980. The progress made in tackling health inequalities, especially child poverty, in the early 2000s slowed down, halted and then went into reverse as the economic crisis gathered pace. The need for joined-up policies which address the wider socioeconomic determinants of health, so strong a feature of the Marmot Report in 2010, are signalled clearly in the Black Report 30 years earlier.

Patchy progress is evident elsewhere as well. There is still a strong adherence to 'behaviour change' and narrow forms of health education, despite evidence that a combination of methods that recognises the complexity of people's health choices is more likely to be successful (NICE, 2007; Boyce and Robertson, 2008). While tobacco regulation has become acceptable across the UK, debates about the regulation of alcohol and food labelling remain strident. For example, the 'responsibility deals' with the food and alcohol industries that the government in England has driven through have been widely criticised. Several major partners, including Alcohol Concern and the Royal College of Physicians, withdrew their support for the 'alcohol deal' on the grounds that a voluntary code with no firm targets or sanctions would allow the drinks industry to continue unchanged (Buck, 2011; and see Chapter 14). Rising rates of obesity-related disease in the UK, along with increasing rates of alcohol-related hospital admissions, indicate that food quality and intake, physical activity levels and alcohol consumption have all become significant public health issues.

General practitioners are still very much focused on clinical work, reluctant to engage in health promotion, and not very cooperative with specialists, other agencies or each other. While responding well to financial stimuli, they are not keen themselves to focus on community-level or population health issues (Boyce et al., 2010; Kennedy, 2011). Meanwhile, spending on acute services across the UK has risen year by year and the financial resources for public health have remained at low levels. In England in 2010–2011, for example, around £4 billion of the £103 billion spend on the NHS was allocated to public health, which represents less than 4 per cent of total health spending (Appleby, 2010).

This snapshot of progress against Ottawa Charter goals suggests that, while there is evidence of progress in some areas, the Wanless (2004) verdict remains justified. The UK is strong on analysis but weaker on delivery. This could be interpreted as a sign and a symptom of the historic dominance of medical public health, with its focus on surveillance and epidemiology, as opposed to health promotion, with its focus on collective, community action and social justice. Alternatively, it could be argued that the persistence of health inequalities over time, in spite of well-intentioned interventions, demonstrates how complex and deep-rooted they are; how bound up with wider society.

1.4 Public health and society

Acheson's definition of public health notes that its achievement depends on the 'organised efforts of society, organisations, public and private, communities and individuals' (1998, p. 4). But who should act? At what level? In which situations? What should its scope and focus be? What type of relationship should exist between public health and the wider society in which it operates? This section notes some of the tensions encountered in working at different levels, stages and types of public health.

Downstream and upstream

Contemporary public health practice focuses on prevention, protection and health improvement. Together, this might be termed 'upstream' work as opposed to 'downstream' clinical medicine. The characterisation of modern medicine as a 'downstream' response to sickness and disease originated with McKinlay (1975) who used the analogy of a river to signify sickness and disease. He argued that health professionals in the USA spent all their time downstream rescuing people from the river of ill health and trying to cure them. This left no time for 'upstream' population health-related activity, which might uncover why so many people were falling into the river in the first place.

In later work, McKinlay and Marceau (2000) focused on tobacco to tease out the tensions between a downstream medical focus and the upstream measures that were needed to halt the disease epidemic. Downstream, health professionals were treating lung cancer patients and trying to persuade individuals to stop smoking whereas upstream, tobacco companies were inducing people to smoke through seductive marketing, reinforcing smoking as normal behaviour and denying and concealing evidence of any negative effects. What was needed was upstream intervention: measures such as taxation, smoke-free zones and regulation of tobacco companies, which could also help to change cultural norms and create a climate in which it was acceptable not to smoke. Public health, they stated, could not divorce itself from the politics and society in which it operated.

> To disregard sociopolitical determinants of health is to relegate public health to prevention and promotion of individual risk behaviors. If public health is to be more successful in the twenty-first century, it must comprehend the magnitude of the forces against it and the strategies used to engineer its defeat. Public health interventions in the new millennium must be appropriate to their sociocultural context.
>
> (McKinlay and Marceau, 2000, p. 49)

This conclusion echoes the one put forward some years earlier in the UK by the epidemiologist Geoffrey Rose, in his classic text on preventive medicine. Rose drew the attention of practitioners to the importance of understanding and finding ways to shift social norms. Arguing that inequalities in health would 'not be much influenced by health education for they reflect the way society is organised', he commented that:

> Social norms rigidly constrain how we live, and individuals who transgress the limits can expect trouble. We may think that our personal life-style represents our own free choice, but that belief is

often mistaken. It is hard to be a non-smoker in a smoking milieu, or vice versa, and it may be impossible to eat very differently from one's family and associates. Social norms set rigid limits on diversity.

(Rose, 1992, p. 56)

Do you think 'downstream' approaches can work, given these wider social influences on health behaviour?

Recent initiatives in behaviour change propose that a downstream approach to changing behaviour is possible, if health messages are subtle enough and incentives are used. 'Nudge theory', which is discussed in Chapter 10, focuses on changing 'choice architecture' to incentivise people to make healthy choices (Thaler and Sunstein, 2008; Halpern, 2011). This might include, for example, encouraging people into last-minute purchases of healthy snacks by moving them to the supermarket checkout area to replace less healthy sweets. Mulgan (2010) reports on pilot interventions in Dundee and Birmingham, where pregnant women were provided with financial incentives in the form of supermarket vouchers if they quit smoking. These had some success, but women in the studies reported that a major reason for quitting was peer support. A key health message about protecting the health of their child was also influential, reflecting the cultural shift the women were making as they recast themselves as 'mothers' with responsibilities for their unborn children (Buck, 2011). This highlights the embedded nature of health decision making and suggests that much behaviour change will involve acting to modify norms and environmental context (House of Lords, 2011). This means moving towards upstream action.

High risk and whole population

In discussing upstream and downstream interventions, we have already begun to consider high-risk and whole-population strategies (Rose, 1992). High-risk strategies identify individuals within a population group who are at higher risk of disease or ill health and offer treatment or programmes aimed at changing their health status and behaviour. In contrast, whole-population strategies focus on interventions aimed at a whole-population group, or in some cases the whole population.

Which focus do you think is most useful – high risk or whole population?

If risk is widely diffused through the population, a whole-population strategy is most appropriate. If risk factors are clearly delineated and confined to particular subgroups, a high-risk strategy may be best. In many cases, whole-population strategies can deliver better outcomes because, although high-risk strategies will help high-risk individuals (if those people can be effectively identified) the overall impact on the disease burden may be low. This is because the much larger population in the middle sectors of the risk distribution curve will generate most of the risk-factor related health problems, even if as individuals they are at lower risk. As Rose stated it:

> The burden of ill health comes more from the many who are exposed to a low inconspicuous risk than from the few who face an obvious problem. This sets a limit to the effectiveness of an individual (high-risk) approach to prevention.
>
> (Rose, 1992, p. 27)

A major British Regional Heart study of 7735 middle-aged men reinforced this view (Emberson et al., 2004). It concluded that if a high-risk multiple drug-based strategy was to have a major impact on cardiovascular disease (CVD), the definition of the high-risk group would need to be extended from 6 per cent to embrace 20 per cent of all middle-aged men. The cost of treating this much bigger high-risk group would then become extremely high. In contrast, a whole-population group approach in which measures were taken to lower cholesterol and systolic blood pressure by 10 per cent across the whole middle-aged male population could reduce the incidence of CVD in middle-aged men by 45 per cent. The authors comment:

> Over one-third of the middle-aged male population without pre-existing CVD would need to be treated with all four drugs to obtain benefits comparable with those following population-wide reductions in blood cholesterol and blood pressure of 10% ... Treating such a large proportion of the 'healthy' population would have considerable financial implications with pharmacological high-risk approaches becoming less cost effective as the absolute risk

threshold is lowered. In comparison, population approaches have been shown to be highly cost effective and more importantly, focus on the determinants of risk factor distributions rather than simply the treatment of risk factors.

(Emberson et al., 2004, pp. 490–91)

A key issue here is determining who should act. In the high-risk approach, the intervention is medical; the treatment is drug therapy-related. In the whole population strategy, by contrast, 'governmental action is likely to be necessary' to reduce total cholesterol and blood pressure levels, 'for instance, through legislation to decrease salt and fat content in processed foods' (p. 491).

Governments in the UK have generally been reluctant to pursue whole-population strategies through legislation or regulation, although in some cases (such as tobacco control or, much earlier, air pollution or seat belt legislation) robust evidence combined with strong lobbying has resulted in such change. Several likely candidates for action exist in food policy (see Chapter 14), including artificial trans-fats in foodstuffs. These are banned in some countries, such as Denmark and parts of the USA (Michels, 2008), but are the subject of voluntary agreements in the UK. This may change if governments are persuaded that the 'obesity epidemic' is as dangerous to health and as intractable as smoking.

Currently, the high-risk approach characterises many public health interventions across the UK. An emphasis on modifying the health behaviour of high-risk individuals is implicit in nudge theory and associated counselling and support services. The use of quality and outcomes frameworks to incentivise general practitioners (GPs) into greater involvement in health promotion could reinforce high-risk approaches, since GPs are only likely to see patients who are already ill and already at high risk.

Socially neutral or social reformers?

The British Regional Heart study raises the question not only of 'Who acts?' but also 'To what end?' Whole-population approaches to cardiovascular disease, for example, would focus on 'the determinants of risk factor distributions rather than simply the treatment of risk factors' (Emberson et al., 2004, p. 409). In other words, interventions aimed at reducing risks for the whole middle-aged male population – such as government regulation of salt and fat content in foodstuffs –

would result in changes to products and production methods, influencing pricing, profits, sourcing and agricultural production more generally. In addition, it would begin to influence public attitudes to salt and fat consumption and perhaps make them less respectable and necessary – social norms might well begin to shift.

In this case, the 'end' in question is socioeconomic reform (of food production) to improve health and prevent disease. Such interventions would benefit the whole population, not just middle-aged men. They can play a part in acting on the causes of ill health because they target and try to modify the socioeconomic, cultural and political infrastructure that shapes and influences health. However, public health work has largely been socially neutral, with a focus on high-risk groups and behaviour change (see Table 1.4). Much of its work has been bound up with clinical interventions, drifting downstream rather than upstream (Hunter et al., 2009).

So should public health be concerned with social reform? The nineteenth-century public health movement certainly thought so. It was highly reformist in its day, persuading governments to legislate and municipal authorities to provide clean water supplies, clear the worst slum housing, and build effective sewage disposal schemes, drainage, municipal housing, street lighting and parks (Jones, 2000b; Sram and Ashton, 2010). A century later, as noted earlier, the Ottawa Charter created a reformist vision for change in the name of health and, in the UK, the New Public Health movement built on the Charter's principles and tried to re-create the spirit and scope of nineteenth-century reform (Ashton and Seymour, 1988).

Alongside this, others developed a blistering critique of individualist approaches, which blame minorities for their own ill health and enable the majority to be socially neutral. In *The Strategy of Preventive Medicine* (1992) Rose argued that:

> The problems of sick minorities are considered as though their existence were independent of the rest of society. Alcoholics, drug addicts, rioters, vandals and criminals, the obese, the handicapped, the mentally ill, the poor, the homeless, the unemployed, and the hungry, whether close at hand or in the Third World – all these are seen as problem groups, different and separate from the rest of their society.

> This position conveniently exonerates the majority from any blame for the deviants, and the remedy can then be to extend charity towards them or to provide special services. This is much less demanding than to admit a need for general or socioeconomic change.
>
> (Rose, 1992, p. 96)

This spirit of social reform is apparent in recent national and international reports on health inequalities. In the WHO's commission report *Closing the Gap in a Generation: Health Equity Through Action on the Social Determinants of Health* (WHO, 2008) health inequality is framed as an issue of social justice. The analysis is very much about reforming the socioeconomic environment to create circumstances in which health can be enjoyed by all. However, some critics have argued that while it is strong on analysis, it is much weaker on recommendations for action (O'Campo et al., 2009; Muntaner et al., 2009).

As noted earlier, *Fair Society, Healthy Lives* (Marmot, 2010) also focuses on socioeconomic inequalities in society and sees these as the underlying causes of inequalities in health. His response to criticisms that an earlier review (WHO, 2008) had produced 'ideology with evidence' was that:

> The same charge could be levelled at the present Review and we accept it gladly. We do have an ideological position: health inequalities that could be avoided by reasonable means are unfair. Putting them right is a matter of social justice. But the evidence matters. Good intentions are not enough.
>
> (Marmot, 2010, p. 3)

It has been unusual in public health to have statements that are quite so social reformist and ideologically charged. In maintaining its credentials as scientific and objective, public health has often projected itself as socially neutral and simply following the evidence. There has been a degree of scepticism about health promotion and its much more overt pursuit of social justice. It is instructive that a report on health inequalities prompted such comment. In this area of public health work, robust evidence and growing consensus about the economic as well as the health consequences of inaction combine to make action more likely.

It remains to be seen how far, and in what ways, the systematic analysis and recommendations for action – such as those proposed in the WHO commission report (WHO, 2008) – become woven into policy across the UK.

Conclusion

In this chapter we have begun to explore the scope and diversity of public health, its political nature and key influences that have shaped its contemporary character. We have noted how the different meanings attached to health can shape views about the relative importance of treating the sick or investing in public health interventions. Some debates have been introduced, such as those between upstream and downstream working, high-risk and whole-population strategies, social neutrality and social reform.

The themes and debates introduced here are developed further in later chapters. For now, it is useful to reflect on where you stand in relation to some of the issues raised. Consider how your own views about health have changed over time and how they influence your approach to public health. Make an initial assessment of your stance on debates about the proper role and function of contemporary public health. Reflect on whether public health is or should become 'everybody's business' in the future.

References

Acheson, D. (1998) *Independent Inquiry into Inequalities in Health*, London, HMSO.

Antonovsky, A. (1979) *Health, Stress and Coping: New Perspectives on Mental and Physical Well-Being*, San Francisco, Jossey-Bass.

Antonovsky, A. (1987) *Unravelling the Mystery of Health*, New York, Wiley.

Antonovsky, A. (1993) 'The sense of coherence as a determinant of health' in Beattie, A. et al. (eds) *Health and Wellbeing: A Reader*, Basingstoke, Macmillan, pp. 202–11.

Appleby, J. (2005) *Independent Review of Health and Social Services Care in Northern Ireland*, Belfast, Department of Health, Social Services and Public Safety, Northern Ireland.

Appleby, J. (2010) 'NHS spending: the numbers keep changing', London, Kings Fund. Available at: www.kingsfund.org.uk/blog/nhs_spending.html (accessed 30 August 2011).

Ashton, J. and Seymour, H. (1988) *The New Public Health*, Milton Keynes, Open University Press.

Blaxter, M. (2004) *Health*, Cambridge, Polity Press.

Bowling, A. (1991) *Measuring Health: A Review of Quality of Life Measurement Scales*, Maidenhead, Open University Press.

Boyce, T. and Robertson, R. (2008) *Commissioning and Behaviour Change: Kicking Bad Habits Final Report*, London, Kings Fund.

Boyce, T., Peckham, S., Hann, A. and Trenholm, S. (2010) *A Pro-active Approach: Health Promotion and Ill-health Prevention*, London, Kings Fund. Available at: www.kingsfund.org.uk/applications/site_search/?term=pro-active +approach+health+promotion&searchreferer_id=0&searchreferer_url=% 2Fapplications%2Fsite_search%2Findex.rm&submit.x=15&submit.y=6 (accessed 8 August 2011).

Buck, D. (2011) *Shove and Nudge: The Tobacco Control Plan and the Responsibility Deal*, London, Kings Fund. Available at: www.kingsfund.org.uk/applications/ site_search/?term=nudge+and+shove&searchreferer_id=0&searchreferer_url= %2Fapplications%2Fsite_search%2Findex.rm&submit.x=5&submit.y=9 (accessed 16 June 2011).

Cox, B.D., Blaxter, M., Buckle, A.L.J., Fenner, N.P., Golding, J.F., Gore, M., Huppert, F.A., Nickson, J., Roth, M., Stark, J., Wadsworth, M.E.J. and Whichelow, M. (1987) *The Health and Lifestyle Survey*, London, Health Promotion Research Trust.

Dahlgren, G. and Whitehead, M. (1991) *Policies and Strategies to Promote Social Equity in Health*, Stockholm, Institute for Future Studies.

Department of Health (DoH) (2010) *Healthy Lives, Healthy People: A Strategy for Public Health in England*, London, HMSO.

Department of Health (DoH) (2011) Healthy Lives, Healthy People, update and way forward, London, HMSO.

Emberson, J., Whinup, P., Morris, M. and Ebrahim, S. (2004) 'Evaluating the impact of population and high risk strategies for the primary prevention of cardiovascular disease', *European Heart Journal*, vol. 25, no. 6, pp. 490–91.

Eriksson, M. and Lindstrom, B. (2005) 'The validity of Antonovsky's sense of coherence scale: a systematic review', *Journal of Epidemiology and Community Health*, vol. 59, pp .460–66.

Eriksson, M. and Lindstrom, B. (2008) 'A salutogenic interpretation of the Ottawa Charter', *Health Promotion International*, vol. 23, no. 2, pp. 190–99.

Faculty of Public Health (2011) 'What is Public Health?'. Available at: www.fph.org.uk/what_is_public_health (accessed 8 August 2011).

Foucault, M. (1973) *The Birth of the Clinic: Archaeology of Medical Perception*, London, Tavistock.

Friedson, E. (1975) *Profession of Medicine*, London, Dodd, Mead and Co.

Griffiths, J. and Dark, P. (2006) *The Future of Public Health: Promoting Health in the NHS*, London, Department of Health.

Halpern, S. (2011) 'Interview with David Halpern: an insight into nudge', *The Psychologist*, vol. 24, no. 6, pp. 432–34.

Health Protection Agency (2010) *Epidemiological Report of Pandemic H1N1 2009 in the UK*, London, Health Protection Agency.

House of Lords Science and Technology Select Committee Report (2011) *Behaviour Change*, House of Lords Paper 179, London, The Stationery Office.

Hughner, R. and Klein, S. (2004) 'Views of health in the lay sector: a complication and review of how individuals think about health', *Health: An Interdisciplinary Journal*, vol. 8, no. 4, pp. 395–422.

Hunter, D., Popay, J., Tannahill, C., Whitehead, M. and Elson, T. (2009) *Learning lessons from the past: shaping a different future*, working committee submission to the Marmot Review. Available at: www.dur.ac.uk/resources/public.health/news/FinalSynthesisedReporttoMarmotReview-WC3subNov09.pdf (accessed 24 August 2011).

Jones, L. (2000a) 'What is health?' in Katz, J., Peberdy, A. and Douglas, J. (eds) *Promoting Health: Knowledge and Practice*, Basingstoke, Macmillan, pp. 18–36.

Jones, L. (2000b) 'Behavioural and environmental influences on health' in Katz, J., Peberdy, A. and Douglas, J. (eds) *Promoting Health: Knowledge and Practice*, Basingstoke, Macmillan, pp. 37–57.

Kelly, M. and Charlton, B. (1995) 'The modern and the post modern in health promotion' in Bunton, R., Nettleton, S. and Burrows, R. (eds) *The Sociology of Health Promotion*, London, Routledge, pp. 78–90.

Kennedy, Sir I. (2011) *The Quality of General Practice in England*, London, Kings Fund.

Lupton, D. (1995) *The Imperative of Health*, London, Sage.

Luthar, S., Cicchetti, D. and Becker, B. (2000) 'The construct of resilience: a critical evaluation and guidelines for future work', *Child Development*, vol. 71, no. 3, pp. 543–62.

Marmot, Sir M. (2010) *Fair Society: Healthy Lives: A Report of the Review of Health Inequalities in England Post-2010*, London, Marmot Review.

McKinlay, J.B. (1975) 'A case for refocusing upstream: the political economy of sickness' in Enelow, A. and Henderson, J.B. (eds) *Behavioral Aspects of Prevention*, Seattle, Washington, American Heart Association, pp. 9–25.

McKinlay, J.B and Marceau, L.D. (2000) 'Upstream healthy public policy: lessons from the battle of tobacco', *International Journal of Health Services*, vol. 30, no. 1, pp. 49–69.

Michels, K.B. (2008) 'The promises and challenges of population strategies of prevention', *International Journal of Epidemiology*, vol. 37, no. 5, pp. 914–16.

Mulgan, G. (2010) *Influencing Public Behaviour to Improve Health and Wellbeing: An Independent Report*, London, The Young Foundation.

Muntaner, L., Sridharan, S., Solar, O. and Benach, J. (2009) 'Community against unjust global distribution of power and money: the report of the WHO Commission on the social determinants of health; global inequality and the future of public health policy', *Health Promotion International*, vol. 30, no. 2, pp. 163–75.

National Institute for Health and Clinical Excellence (NICE) (2007) 'Guidance on behaviour change (PH6)'. Available at: http://guidance.nice.org.uk/PH6 (accessed 9 August 2011).

National Institute for Health and Clinical Excellence (NICE) website. Available at: http://guidance.nice.org.uk (accessed 21 August 2011).

O'Brien, M. (1995) 'Health and lifestyles: a critical mess? Notes on the dedifferentiation of health' in Bunton, R., Nettleton, S. and Burrows, R. (eds) *The Sociology of Health Promotion*, London, Routledge, pp. 90–105.

O'Campo, P., Kirst, M., Shankardass, K. and Lofters, A. (2009) 'Closing the gap in urban inequities', *Journal of Public Health Policy*, vol. 30, pp. 183–88.

Platform 51 (ex-YWCA) (2011) *Women Like Me: Supporting Wellbeing in Women and Girls*, London, Platform 51. Available at: www.platform51.org/downloads/resources/reports/mentalhealthreport.pdf (accessed 9 August 2011).

Popay, J., Bennett, S., Thomas, C., Williams, G., Gatrell, A. and Bostock, L. (2003) 'Beyond "beer, fags, eggs and chips"? Exploring lay understandings of social inequalities in health', *Sociology of Health and Illness*, vol. 25, no. 1, pp. 1–23.

Rose, G. (1992) *The Strategy of Preventive Medicine*, London, Ballière Tindall.

Scottish Government (2011) 'Patients' Rights Act (SP Bill 42) summary'. Available at: www.scottish.parliament.uk/s3/bills/42-PatientRights/ (accessed 8 August 2011).

Sidell, M. (2007) 'Older people's health: applying Antonovsky's salutogenic paradigm' in Douglas, J., Earle, S., Handsley, S., Jones, L., Lloyd, C.E. and Spurr, S. (eds) *A Reader in Promoting Public Health*, London, Sage, pp. 27–32.

Sram, I. and Ashton, J.R. (2010) 'Millennium report to Sir Edwin Chadwick' in Douglas, J., Earle, S., Handsley, S., Jones, L., Lloyd, C.E. and Spurr, S. (eds) *A Reader in Promoting Public Health* (2nd edition), London, Sage, pp. 15–19.

Stainton Rogers, W. (1991) *Explaining Health and Illness: An Exploration of Diversity*, Hemel Hempstead, Harvester Wheatsheaf.

Thaler, R.H. and Sunstein, C. (2008) *Nudge: Improving Decisions about Health, Wellbeing and Happiness*, London, Penguin.

The Open University (1992) K258 *Health and Wellbeing*, Milton Keynes, The Open University.

Townsend, P. and Davidson, N. (1982) *Inequalities in Health: The Black Report*, London, Penguin.

Ungar, M. (2008) 'Resilience across cultures', *British Journal of Social Work*, vol. 38, no. 2, pp. 218–35.

Wanless, Sir D. (2004) *Securing Health for the Whole Population*, London, HMSO.

Wills, J. (2010) 'Health promotion: not drowning but waving?' in Douglas, J., Earle, S., Handsley. S., Jones, L., Lloyd, C.E. and Spurr, S. (eds) *A Reader in Promoting Public Health*, London, Sage, pp. 62–67.

World Health Organization (WHO) (1946) *Preamble to the Constitution of the World Health Organization*, Geneva, WHO.

World Health Organization (WHO) (1984) *Report of the WHO Working Group on Health Promotion*, Geneva, WHO.

World Health Organization (WHO) (1986) *The Ottawa Charter for Health Promotion*, Geneva, WHO.

World Health Organization (WHO) (1997) *The Jakarta Declaration on Health Promotion into the 21st Century*, Geneva, WHO.

World Health Organization (WHO) (2005) *The Bangkok Charter for Health Promotion in a Globalised World*, Bangkok, WHO.

World Health Organization (WHO) (2008) *Closing the Gap in a Generation: Health Equity Through Action on the Social Determinants of Health*, Geneva, WHO.

Chapter 2: The public health challenge

Philippa Bird and Margaret Whitehead

Introduction

The conditions into which people are born, and in which they grow up and live their adult lives, have a powerful influence on how healthy they are and how long they live. In this chapter we begin by considering international and UK trends in mortality and morbidity, identifying that mortality rates are higher and life expectancy is lower among people in deprived circumstances. We then investigate the complex role and interaction of social determinants at all levels in shaping people's health before setting out some key principles for public health action.

2.1 International trends in health and disease

Over the last century there has been a dramatic increase in life expectancy in most countries in the world. Between 1970 and 2009 life expectancy increased significantly (see Figures 2.1a and 2.1b on pages 41 and 42) However, these improvements have not been experienced equally and there are large and growing differences between countries. A child born in Japan is expected to live to 83 years of age. In contrast, a child born in Zambia will live to little over half of this age – life expectancy is currently only 46 years.

Trends in life expectancy

Several countries stand out as having achieved particularly striking improvements in life expectancy, given their level of economic development. In 2009, while Vietnam and India had a similar national income per capita, life expectancy was 11 years higher in Vietnam (75 years) than in India (64 years). In contrast, the United States population had a life expectancy of 79 years, compared with 81 in Sweden and Canada, although the USA had a higher national income per capita.

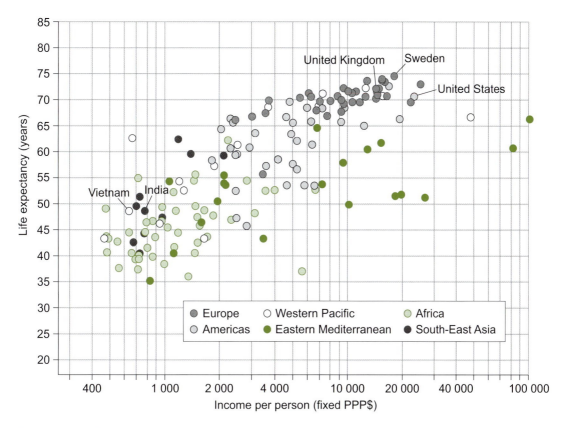

Figure 2.1a Life expectancy in relation to gross national income per capita*,
by country in 1970

* Gross national income per capita is measured using purchasing power
parity (PPP), which adjusts for differences in prices and inflation.

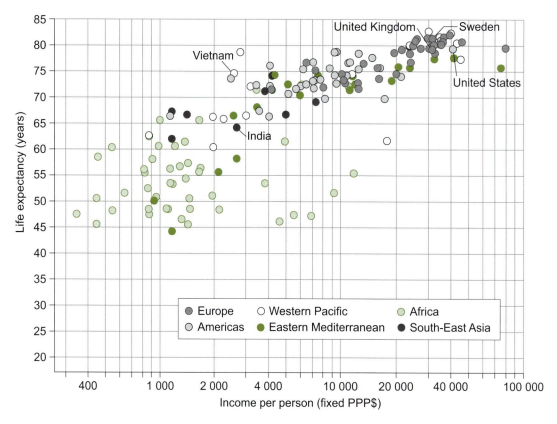

Figure 2.1b Life expectancy in relation to gross national income per capita*, by country in 2009
* Gross national income per capita is measured using purchasing power parity (PPP), which adjusts for differences in prices and inflation.

 In which region, according to Figure 2.1, is life expectancy and personal income lowest?

In southern and eastern Africa, life expectancy is low and has been falling since the 1980s in several countries, largely as a result of the AIDS epidemic and armed conflicts. In South Africa, life expectancy fell to 51 years between 1970 and 2009 and in Lesotho, Zambia, Zimbabwe and Swaziland, it fell to 46 years. In the whole of the African region, people live to only 54 years on average (World Health Organization [WHO], 2011a).

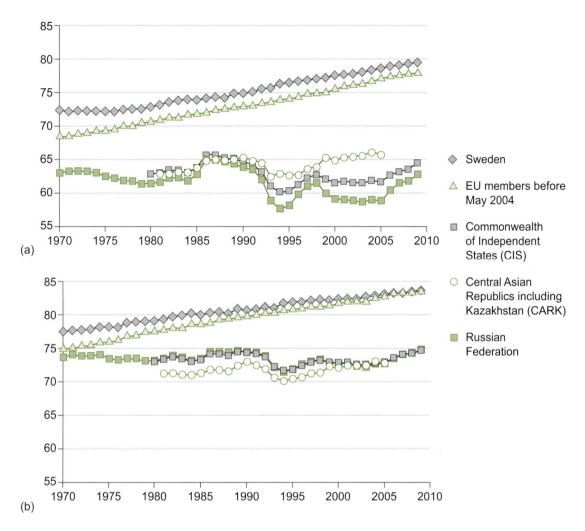

Figure 2.2 European trends in life expectancy at birth, for males (a) and females (b) (1970–2009) (Source: adapted from WHO, 2011b)

Within Europe, several central and eastern European countries have also experienced an unprecedented decline in life expectancy since 1990 – following the break-up of the former Soviet Union – but are now showing signs of recovery (Figure 2.2). In these countries, men in more disadvantaged social groups have been hardest hit. In Europe, male mortality is now 2.7 times as high as female mortality (WHO, 2008a).

The *Global Burden of Disease* study (WHO, 2008a) estimated that of the almost 59 million deaths that occurred worldwide in 2004, 35 million (60 per cent) were due to non-communicable diseases (including ischaemic heart disease, stroke, cancers and diabetes), 18 million (30 per cent) were due to communicable diseases, reproductive or nutritional conditions (including respiratory infections, HIV/AIDS, tuberculosis and diarrhoeal diseases and neonatal conditions) and almost 6 million (10 per cent) were as a result of injuries. The age of death varies considerably. In the African region, almost half of all deaths occur in children under the age of 15, compared with only 1 per cent of deaths in high income countries.

Morbidity and the burden of disease

There are dramatic inequalities between countries in both the prevalence of morbidity and the main causes of ill health. In Europe, the Americas and the Western Pacific, the twentieth century saw falls in infectious and parasitic diseases and a rise in non-communicable diseases. Unipolar depression, ischaemic heart disease and cerebrovascular disease are now leading causes of the burden of disease in these regions (Table 2.1).

Table 2.1 The burden of disease in disability-adjusted life years (DALYs*) by WHO region (2004)

African region	% of DALYs	Region of the Americas	% of DALYs
1 HIV/AIDS	12.4	1 Unipolar depressive disorders	7.5
2 Lower respiratory infections	11.2	2 Violence	4.6
3 Diarrhoeal diseases	8.6	3 Ischaemic heart disease	4.6
4 Malaria	8.2	4 Alcohol use disorders	3.4
5 Neonatal infections and other	3.6	5 Road traffic accidents	3.2
6 Birth asphyxia and birth trauma	3.6	6 Diabetes mellitus	2.9
7 Prematurity and low birth weight	3.0	7 Cerebrovascular disease	2.8
8 Tuberculosis	2.9	8 Lower respiratory infections	2.5
9 Road traffic accidents	1.9	9 Chronic obstructive pulmonary disease	2.2
10 Protein-energy malnutrition	1.9	10 Congenital anomalies	2.1

Eastern Mediterranean region	% of DALYs	European region	% of DALYs
1 Lower respiratory infections	8.5	1 Ischaemic heart disease	11.1
2 Diarrhoeal diseases	5.9	2 Cerebrovascular disease	6.3
3 Ischaemic heart disease	4.3	3 Unipolar depressive disorders	5.6
4 Neonatal infections and other	4.3	4 Alcohol use disorders	3.3
5 Birth asphyxia and birth trauma	3.9	5 Hearing loss, adult onset	2.6
6 Prematurity and low birth weight	3.8	6 Road traffic accidents	2.4
7 Unipolar depressive disorders	3.7	7 Trachea, bronchus, lung cancers	2.2
8 Road traffic accidents	3.6	8 Osteoarthritis	2.1
9 War and conflict	2.7	9 Cirrhosis of the liver	2.0
10 Congenital anomalies	2.6	10 Self-inflicted injuries	2.0

South-East Asia region	% of DALYs	Western Pacific region	% of DALYs
1 Lower respiratory infections	6.4	1 Cerebrovascular disease	6.0
2 Diarrhoeal diseases	5.2	2 Unipolar depressive disorders	5.7
3 Ischaemic heart disease	4.9	3 Chronic obstructive pulmonary disease	4.5
4 Unipolar depressive disorders	4.8	4 Refractive errors	4.0
5 Prematurity and low birth weight	4.1	5 Road traffic accidents	3.6
6 Neonatal infections and other	3.2	6 Alcohol use disorders	3.2
7 Birth asphyxia and birth trauma	3.1	7 Ischaemic heart disease	3.0
8 Tuberculosis	2.8	8 Hearing loss, adult onset	2.6
9 Road traffic accidents	2.5	9 Birth asphyxia and birth trauma	2.1
10 Cerebrovascular disease	2.2	10 Tuberculosis	2.1

* DALYS are used to measure and compare the burden of disease, in terms of healthy years of life lost due to death and living in an unhealthy state due to disease or injury. One DALY equates to the loss of one year of healthy life.

(Source: WHO, 2008a, p. 45)

Non-communicable diseases have also become more prevalent in low- and middle-income countries, and now account for 50 per cent of the burden of disease (WHO, 2008a). In Africa, South-East Asia and the Eastern Mediterranean, the rise in non-communicable diseases has occurred alongside a continued high burden of communicable disease, in particular respiratory infections and diarrhoeal diseases, and HIV/ AIDs in Africa (Table 2.1). This has resulted in poorer countries facing a 'double burden' of disease.

2.2 Social gradients in health

Within countries, people who are less advantaged live shorter lives and suffer more ill health. In other words, there is a social gradient in health and wellbeing. This means that it is not only the poorest whose health is affected; rather people across the rest of the social hierarchy experience worse health than those in the most advantaged social and economic circumstances. Social position refers to a person's place in this social hierarchy. Commonly used indicators of an individual's social position include income, educational level, type of occupation and area of residence. A person's social position influences the degree of exposure to important health risks, such as poverty, nutritional deficiencies, health-damaging behaviours, dangerous working conditions, degree of powerlessness, and so on.

What advantages and drawbacks might there be in using area of residence as an indicator of health risk?

Area-based indicators, such as the unemployment rate within a defined geographic area, can be valuable in assessing health risks. Deprivation indexes which combine several indicators – such as the Townsend Index, Carstairs Index and Index of Multiple Deprivation (IMD) – can provide key insights into the extent of deprivation. These area-based indicators are useful, but it should be remembered that they may suffer from the 'ecological fallacy'; that is, not all people who live in disadvantaged areas are poor – and not all poor people live in disadvantaged areas.

The extent of health inequalities

Although life expectancy in the UK has improved over time, inequalities have remained and slightly increased. In 2001–2006, men in England and Wales with higher managerial and professional occupations lived almost 5 years longer and women from the same occupations lived over 2 years longer than those in routine and manual occupations (Figure 2.3).

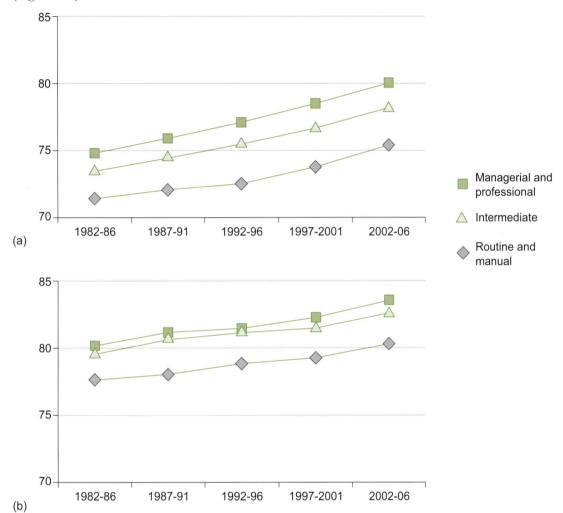

(a)

(b)

Figure 2.3 Life expectancy at birth by social class* among men (a) and women (b) in England and Wales (1982–2006)
* Grouped by condensed Nation Statistics Socio-economic Classification (NS-SeC)

(Source: adapted from Office for National Statistics, 2010)

Inequality is also highlighted in comparisons between areas. In all four countries in 2004–2006 the life expectancy of people living in the 'most deprived' areas was lower than for people living in the 'least deprived' areas. It can be difficult to make direct comparisons between studies due to differences in methods, including the cut-off points for comparison and the size of areas. In Scotland, people living in the 10 per cent most deprived areas had a reduced life expectancy of 13 years for men and 8.6 years for women, compared with the 10 per cent least deprived areas (Scottish Government, 2008). In Northern Ireland, the gap between the most and least deprived 20 per cent of areas was 3.8 years for men and 2.6 years for women (Department of Health, Social Services and Public Safety Northern Ireland [DHSSPSNI], 2007). A particularly striking illustration of the extent of inequality was given by the then UK Minister of Health, Patricia Hewitt, relating it to a journey on the London Underground:

> Travel just eight tube stations from where we are here, in central London, to Canning Town in east London and, for every stop in the Underground, male life expectancy drops by roughly one year.
>
> (Hewitt, 2005)

Such systematic inequalities in health are evident at birth, exist in childhood for some outcomes and persist into adulthood. Evidence on health inequalities is extensive and has described gradients in high-, low- and middle-income countries. In Scotland, for example, 9 per cent of mothers in the most deprived fifth of the population had babies with low birth weight in 2004–2005, compared with only 5 per cent of mothers in the most affluent fifth of the population (Scottish Government, 2008). In England and Wales, infants born in the most deprived 20 per cent of wards are twice as likely to die before the age of 1 than infants born in the least deprived 20 per cent of areas (see Figure 2.4, page 49).

Children living in disadvantaged households are at greater risk of ill health and mortality. In India, children from the poorest fifth of households are almost three times more likely to die before their fifth birthday than those from the richest fifth, and there is a gradient in mortality in the intermediate groups (Houweling and Kunst, 2010). Child height is associated with socioeconomic advantage; at the age of 10 the height gap between children whose mothers had university education and those whose mothers had the lowest education level was 1.7 cm (girls) or 1.4 cm (boys) in England (Howe et al., 2010).

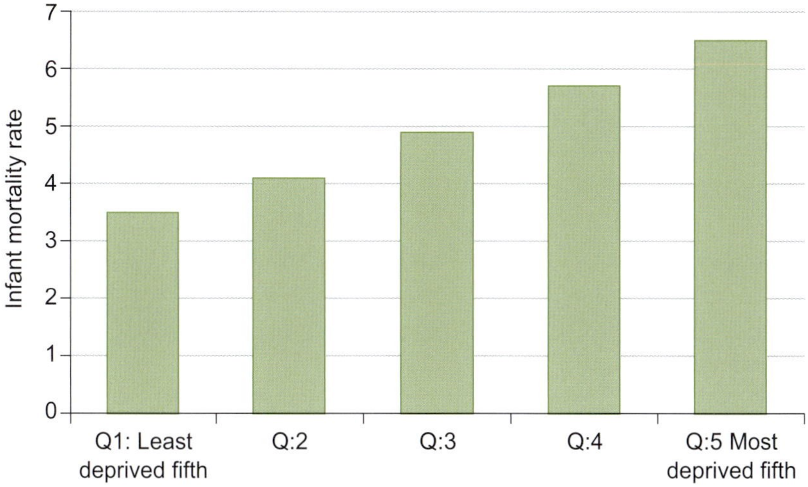

Figure 2.4 Infant mortality rates by area deprivation quintile using the Townsend Index of Material Deprivation, England and Wales (2004–2006)

(Source: adapted from Norman et al., 2008, p. 26)

In adulthood, the social gradient in health continues to be evident. Throughout Europe, lower socioeconomic status groups experience poorer self-assessed health and have higher mortality rates (Mackenbach et al., 2008). There is also a gradient in mental health. In Wales, 27 per cent of people who have never worked or who have experienced long-term unemployment have mental health problems compared with 11 per cent of the employed routine and manual workforce and 7 per cent of those with managerial and professional occupations (Welsh Assembly Government, 2008).

Measuring health inequalities

Health inequalities are often presented as absolute or relative differences between groups. It is important to note that these two measures can give different information about the size and direction of changes in inequalities, as shown in Table 2.2 (page 50). An example of an absolute inequality is the *difference between* the death rate for the most disadvantaged group in a population and the death rate for the population on average. An example of a relative difference is the *ratio between* the death rate for the most disadvantaged group in a population and the death rate for the population on average. If rates of disease are falling in both groups, it is possible for the relative difference to increase, even if the absolute difference stays the same or falls slightly (see Table 2.2). There are advantages and disadvantages to both measures and it is useful to report and consider both.

Table 2.2 Absolute and relative health inequality in England (1995/1997–2002/2003)

Rates and gaps	1995–1997	2002–2003	Change in inequity
Death rate for the 20 per cent most deprived local authorities (in deaths per 100,000 population)	173	129	–
Death rate for England as a whole (in deaths per 100,000 population)	141	103	–
Absolute gap (difference) between disadvantaged and England as a whole (in deaths per 100,000 population)	173–141 = 32	129–103 = 26	Reduction
Relative gap (ratio) between disadvantaged and England as a whole	173/141 = 1.22	129/103 = 1.25	Increase

(Source: adapted from Department of Health [DoH], 2005)

2.3 The social determinants of population health

In order to develop effective responses to promote health and reduce health inequalities, it is important to understand the root causes – or 'determinants' – of population health in general and inequalities in health in particular. Figure 2.5 (page 51) conceptualises the determinants of population health in general as rainbow-like layers of influence. Individuals possess age, sex and other constitutional factors that influence their health but are largely fixed and therefore depicted at the core of the diagram. The surrounding layers of factors that influence health may be modifiable by policy or practice: Layer 1 – the general socioeconomic, cultural and environmental conditions; Layer 2 – the conditions in which people live and work; Layer 3 – people's interactions with their family, peers and community; and Layer 4 – individual lifestyle factors.

What does Figure 2.5 reveal about the determinants of population health?

This model of the determinants of health emphasises interactions between the layers and between factors within the layers. Individual lifestyles are embedded in social networks and communities, and in

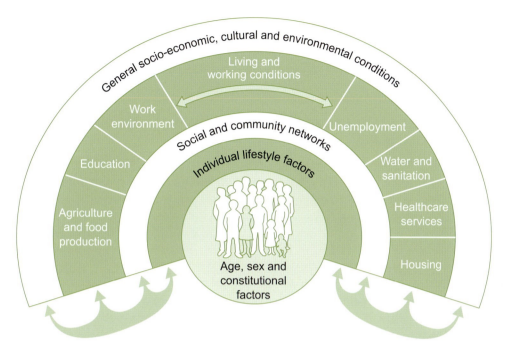

Figure 2.5 The main determinants of health

(Source: Dahlgren and Whitehead, 1993, reproduced in Dahlgren and Whitehead, 2007)

living conditions and working conditions, which in turn are related to the wider socioeconomic and cultural environment (Dahlgren and Whitehead, 2007). Access to effective health services is one of the many diverse determinants of health.

The determinants of health may have a positive or protective effect on health or may be risk factors for ill health. Positive health factors – such as economic and food security, good quality social relationships and adequate housing – contribute to the maintenance of health. Protective factors are ones that eliminate the risk of disease or facilitate resistance to disease. The classic example is immunisation against a variety of diseases, but there are also protective effects of healthy diets and psychosocial factors, such as a sense of purpose and direction in life. In contrast, risk factors or risk conditions, such as smoking or poor-quality housing, increase the likelihood of health problems and diseases that are potentially preventable. The focus of public health and medical research is often on risk factors, although it is also useful to understand the positive and protective factors that enable people to remain healthy even when they are exposed to risks (Dahlgren and

Whitehead, 2007). Positive, protective and risk factors/risk conditions shape people's health throughout their lives. They may have immediate effects on health, or there may be time lags or even effects across generations.

Layer 1: The outer layer of the rainbow – the macro-policy environment

The driving forces that shape the layers of the rainbow and population health are, to a large extent, related to the macro-policy environment (Figure 2.5). This includes the structures and processes that determine the distribution of power and resources.

Over time, the health of populations has improved with the economic development of countries. Yet we noted variation in the life expectancy achieved by countries at the same level of development (Figure 2.1); economic development does not automatically translate to better health. The extent to which the economic resources generated raise the living standards of low income groups and are invested in public systems for health and education determines improvements in health (Anand and Ravallion, 1993). If economic growth primarily increases the income of the groups that are already affluent and public health services are drastically underfunded, then the positive links between economic growth and improved health are reduced or even eliminated (Sen, 2001). Above a certain level of economic growth, there is little relationship between country-level wealth and health. Among these wealthier countries, there is increasing evidence of a relationship between the level of social inequality and health. Countries with more equal income distribution (including Sweden and Norway) tend to have better health, including higher life expectancy and lower infant mortality rates (Wilkinson and Pickett, 2006). Countries with unequal wealth distribution may have worse health due to unhealthy public policies and limited investments in health, education and welfare systems (Lynch et al., 2000), the psychological and social effects of living in an unequal society (Wilkinson and Pickett, 2006) and an increased burden of poverty.

In what ways might poverty influence people's health?

Poverty can be both a determinant of ill health and (particularly in low- and middle-income countries) a consequence of ill health. People who live in relative poverty 'lack the resources to obtain the types of diet, participate in the activities and have the living conditions which are customary, or at least widely encouraged or approved, in societies to which they belong' (Townsend, 1979, p. 31). Living in relative poverty means that you may live in poorer quality housing compared with others and be less able to access essential services. It also means that, in comparison to others, you may have less power to protect your health or feel that you have low status in society. Both of these factors are important for health.

The proportion of people living in poverty in the UK rose during the 1980s. It has since fallen to a level where 17 per cent of the population live with below 60 per cent median income (Department for Work and Pensions, 2011). Living in poverty is particularly harmful to children, in terms of both their current health and development and their long-term socioeconomic and health prospects. Children in the UK are more likely to live in poverty than in any other country in the Organisation for Economic Co-operation and Development (OECD), except for the United States (UNICEF, 2007). While all UK nations made progress in reducing relative child poverty up until 2005, the downward trend faltered with the onset of recession. In England in 2009–2010, 2.6 million children (20 per cent of all children) were still living in poverty before housing costs (Department for Work and Pensions, 2011).

The tax and benefit system in a country can have a profound impact on the prevalence and depth of poverty experienced by different groups in the population. Figure 2.6 (page 54), shows similar poverty levels in Sweden and selected European countries compared with the United States, before transfers through the respective tax and benefit systems. Once transfers have taken place, however, poverty is reduced in all countries, but to a much greater degree in Sweden and the UK than in the United States and Spain. This shows that national governments can, and do, have a great influence on poverty within their borders, through the fiscal and social protection levers they have at their disposal.

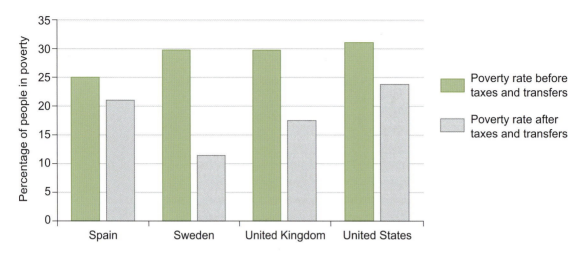

Figure 2.6 Proportion of people in relative poverty (below 60 per cent median income) before and after taxes and transfers, selected countries in the mid 2000s
(Source: adapted from OECD, 2008)

Layer 2: Living and working conditions

Developments in Europe over the past century have shown how population health can be promoted by improvements in living and working conditions, and access to essential goods and services such as safe and affordable food, education and healthcare. Actions on this layer of determinants have been very important historically, and there are strong social gradients in these factors.

The conditions of early life have a close association with child health and lay the foundations for health later in life. For example, children who grow up in disadvantaged circumstances are at greater risk of premature mortality in adulthood, including due to coronary heart disease and stroke (Galobardes et al., 2008). Early childhood is an important period for social, cognitive and physical development, as well as for the development of behaviours and lifestyles. The conditions of early life influence child development, with direct influences on health. They also have a powerful influence on adult socioeconomic position, with an indirect effect on adult health.

Pregnancy has been identified as a critical period for child development. Poor foetal development as a result of poor nutrition during pregnancy or maternal stress is a risk for ill health later in life, including diabetes risk (Barker, 1998). In the first years of life, children need to grow up in environments that are safe, caring and healthy. In the first years of life, children acquire psychological and social skills particularly fast and missing out on the development of these skills can have long-term effects on health (Kuh and Hardy, 2002). Pre-school schemes and education play an important role; education is one of the most important links between child socioeconomic circumstances and adult health (Galobardes et al., 2008). Ensuring good quality and equitable schooling and improving educational achievement among disadvantaged children would improve their pathways into adult circumstances and health.

The work environment has long been recognised as an important influence on health. In England today, over two million people suffer from illnesses that they believe are caused or made worse by their current or past work, and occupational injury and illness causes the loss of over 28 million working days each year (Health and Safety Executive, 2010).

Although there have been significant improvements in physical working conditions in many European countries, there is growing evidence of social and psychological issues in the workplace and their health impacts. People who have a lower social status, do monotonous work, have inadequate social support and have financial worries experience psychosocial stress (Brunner and Marmot, 2006). Numerous studies have demonstrated that a high level of demand with little control at work, or high effort and low reward, are important risk factors for poor health (Karasek et al., 1988; Marmot et al., 1997).

Health services are essential for people to maintain good health. However, there continue to be inequalities in access to healthcare, the quality of healthcare received and the social and economic impacts of accessing healthcare.

Layer 3: Social and community relationships

There has been growing interest in the role of social and community relationships, social capital and social cohesion for health. At the individual level, there is good evidence that having supporting relationships and being part of social networks is good for health, and being socially isolated puts people at increased risk of premature death (Berkman and Glass, 2000). At the population level, the term 'social capital' refers to the 'quality and quantity of social interactions and social institutions' in populations or areas (McKenzie et al., 2002, p. 280). Despite difficulties in definitions and measurement (Baum, 1999), there is some evidence that social capital has health benefits, including mental health (McKenzie et al., 2002), although findings have been inconsistent. However, there remains considerable debate on the relative importance of these factors (Wilkinson and Pickett, 2006; Lynch et al., 2000). Furthermore, the potential dangers of focusing on social cohesion have also been raised. There is concern that disadvantaged groups could be 'victim blamed' for bringing about their own poor health due to a lack of social networks and cohesion (Lynch et al., 2000).

Layer 4: Lifestyle factors

Individual lifestyle factors – such as smoking, diet and physical activity – are shaped by the outer layers of the rainbow and, in turn, affect health. Many of these factors are particularly important in light of the growing burden of non-communicable disease in high, low and middle income countries. Much of the research has focused on adult lifestyles, although there is growing concern about the development of unhealthy lifestyles in childhood and adolescence, which may persevere into adulthood.

What factors do you think shape people's behaviours and lifestyle choices?

Personal behaviours are shaped by wider determinants of health. We need to understand the social circumstances that lead to unhealthy behaviours; that is, why people behave the way they do. This is sometimes termed understanding 'the causes of the causes'. However, while differences in behaviours between different social groups may contribute to the observed inequalities in health between social groups, they do not completely explain them. Even after taking behaviours such as smoking into account, there remains an unexplained gradient in ill health, such as coronary heart disease and child health, which raises questions about underlying causes (Marmot et al., 1978; Dowd, 2007). Both of these issues show that policy and practice responses need to tackle health behaviours in combination with action on other determinants of health in order to build supportive environments for behaviour change.

Smoking can be taken as an example. Every year, an estimated five million deaths worldwide are caused by tobacco use or second-hand smoke (WHO, 2009). In the UK, the prevalence of smoking has been falling since the 1970s and has now levelled out. The fall in smoking has not been uniform across the population, and has been slower among women and disadvantaged groups (Graham et al., 2006). In other countries in northern Europe smoking has a similar negative gradient. However, there is some evidence that the opposite pattern exists in countries in southern Europe, with higher smoking rates among more advantaged groups, likely to be related to the stage of the smoking epidemic (Cavelaars et al., 2000). Smoking prevalence is increasing in low and middle income countries, with poor men most likely to smoke (Hosseinpoor et al., 2011). Although smoking-related mortality rates are currently lower than in high income countries, they are likely to rise over the coming decades as a result of the time lag in health effects (WHO, 2009).

In order to understand inequalities in smoking, it is necessary to consider the wider determinants of smoking. People living in disadvantaged circumstances are more likely to start smoking and less likely to be able to quit. Table 2.3 shows the effects of cumulative deprivation throughout the life course on smoking. Each additional type of disadvantage is associated with a greater chance of having ever smoked and a decreased likelihood of having quit smoking. Action to tackle smoking needs to recognise such contextual constraints on people's behaviours and lifestyles, and address the poverty and disadvantage of affected groups, not just the smoking behaviour (Graham et al., 2006).

Table 2.3 Disadvantaged trajectories and smoking status of women aged 22–34, England (1998–2002)

	Number	Ever smoked (%)	Former smoker (as % of ever smokers)
Whole sample	9936	45.6	34.6
Sample with:			
childhood disadvantage	3800	51.6	30.4
plus left full-time education ≤16	2081	61.0	27.7
plus a mother <22	744	70.3	22.4
plus adult disadvantage	405	75.6	17.3
none of these	3614	33.3	45.1

(Source: adapted from Graham et al., 2006)

2.4 How do the social determinants generate social inequalities in health?

The social determinants described above shape everyone's health, but diverse experiences of these determinants by different groups in society give rise to health inequalities. Five pathways between the determinants of health and the generation of health inequalities have been put forward (Dahlgren and Whitehead, 2007). These pathways summarise how people's experiences differ according to their social position. The effects of these pathways accumulate to generate and perpetuate health inequalities. The pathways are summarised below (adapted from Dahlgren and Whitehead, 2007).

Pathway 1: Different levels of power and resources

Groups that are better off in terms of education, income or occupation typically have more power and opportunities to live a healthy life than those who are disadvantaged. First, people in less advantaged groups lack the power to avoid exposure to unhealthy living and working conditions (outlined in pathway 2 below). Second, socioeconomic position can also have direct psychological effects on health in its own right, having a 'huge impact on whether people feel valued, appreciated and needed or on the other hand looked down on, treated as insignificant, disrespected, stigmatised and humiliated' (Wilkinson, 2005, p. 26). These psychological effects can influence health directly through the endocrine and immune systems, and influence the development and persistence of unhealthy behaviours. Thus, efforts to reduce differences in power and resources, for example through reducing inequalities in educational attainment and income, are likely to have a positive effect on health inequalities.

Pathway 2: Different levels of exposure to health hazards

Exposure to almost all risk factors is inversely related to social position – that is, the lower the social position, the greater the exposure to different material, psychosocial and behavioural risks. While some risk factors may be relatively unimportant for the overall health of the population, they may play a larger role in explaining health inequalities. For example, a French report showed that work-related risk factors accounted for only 5 per cent of cancers in the whole population, but accounted for 20 per cent among people in manual occupations (Haut Comité de la Santé Publique, 1998). It is therefore important to identify the most important risk factors for each group in society in a particular country in order to tackle inequalities. It is also important to understand why there is a social gradient in risk factors, in order to address the root causes. This is likely to require action across the levels of the social determinants, addressing unequal exposure to risks through living and working conditions and social and community factors, but also considering behavioural factors and the general socioeconomic conditions.

Pathway 3: The same level of exposure leading to differential impacts

In some cases, the same level of exposure may have different effects on different socioeconomic groups. For example, prolonged stress may suppress the immune system, increasing susceptibility to and severity of respiratory infections (Brunner, 1997). Health inequalities are shaped by the combined, interrelated effects of multiple factors. Risk factors such as low income, stress and poor housing may reinforce each other, or be moderated by protective or promotive factors such as social support or access to healthcare. The focus for action should therefore include people's wider social, economic and cultural environments, as well as individual risk factors. Risk factors tend to cluster together, for example a person with low income is likely to live in poor-quality housing and more likely to smoke or have family members who smoke. Interventions therefore need to identify appropriate entry points to reduce their reinforcing effects on health inequalities.

Pathway 4: Different social and economic effects of being sick

Being in poor health may lead to loss of earnings or social isolation. There is evidence that people in high socioeconomic groups are more likely to keep their jobs if they become ill, in comparison with people in lower socioeconomic groups (Lindholm et al., 2002). Childhood ill health may affect education and lifelong socioeconomic prospects. At the same time, sick people may face additional financial costs from accessing healthcare. Together, these could result in downward social drift of unhealthy individuals. There is some evidence that chronic illness, including mental illness, may lead to social drift into lower socioeconomic groups. In the UK, socioeconomic disadvantage mostly occurs before poor health (Blane et al., 1993). However, in countries where the costs of healthcare are high and welfare safety nets are less comprehensive, as is the case in many low- and middle-income countries, the financial burden of ill health can lead to households falling into poverty – the 'medical poverty trap' (Whitehead et al., 2001). Policy and practice implications include the need to improve financial and social support systems and effective rehabilitation for people who suffer ill health.

Pathway 5: Life course effects

The pathways identified above operate throughout the life course. Experiences and circumstances at different times in the life course affect health later in life and even across generations (Kuh et al., 2003). Social position in childhood has been shown to affect mortality in adulthood, independently of adult socioeconomic position (Galobardes et al., 2008). There is evidence of critical periods, in which people are particularly susceptible to risks, with long-term effects on health.

 What do you think might be a critical period of health risk, based on your reading so far in this chapter?

We noted foetal development as being a critical period in the life course. Poor foetal growth has been shown to be associated with coronary heart disease, stroke, diabetes and respiratory disease in adulthood (Barker, 1998). Poor foetal growth has a social gradient (Spencer and Logan, 2002), so this is likely to contribute to adult health inequalities. Risks (or protective or promotive factors) may accumulate throughout the lifetime or trigger chains of risk, in which one exposure leads to another in a chain. Effects may be passed from parents to children. Understanding of life-course effects informs both how and when to intervene to tackle inequalities. Recognition of critical periods, accumulation and chains of risk allows the development of interventions targeted at the key points in the life course, in particular interventions during pregnancy or childhood, to reduce the risk of ill health later in life.

2.5 Taking action on health inequalities

Building national and international consensus

Over the past 30 years, there has been a series of landmark inquiries into the causes of and solutions to social inequalities in health, starting with the seminal Black Report of 1980 (Black et al., 1980), through to the Acheson Inquiry of the 1990s (Acheson et al., 1998) in the UK, and the more recent WHO Global Commission on Social Determinants of Health (WHO, 2008b) and the Strategic Review of Health Inequalities in England Post-2010 (Marmot, 2010). They all come to similar conclusions:

- the reduction of health inequalities is a matter of fairness and social justice
- they result from social inequalities in society ultimately caused by 'bad politics' and inequalities in power
- to reduce health inequalities therefore requires action on inequalities in wider social determinants operating outside the health system;
- there is a need to tackle ill health across the whole social gradient in health, not solely concentrate on reducing the gap between the most disadvantaged and others, if the goal is to make an impact on the observed health inequalities.

(Whitehead and Popay, 2010, p. 1234)

Given this analysis, what are the key priority areas for action?

The reports reach a consensus on common remedies and priority groups. Based on the best available evidence, they seek to:

- give a high priority to providing all children with a better start in life
- take steps to improve the living standards of poorer households
- improve conditions of daily life, including housing and working conditions and fair employment
- redress the balance of healthcare systems towards prevention, primary care and community health
- tackle the inequitable distribution of power, money and resources
- develop an evaluation and monitoring system that assesses all policies likely to have an impact on health for their impact on health inequalities.

Although the Black Report of 1980 did not have the benefit of the much greater accumulation of evidence over subsequent years, it was sufficiently far-sighted to identify the crux of the matter: tackling the social determinants of health. It is unfortunate that over 30 years later the message is still largely falling on deaf ears – although there are signs of an emerging understanding globally that something needs to be done.

Implications for public health action

The concepts of the wider determinants of health and pathways to health inequalities imply a number of principles for action to reduce health inequalities from the perspective of public health practitioners working at the national or local level. Eight principles for public health action are set out below (adapted from Whitehead and Dahlgren, 2007).

Principle 1: Policies and interventions should strive to level up

The fact that people with lower levels of power and resources experience poorer health is unfair. Action to improve the health of those who are less advantaged to the level enjoyed by the most advantaged group is needed as 'a matter of fairness and social justice' (Marmot, 2010, p. 15). Differences in the magnitude of health inequalities between countries suggest that reductions in health inequalities are feasible. Levelling-down the healthiest to the level of the least healthy would be inequitable and is not an option.

Principle 2: Action should focus on levelling up the gradient as well as closing the gap

Many policies to reduce inequalities have focused on closing the gap between the worst off and either the best off group or the population average. This approach targets interventions at the least healthy groups, with the aim of improving their health at a faster rate than the rest of the population. This is an important step to reducing inequalities, but targeting the worst off alone is not sufficient to tackle the social gradient in health. Alternatively, approaches to reduce the social gradient seek to improve the health of the whole population, including middle-income groups, to the level enjoyed by the best off.

In practice, a combination of both approaches is required. The *Strategic Review of Health Inequalities in England Post-2010* recommended that actions to tackle the social gradient in health need to be universal – to cover everyone – but that the scale and intensity of the universal policies should be matched to the level of disadvantage of different groups in the population. The Review calls this approach 'proportionate universalism' (Marmot, 2010, p. 15).

Principle 3: Population health policies and interventions should have the dual purpose of promoting health gains in the population as a whole and reducing health inequalities

Policies and interventions to improve overall population health and to reduce inequalities in health are sometimes portrayed as conflicting. However, these two goals go hand in hand (Whitehead and Dahlgren, 2007). Reducing health inequalities is a key objective for health systems. Furthermore, overall population health targets are more likely to be achieved when efforts are made to reduce inequalities.

Principle 4: Actions should be concerned with tackling the determinants of health and the pathways to health inequalities

Actions need to acknowledge both the determinants of health and the pathways that generate and maintain health inequalities. There is a need to consider the 'causes of the causes' of ill health (Marmot, 2010). Lifestyle issues need to be understood in the context of social and community factors and living and working conditions. These factors need to be understood in the context of upstream issues, such as the political context. This insight points to action across all the levels of the determinants of health.

Factors that may not be a key cause of ill health at the population level may be important causes of poor health in particular groups. Action to tackle health inequalities needs to identify the determinants of health in different groups and identify pathways that maintain and generate health inequalities in order to intervene in the most effective way (Whitehead and Dahlgren, 2007).

Principle 5: Actions need to have appropriate timing and timeframes

Policies and interventions need to identify appropriate times in the life course for action on health inequalities. While it is important to address the determinants of health and health inequalities throughout people's lives, pregnancy and early childhood should be a particular focus. Furthermore, interventions need to be sustainable and implemented for a sufficient period of time.

Principle 6: Policy and interventions need to take a participatory approach

This principle entails involving communities and marginalised groups in the development and implementation of policy and interventions (Whitehead and Dahlgren, 2007). Furthermore, health professionals need to collaborate with other sectors, including education, social services and work and pensions, to address the wider determinants of health. Collaboration should include improved communication, participatory decision making and partnership working.

Principle 7: The extent of inequalities, progress towards goals and equity impacts should be measured

The evidence base on the extent and types of inequalities needs to be strengthened in order to inform action. Differences in health need to be measured in terms of socioeconomic position (education, income or occupation), geographic area, ethnicity and gender. Where ethnic or geographical inequalities are identified, they should be understood in the context of differences in socioeconomic position (Whitehead and Dahlgren, 2007).

This principle also entails monitoring progress towards goals and evaluation of policies and interventions. It is important to measure both absolute and relative differences in inequalities (see Table 2.1, pages 44-45). Actions may have time lags before health effects are felt, therefore long follow-up periods are useful.

Policies in the health sector or other sectors may have differential effects on groups in the population, with implications for health inequalities. It is important to measure differential effects, not just average effects, for example using health equity impact assessments (Whitehead and Dahlgren, 2007).

Principle 8: Health systems should be built on equity principles

Equity principles include: the provision of services according to need (not ability to pay); ensuring that all members of the population receive the same high standard of care (without discrimination by age, gender, ethnic origin or socioeconomic position); ensuring that public health services are not driven by profit; and explicitly stating and monitoring achievement towards the underlying values and equity objectives of the health system (Whitehead and Dahlgren, 2007).

Conclusion

In the twenty-first century, addressing the social determinants of health and reducing health inequalities are among the most pressing challenges for policies that aim to promote and sustain population health. The large, and in some cases widening, gaps between high and low income countries and between privileged and disadvantaged groups within societies are unacceptable and unfair, given that they are not governed by some law of nature, but are modifiable by purposeful actions.

The challenge for people working in public health is not to be discouraged by the sheer scale of the problem into concluding that there is nothing that they can do because the solutions are all at the macro-level. Nothing could be further from the truth. To tackle the problem requires action on the many different layers of the rainbow, by people making efforts in their own sphere of influence – whatever that may be. The renewed global interest in this challenge, stimulated by such initiatives as the Commission on Social Determinants of Health (WHO, 2008b), has spurred the public health community to examine what contributions they can make in their day-to-day work, including how they can work together with other sectors to bring about the necessary changes. A shared understanding of the wider influences on population health and recognition that everyone has a role to play, however modest, will be the keys to meeting this challenge head on.

References

Acheson, D.C., Barker, D., Chambers, J., Graham, H., Marmot, M. and Whitehead, M. (1998) *Report of the Independent Inquiry into Inequalities in Health*, London, The Stationery Office.

Anand, S. and Ravallion, M. (1993) 'Human development in poor countries: on the role of private incomes and public services', *The Journal of Economic Perspectives*, vol. 7, pp. 133–50.

Barker, D. (1998) *Mothers, Babies and Health in Later Life*, Edinburgh, Churchill Livingstone.

Baum, F. (1999) 'Social capital: is it good for your health? Issues for a public health agenda', *Journal of Epidemiology and Community Health*, vol. 53, pp. 195–96.

Berkman, L.F. and Glass, T. (2000) 'Social integration, social networks, social support, and health' in Berkman, L.F. and Kawachi, I. (eds) *Social Epidemiology*, New York, Oxford University Press.

Black, D., Morris, J., Smith, C. and Townsend, P. (1980) *Black Report. Inequalities in Health: Report of a Research Working Group*, London, Department of Health and Social Security.

Blane, D., Smith, G.D. and Bartley, M. (1993) 'Social selection: what does it contribute to social class differences in health?', *Sociology of Health and Illness*, vol. 15, pp. 1–15.

Brunner, E. (1997) 'Stress and the biology of inequality', *British Medical Journal*, vol. 314, pp. 1472–76.

Brunner, E. and Marmot, M. (2006) 'Social organization, stress, and health' in Marmot, M. and Wilkinson, R.G. (eds) *Social Determinants of Health* (2nd edition), Oxford, Oxford University Press.

Cavelaars, A.E.J.M., Kunst, A.E., Geurts, J.J.M., Crialesi, R., Grötvedt, L., Helmert, U., Lahelma, E., Lundberg, O., Matheson, J., Mielck, A., Rasmussen, N.K., Regidor, E., Rosário-Giraldes, M., Spuhler, T. and Mackenbach, J.P. (2000) 'Educational differences in smoking: international comparison', *British Medical Journal*, vol. 320, pp. 1102–7.

Dahlgren, G. and Whitehead, M. (1993) *Tackling Inequalities in Health: What Can We Learn From What Has Been Tried? Working Paper Prepared for the King's Fund International Seminar on Tackling Inequalities in Health*, Oxfordshire, King's Fund.

Dahlgren, G. and Whitehead, M. (2007) *European Strategies for Tackling Social Inequities in Health: Levelling Up Part 2*, Copenhagen, World Health Organization Regional Office for Europe.

Department for Work and Pensions (2011) *Households Below Average Income (HBAI) 1994/95–2009/10*, London, Department for Work and Pensions. Available at: http://research.dwp.gov.uk/asd/hbai/hbai2010/pdf_files/full_hbai11.pdf (accessed 11 September 2011).

Department of Health (DoH) (2005) *Tackling Health Inequalities: Status Report on the Programme for Action*, London, Department of Health. Available at: www.dh.gov.uk/en/Publicationsandstatistics/Publications/PublicationsPolicyAndGuidance/DH_4117696 (accessed 11 September 2011).

Department of Health, Social Services and Public Safety Northern Ireland (DHSSPSNI) (2007) *Health and Social Care Monitoring System: Changes in the NI Life Expectancy Gap, 1999/01–2004/6*, Belfast, DHSSPSNI.

Dowd, J.B. (2007) 'Early childhood origins of the income/health gradient: the role of maternal health behaviors', *Social Science and Medicine*, vol. 65, pp. 1202–13.

Galobardes, B., Lynch, J.W. and Davey Smith, G. (2008) 'Is the association between childhood socio-economic circumstances and cause-specific mortality established? Update of a systematic review', *Journal of Epidemiology and Community Health*, vol. 62, pp. 387–90.

Graham, H., Inskip, H.M., Francis, B. and Harman, J. (2006) 'Pathways of disadvantage and smoking careers: evidence and policy implications', *Journal of Epidemiology and Community Health*, vol. 60, pp. ii7–ii12.

Haut Comité de La Santé Publique (1998) *La santé en France 1994–8 [Health in France 1994–8]*, Paris, La Documentation Francaise.

Health and Safety Executive (2010) *The Health and Safety Executive Statistics 2009/10*, Sudbury, The Health and Safety Executive. Available at: www.hse.gov.uk/statistics/overall/hssh0910.pdf (accessed 11 September 2011).

Hewitt, P. (2005) *Annual health and social care lecture – Investment and reform: transforming health and healthcare*, Speech by Rt Hon Patricia Hewitt MP, Secretary of State for Health, 13 December 2005. Available at: http://webarchive.nationalarchives.gov.uk/+/www.dh.gov.uk/en/MediaCentre/Speeches/Speecheslist/DH_4124484 (accessed 30 October, 2011).

Hosseinpoor, A.R., Parker, L.A., Tursan d'Espaignet, E. and Chatterji, S. (2011) 'Social determinants of smoking in low- and middle-income countries: results from the World Health Survey', *PLoS ONE*, vol. 6, no. 5, e20331.

Houweling, T.A.J. and Kunst, A.E. (2010) 'Socio-economic inequalities in childhood mortality in low- and middle-income countries: a review of the international evidence', *British Medical Bulletin*, vol. 93, pp. 7–26.

Howe, L.D., Tilling, K., Galobardes, B., Davey-Smith, G., Gunnell, D. and Lawlor, D.A. (2010) 'Socio-economic differences in childhood growth trajectories: at what age do height inequalities emerge?', *Journal of Epidemiology and Community Health*, doi:10.1136/jech.2010.113068.

Karasek, R.A., Theorell, T., Schwartz, J.E., Schnall, P.L., Pieper, C.F. and Michela, J.L. (1988) 'Job characteristics in relation to the prevalence of myocardial infarction in the US Health Examination Survey (HES) and the Health and Nutrition Examination Survey (HANES)', *American Journal of Public Health*, vol. 78, pp. 910–18.

Kuh, D., Ben-Shlomo, Y., Lynch, J., Hallqvist, J. and Power, C. (2003) 'Life course epidemiology', *Journal of Epidemiology and Community Health*, vol. 57, pp. 778–83.

Kuh, D. and Hardy, R. (2002) 'A life course approach to women's health: does the past predict the present?' in Kuh, D. and Hardy, R. (eds) *A Life Course Approach to Women's Health*, Oxford, Oxford University Press.

Lindholm, C., Burstrom, B. and Diderichsen, F. (2002) 'Class differences in the social consequences of illness?', *Journal of Epidemiology and Community Health*, vol. 56, pp. 188–92.

Lynch, J.W., Davey Smith, G., Kaplan, G.A. and House, J.S. (2000) 'Income inequality and mortality: importance to health of individual income, psychosocial environment, or material conditions', *British Medical Journal*, vol. 320, pp. 1200–04.

Mackenbach, J.P., Stirbu, I., Roskam, A-J.R., Schaap, M.M., Menvielle, G., Leinsalu, M. and Kunst, A.E. (2008) 'Socio-economic inequalities in health in 22 European countries', *New England Journal of Medicine*, vol. 358, pp. 2468–81.

Marmot, M. (chair) (2010) *Fair Society, Healthy Lives: Strategic Review of Health Inequalities in England Post-2010*, London, The Marmot Review. Available at: www.marmotreview.org/AssetLibrary/pdfs/Reports/FairSocietyHealthyLives. pdf (accessed 10 September 2011).

Marmot, M.G., Bosma, H., Hemingway, H., Brunner, E. and Stansfeld, S. (1997) 'Contribution of job control and other risk factors to social variations in coronary heart disease incidence', *The Lancet*, vol. 350, pp. 235–39.

Marmot, M.G., Rose, G., Shipley, M. and Hamilton, P.J. (1978) 'Employment grade and coronary heart disease in British civil servants', *Journal of Epidemiology and Community Health*, vol. 32, pp. 244–49.

McKenzie, K., Whitley, R. and Weich, S. (2002) 'Social capital and mental health', *The British Journal of Psychiatry*, vol. 181, pp. 280–83.

Norman, P., Gregory, I., Dorling, D. and Baker, A. (2008) 'Geographical trends in infant mortality: England and Wales, 1970–2006', *Health Statistics Quarterly*, vol. 40, pp. 18–29.

Office for National Statistics (2010) 'Trends in life expectancy by the national statistics socio-economic classification 1982–2006' *Health Statistics Quarterly*, 22 February. Available at: www.ons.gov.uk/ons/rel/hsq/health-statistics-quarterly/ trends-in-life-expectancy-by-the-national-statistics-socio-economic-classification-1982-2006/index.html (accessed 2 October 2011).

Organisation for Economic Co-operation and Development (OECD) (2008) 'OECD.statsextracts'. Available at: http://stats.oecd.org/Index.aspx? QueryId=9909&QueryType=View (accessed 2 October 2011).

Scottish Government (2008) *Equally Well: Report of the Ministerial Task Force on Health Inequalities 2008*, Edinburgh, Scottish Government. Available at: http://scotland.gov.uk/Publications/2008/06/25104032/0 (accessed 11 September 2011).

Sen, A. (2001) 'Economic progress and health' in Leon, D. and Walt, G. (eds) *Poverty, Inequality and Health: An International Perspective*, Oxford, Oxford University Press.

Spencer, N. and Logan, S. (2002) 'Social influences on birth weight', *Journal of Epidemiology and Community Health*, vol. 56, pp. 326–27.

Townsend, P. (1979) *Poverty in the United Kingdom: A Survey of Household Resources and Standards of Living*, London, Penguin.

UNICEF (2007) *Child Poverty in Perspective: An Overview of Child Well-being in Rich Countries, Innocenti Report Card 7*, Florence, UNICEF Innocenti Research Centre. Available at: www.unicef-irc.org/publications/pdf/rc7_eng.pdf (accessed 11 September 2011).

Welsh Assembly Government (2008) *Chief Medical Officer of Health Annual Report*, Cardiff, Welsh Assembly Government.

Whitehead, M. and Dahlgren, G. (2007) *Concepts and Principles for Tackling Social Inequities in Health: Levelling Up Part 1*, Copenhagen, World Health Organization Regional Office for Europe.

Whitehead, M., Dahlgren, G. and Evans, T. (2001) 'Equity and health sector reforms: can low-income countries escape the medical poverty trap?', *The Lancet*, vol. 358, pp. 833–6.

Whitehead, M. and Popay, J. (2010) 'Swimming upstream? Taking action on the social determinants of health inequalities', *Social Science and Medicine*, vol. 71, pp. 1234–6.

Wilkinson, R. (2005) *The Impact of Inequality: How to Make Sick Societies Healthier*, London, Routledge.

Wilkinson, R.G. and Pickett, K.E. (2006) 'Income inequality and population health: a review and explanation of the evidence', *Social Science and Medicine*, vol. 62, pp. 1768–84.

World Health Organization (WHO) (2011a) *World Health Statistics 2011*, Geneva, World Health Organization. Available at: www.who.int/whosis/whostat/EN_WHS2011_Full.pdf (accessed 11 September 2011).

World Health Organization (WHO) (2011b) 'European health for all database'. Available at: http://data.euro.who.int/hfadb/ (accessed 2 October 2011).

World Health Organization (WHO) (2009) *Global Health Risks. Mortality and Burden of Disease Attributable to Selected Major Risks*, Geneva, World Health Organization. Available at: www.who.int/healthinfo/global_burden_disease/GlobalHealthRisks_report_full.pdf (accessed 11 September 2011).

World Health Organization (WHO) (2008a) *Global Burden of Disease – 2004 Update*, Geneva, World Health Organization. Available at: www.who.int/healthinfo/global_burden_disease/GBD_report_2004update_full.pdf (accessed 11 September 2011).

World Health Organization (WHO) (2008b) *Closing the Gap in a Generation. Report of the WHO Commission on the Social Determinants of Health*, Geneva, World Health Organization. Available at: http://whqlibdoc.who.int/publications/2008/9789241563703_eng.pdf (accessed 10 September 2011).

Chapter 3: Working in organisations: skills and approaches

Ian Bowns and Jenny Griffiths, with Linda Jones and Mike Lucas

Introduction

Major reviews of public health in the UK have highlighted the need to strengthen leadership and management across public health in both the National Health Service (NHS) and local government (Department of Health [DoH], 2001; Wanless, 2004). The 2001 review of the public health function in England concluded that public health leadership 'requires a facilitative, influencing style that can make use of horizontal networks in addition to vertical "command and control" networks' (DoH, 2001, p. 32). In other words, public health involves not only transmitting public health knowledge but also influencing and persuading others – in organisations, committees and so on – to adopt public health priorities. It demands action, therefore, not just in controlled organisational environments but also in less manageable, more risky settings. This signals the need for teamwork, collaboration, leadership and management skills to be developed at all levels, both within and across organisations.

This chapter explores three key skill areas: building and leading teams, cross-boundary working and leading and managing change. It introduces concepts and skills that practitioners will find valuable in their managerial practice within public health teams and organisations in any setting, including skills to optimise team working and management across organisational interfaces. It discusses the challenges presented by organisational change and development and offers some understanding of different approaches. In doing so, it draws on a well-established body of leadership and management theory and reflects on how the application of this can develop public health practice.

3.1 Building and leading teams

Not every group is a team. Teams share at least one common goal or purpose, whereas groups characteristically do not. Superficially, this seems to be an adequate distinction, until tested against examples. We would not usually describe a group of people on a plane as a team, although they do share a goal of reaching the destination. The dividing line between a group and a team is that the goals of a team are longer term, the team has at least some level of persistent organisation, and the team's members have some level of commitment to the team and its individual members. A large group of people (say, more than 12) will probably be too big to function as a team, but the size of effective teams is very variable.

Different types of social groupings exist in organisations and not all of them will require a team approach. A committee, for example, is part of a governance structure: a group of people appointed for a specific function, typically consisting of representatives of a larger group. Although committees can also be teams (and teams can meet in committee), they rarely share the level of interpersonal commitment expected from a team. Other typical organisational groupings may exhibit some team characteristics. Steering groups or working groups, for example, could find it difficult to achieve their ends without some shared goals and commitment.

Why have teams?

There are both business and human reasons for having teams. Human reasons include the psychological need for belonging and affiliation. Teams can motivate individuals and, in doing so, support their learning development.

Business reasons include the management of complex work, which may have uncertain processes or outcomes, and solving multifaceted problems, when the combined resources of the group are potentially more effective than any individual. Teams developed with partner organisations may accomplish tasks that cannot be achieved by a single department or organisation alone. Such teams are particularly common in public health practice to address complex social and health problems where a range of agencies make significant contributions, such as tobacco control, alcohol and other substance misuse strategies, domestic violence, and mental health promotion and care. Box 3.1 highlights the skills that might be deployed by a team to help vulnerable young people.

Box 3.1 Multi-professional service teams

Local authorities establish service teams consisting of a range of professional staff with the aim of improving outcomes for vulnerable young people by:

- promoting their health
- increasing educational attainment and participation in the labour market
- reducing offending and anti-social behaviour.

Such teams need multidisciplinary membership and expertise from: the NHS (services for mental health, substance and alcohol misuse, and sexual health); social work (help with homelessness, family and relationship problems); special educational services and schools; and possibly youth justice services and the police.

What are your views on the strengths and weaknesses of this type of multi-professional team?

One strength is its multidisciplinary membership, which brings together expertise from a range of services to provide a coordinated response. The team has a welcome focus on outcomes for young people, and the ability to measure performance by reducing numbers of young people not in education, employment or training (the so-called NEET groups), anti-social behaviour and offending. But there may also be weaknesses, such as conflicting values among team members (e.g. educational and remedial principles are very different) and the potential for competition.

Teams can encounter problems, some of which are inherent in their nature. All teams take time and effort to develop, because they require mutual understanding about beliefs and ways of working. Strong teams tend to be clear about their purpose, have broadly shared values and clarity about the roles of team members, who are supportive of each other. They identify the most appropriate method of working and regularly review how they are doing. Weaker teams may be too large, encompass a range of potentially conflicting values, emphasise individuals and have a competitive culture. They may not measure their performance or use the skills of members appropriately. In complex multi-agency, multidisciplinary teams such as the team in Box 3.1, the 'leader' of the team may not have much control over membership or management. These issues are explored further below.

Team building and dynamics

Although very often teams will be composed of current staff or the given representatives of partner directorates or organisations, there are many situations where there remains at least an element of choice regarding team membership. Team cohesion and performance is important, as well as expertise and representation. Potential team members need to 'fit' with vacant roles and subscribe to team working. A frequent trade-off is between representation, where seniority within a department or organisation is valuable, and technical expertise, which might suggest a specific, though less senior member of staff.

All too often teams are recruited to be representative of the different professional or occupational groups and/or skills and competencies required, without consideration of whether the people in a team will complement each other or manage to work together effectively. Since most teams will need leadership, operational support, coordination and technical expertise (Handy, 1990), an understanding of the roles that different members might play within a team setting can be very useful.

A pioneer in this field (Belbin, 1981) developed a team role inventory to assess how an individual behaves in a team environment. He delineated nine role types in three role clusters against which an individual's behavioural traits could be measured. These were: people-oriented roles (coordinating, team working and resource gathering); action-oriented roles (shaping, implementing, finishing); and cerebral-oriented roles (creating, evaluating, specialist). Belbin's team roles are widely used as an aid to discussing effective team behaviour, despite some concerns about their validity and reliability. The roles are described in Box 3.2.

Box 3.2 Belbin's team roles

1 **Coordinator** – keeps the team operating effectively at an operational level, focusing effort and allocating tasks.

2 **Shaper** – develops the broad strategic approach.

3 **Plant** – creative mind, generating novel ideas and insights.

4 **Monitor evaluator** – constantly assesses team progress.

5 **Resource investigator** – the link to the organisation beyond the team, securing resources (often information).

6 **Specialist** – brings specific technical expertise relevant to the particular work at hand.

7 **Team worker** – attends to the 'people' issues between team members.

8 **Implementer** – ensures that proposed solutions are practicable.

9 **Finisher** – ensures that the team actually cross the finishing line.

(Belbin, 2010)

How far does Belbin's work on role types in Box 3.2 relate to your experience of working in teams?

An appreciation of the requirements of team roles assists team selection and ongoing management and helps you to know what role you are performing in a team. In smaller teams especially, one individual often fulfils more than one role, and this may have been your experience. However, where the volume of work may be manageable but the number and diversity of roles an individual is called on to fulfil is not, there is a risk of role overload. Teams need to be balanced to be effective. For example, teams can have several 'shapers' and 'plants' but lack people fulfilling operational roles – in which case the team is unlikely to deliver on its outcomes.

The focus on behavioural traits in teams is quite widespread. You may have encountered the Myers Briggs Type Indicator (MBTI), which is a widely used psychometric approach to identifying personality and leadership types that is not without its critics. The MBTI tool focuses on eliciting individual preferences in four key areas for team working:

relating to others, working within structures, making decisions and using information. Emotional intelligence (EI) (Goleman, 1998) also focuses on behavioural traits, starting from the premise that IQ is too narrow a measure of intelligence. Successful leaders and team members, it is argued, also possess EI. They are able to understand and manage their own emotions while also recognising, understanding and managing the emotions of others. There have been various attempts to test this, including the Emotional Quotient Inventory Test (Bar-On, 2006). Some critics have dismissed claims that EI is a type of intelligence analogous to IQ and that it can be assessed through testing (Landy, 2005), but others have seen it as a useful delineation of competencies and skills that can drive high performance. EI is usually linked with 'soft skills' such as empathy and reflexivity, which are essential to create successful interpersonal relationships (Checkland and Poulter, 2006).

Tuckman (1965) observed that team building and dynamics change over time. He described four archetypal stages in the formation of successful teams in terms of the feelings experienced by team members at the time, the typical behaviours exhibited, and the tasks they are likely to be engaged in.

- **Forming** – where individuals want to avoid conflict and be accepted; they gather information about each other and the project but serious issues are avoided, so not much gets done.
- **Storming** – moving out of the comfort zone, with more confrontations as key challenges and issues are exposed; there are winners and losers at this stage and pressure for rules to manage conflict.
- **Norming** – tasks and responsibilities are agreed; understanding and appreciation of each other grows with group cohesion, mutual support and resistance to outside pressures.
- **Performing** – team is interdependent; energy is focused on the task with high levels of trust, flexibility of roles, loyalty and high morale.

These stages characteristically progress sequentially, although teams can 'regress' to an earlier stage of development under certain circumstances, notably internal or external stress or change. Tuckman's observations have proved durable and in 1977 he added a fifth stage 'adjourning' – that is, completion and disengagement (Tuckman and Jensen, 1977). His key insight is that conflict is normal in developing social relationships and that the 'storming' phase is a necessary part of creating a team. The extent to which any particular team needs to go through the process of team development in depth will depend on many factors, particularly the perceived scale and importance of the team's work to its members. But no group of individuals, with varying pre-existing relationships, can be expected to achieve peak performance without establishing a modus operandi – a way of working. This is a key responsibility for anyone who forms or leads a team.

3.2 Roles and identities

Group membership involves the construction of social identity: part of people's self-concept derives from their membership of social groups. Teams, as we have noted, provide opportunities for such identity building through relating to others, adopting roles and becoming integrated. Alvesson (2000) suggests that building identity is an embedded feature of knowledge-intensive industries, where often well-qualified employees work intensively and with little supervision. While intrinsic motivation to 'do a good job' and be a reliable employee and team member may partly explain their dedication, he argues that people also co-create a group social identity. For example, he suggests that 'working a lot is, apart from everything else, identity work; through long hours one confirms who one is' (p. 1108). People's loyalty is to their professional peer group, with a shared ethos of dedication, cooperation and reciprocity, rather than to a corporate organisational ethic.

Such ideas are thought-provoking in the context of public health, which is also a knowledge-intensive enterprise. Practitioners often work fairly autonomously, at a distance from each other, in a variety of settings and may be driven more by intrinsic motivation than extrinsic rewards. Many also work across professional groups and boundaries. In such indeterminate and 'risky' situations their loyalties may lie more with their professional peer group than their wider organisation or project team. Moulding together different professional groups, such as those identified in Box 3.1, to create an effective team is a key challenge.

Building in flexibility

Communication and leadership are obviously central to moulding a team and a flexible approach in both areas is important. Team communications can embrace telephone, video and web-based technologies that facilitate collaborative working within and across organisations. Email, instant messaging and interaction using social media might all be valuable at different times.

Our own communication and behaviour is possibly our most important tool in achieving change in others. Adapting communications to suit the preferences and styles of other people is advantageous but challenging, especially when communicating one-to-many, such as in team meetings. Public health teams are composed of disparate individuals, so time is needed to think about the nature of the audience. Many people respond to visual messages and the narrative aspects of an argument, rather than numbers and statistical methods of communication. This may challenge the prevailing culture in public health, as anecdote sits uneasily with perceptions of factual, evidence-based practice. However, flexibility in presentation – using stories, words and images, for example – may convey a point more effectively than a rigid approach (see Box 3.3).

> **Box 3.3 Behavioural flexibility**
>
> A director of public health (DPH) was attempting to persuade a clinician to participate in a quality improvement programme that had high aspirations. Initial attempts were greeted without much enthusiasm until the clinician's level of anxiety regarding complaints and litigation brought their risk aversion to the DPH's attention. Future discussions regarding quality improvement were subsequently couched more in terms of the avoidance of risk and complaints, with greater success. The underlying message and objectives had not changed, although they were expressed rather differently.

Flexibility in leadership is also highlighted in the classic theory of situational leadership (Hersey and Blanchard, 1977). This is one of a family of leadership theories that suggest there is not a single best style of leadership, but that a range of styles should be employed by the leader to fit the situation and the followers. They proposed four styles of team leadership.

- **Telling** – one-way communication from the leader defines the roles of the individual or group and micro-manages the detailed operation of the team.
- **Selling** – the leader remains the main decision maker, but there is greater communication. An attempt is made to persuade followers that the course of action is best.

- **Participating** – shared decision making about both the 'what' and the 'how' of the tasks, with less management of detail and higher support for team relationships.
- **Delegating** – the leader is involved in relevant decisions but more responsibility is passed to the team, particularly on process matters, which the leader monitors, potentially on an exception basis.

Which style would you see as most relevant to public health practice?

Professional cultures, such as public health practice, are predominantly based on assumptions of a delegating style of leadership, and a mature followership. This may not be appropriate to every situation. Crucially, this approach to management proposes that the leadership style to be adopted in particular circumstances will be adapted to the situation by a leader capable of leading in any of these styles. The level of decision making should also relate to the nature of the decision itself. Simple decisions, with limited consequences, can simply be taken at the appropriate level, even where the leader and team are capable of much more complex decision making.

Building in learning

The most effective teams are those that learn. Wenger (2000) has drawn attention to what he terms 'communities of practice' and their role in social learning. Communities of practice are bound together by a 'collectively developed understanding of what their community is about and hold each other accountable to this sense of joint enterprise' (p. 229). Members become competent through building and sharing resources (language, routines, styles, tools, etc.) which define them as members of the community. The key message from Wenger's research is the importance of learning as a social process and the rich learning process that can be built into work groups and organisations. As the public health workforce becomes more diverse, there may be opportunities to create new 'communities of practice' that harness learning from its teams and initiatives to enhance future practice.

However, Wenger also drew attention to the potential drawbacks of communities of learning. If the level of learning energy falls away and trust and self-awareness are not maintained, communities 'can learn not to learn. They are the cradles of the human spirit but they can also be its cages' (p. 230). This aligns with earlier work highlighting the dangers for teams of members over-identifying with the team. If 'norming' is too successful the result could be 'groupthink' (Janis, 1972). In groupthink the varied views of the individual members are suppressed in the interests of group cohesion, impairing the team's ability to identify when it is collectively making mistakes. Janis describes it as:

> a mode of thinking that people engage in when they are deeply involved in a cohesive in-group, when the members' strivings for unanimity override their motivation to realistically appraise alternative courses of action.
>
> (Janis, 1972, p. 9)

The most senior or, in flatter teams, the most assertive members may enforce groupthink, with others getting swept along by them. This can lead to serious errors, which later appear obvious or rudimentary. It is possible to adopt behaviours that avoid these risks, particularly by encouraging critical appraisal at every stage of assumptions, beliefs and even knowledge that the team has been taking for granted. A truly mature team may be one that prevents the dangers of groupthink by preserving a healthy degree of challenge internally and externally and, Wenger would add, by continuing to learn, interact and reflect in a productive way.

3.3 Working across boundaries

Much public health work is collaborative. Intractable health challenges, such as child poverty, low educational attainment or obesity, are interconnected and unlikely to be resolved without agencies and communities working together. The ability to work comfortably across boundaries is therefore essential. Boundaries come in many forms; for example, organisational, institutional, cultural, political, faith-based and linguistic. Each of these ways in which people organise themselves creates boundaries and each of these groups will, to a greater or lesser extent, have its own culture. While boundaries may be fairly fluid, 'shared practice by its very nature creates boundaries' (Wenger, 2000, p. 232). At the same time, boundaries create new opportunities for learning: for open engagement with new ideas and new ways of doing things.

Organisational cultures

Culture, in brief, is 'the way we do things around here' and it has a huge impact on the effectiveness of organisations, teams and individuals. Handy (1985) defined four main types of organisational and team culture, including power culture, with decisions largely made by one person, and role culture, dominated by bureaucratic hierarchies. His two other types were task culture – team focused, with flexible lines of communication and minimal direction from above – and person culture, with high levels of autonomy and individual working. But this focuses attention on visible structures, whereas culture arguably constitutes the informal social aspects of an organisation that influence how people think, what they regard as important and how they behave and interact (Mannion et al., 2005).

Most organisations of any significant size have a range of cultures (Mintzberg, 1989), but these are not always immediately observable, because they can be cognitive. Schein (2004, p. 1) argues that in groups and organisations culture exists at different levels. It may seem to manifest itself in 'very tangible' visible structures, but attention must also be paid to beliefs and values expressed in strategies and goals and to the 'deeply embedded, unconscious basic assumptions' that constitute the 'essence of culture'. Schein's 'levels of culture' are set out in Figure 3.1.

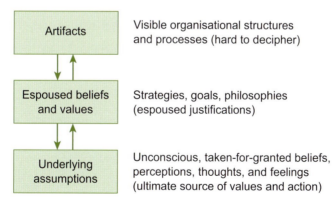

Figure 3.1 Levels of culture

(Source: Schein, 2004)

Figure 3.1 highlights that even visible structures may be hard to decipher, although Schein suggests that over time their meaning becomes clearer. To gain further insight one must understand the espoused values that underpin goals and philosophies. However, 'espoused beliefs and values often leave large areas of behaviour unexplained', especially if values are very abstract or contradictory (p. 4). Underneath the espoused beliefs and values lurk underlying assumptions – the taken-for-granted patterns that are never discussed or challenged, and are therefore very difficult to change.

Large, complex organisational structures, such as a public health or health and social care organisation or system, exhibit highly differentiated cultures in which different groups or parts may espouse different, and perhaps conflicting, values and underlying assumptions. Careful management is required either to integrate these different cultures effectively or, more likely, to ensure suitable interfaces between the cultures to enable effective working relationships.

What would you identify as the different levels of culture (Figure 3.1) that exist in public health?

It is difficult to pin down the culture (or cultures) of public health. Handy's description of a 'task culture' may best describe the artifact level, as much work is team-based and task-focused. The term 'matrix management' is often used to describe the composition and horizontal management of such teams drawn from different groups and organisations. Public health's self-perception might be that it espouses a set of principles based on justice, fairness and evidence-based rationality. But other espoused values may conflict with these:

- independence, which sits uncomfortably in any corporate culture
- passion (e.g. about reducing health inequities), which may conflict with rationality.

Underlying assumptions about the social nature and wider determinants of health may form the unconscious bedrock of much public health practice.

If progress is to be made in health improvement and reducing health inequalities, it is also important to understand the artifacts, values and assumptions of other agencies and systems with which public health needs to work. For example, local authorities are bureaucratic and procedural at the artifact level and democratically accountable to their electorates, making them subject to very different pressures, values and underlying assumptions. In the majority of organisations concerned with the delivery of healthcare, a biomedical understanding of health and illness dominates and this assumption challenges public health practitioners working in them or across their boundaries (Dooris and Hunter, 2007). Working in partnership with community groups, voluntary organisations or private companies may reveal other, very different and possibly disrupting values and assumptions (Coulson, 2005). Partnership working is discussed further in Chapter 13.

Lack of understanding of differing cultures in organisations and communities can often stifle attempts to work effectively across boundaries, hence the saying 'culture destroys strategy'. With an understanding of the similarities and differences between them, it is possible to manage interactions with different groups and their members more effectively. It is valuable to work with organisational or community leaders in positions of power and influence, for example, non-executive directors, trustees, religious leaders and chairs of community groups. These leaders explicitly and deliberately develop an understanding of different cultures and seek to modify cultures and provide a bridge between different groups.

Boundary-spanning roles

Because of the complexity of public health challenges and the differences in their cultures, the NHS, local government and other sectors have all created job roles – such as partnership and alliance coordinators, and community development practitioners – with the specific responsibility of working collaboratively in multi-sectoral settings. Many practitioners undertake 'boundary-spanning' activities within one organisation; for example, leading on collaborative working on complex health topics such as obesity or tobacco control. Boundary spanning occurs at all levels – from front-line practitioners through to middle levels and to senior management (Hutt et al., 2000). Box 3.4 (page 84) gives an example of what might be achievable through boundary spanning.

Box 3.4 Value of cross-organisational experience

The officers of a local health authority had reasonable relationships
with their counterparts in its coterminous local authority, but there
were tensions between the appointed health authority board and
the elected councillors. This was partly exacerbated by the fact that
the national government, which indirectly appointed the health
board, had a very different political complexion from the particular
council. An NHS assistant director within public health had
previously worked within local authorities and was able to support
the management and board members to negotiate the potential
pitfalls of working with both officers and elected members.

Boundary spanners can have a major impact, in particular where they
have developed strong working relationships and understand the visible
and hidden culture of the partner organisation. Formal collaborative
structures that are dependent on roles may not be effective without the
life blood of interpersonal relationships, which help to share learning,
build trust, resolve conflict and enhance decision making. At the same
time, Adobor (2006) points to the need to guard against the
disadvantages of over-reliance on interpersonal relationships, such as the
risk of relationship breakdown, conflicts of personal interest, the
formation of 'cliques' which exclude others, and the risk of instability or
failure when key individuals move to a new position.

Working across organisations requires good organisational skills,
including programme and project management. Because much public
health work lies at the interface between organisations and is usually
undertaken by a team of practitioners from different backgrounds, it
will require skilled and robust project management (see Chapter 13).
Public health practitioners may lack authority if their professional
expertise is not perceived as relevant in the agencies or communities
with which they are collaborating. They may have to live with tension
and ambiguity associated with managing without 'positional power'; that
is, without the authority derived from their professional role and related
status (Williams, 2010). Personal power, demonstrated through well-
developed interpersonal skills, particularly the ability to attract others
and build loyalty, may counterbalance a lack of positional power.

Williams (2002) identifies three roles that work across and between organisations: the reticulist, the entrepreneur and the interpreter or communicator, with associated skills and competencies. He notes that research highlights a high degree of connectivity and interplay between these roles and competencies, all of which are, to a greater or lesser degree, likely to be beneficial to practitioners. These three roles are discussed below.

Reticulists – creators and managers of networks

Most effective public health practitioners possess some reticulist skills. Reticulism means the creation, activation or refashioning of decision networks to address issues. Reticulists are 'individuals who are especially sensitive to and skilled in bridging interests, professions and organisations' (Webb, 1991). They help establish a common set of goals and facilitate better coordination by recruiting and building coalitions. Reticulist skills include an appreciation of political and organisational context and an ability to cultivate a network of formal and informal relationships. Reticulists have strong political and diplomatic skills and know how and when to adopt appropriate types of behaviour; for example, bargaining, persuasion or even (on occasion and when effective) confrontation (Friend et al., 1974). Because there is less control and direct accountability in network management than in hierarchies, reticulists are skilled in managing the inherent uncertainties of multiple accountabilities and appreciating and respecting the different modes of governance that exist within organisations.

Public entrepreneurs

A second type of boundary spanner is the 'public entrepreneur' – someone who introduces and implements innovative ideas into public practice (Roberts and King, 1996). Entrepreneurs are creative, have effective problem-solving skills, can think across whole systems, are able to tolerate and take risks and are focused and tenacious. They are catalysts and brokers who bring new ideas and people into organisations and communities from outside, and find ways around bureaucracy. For example, in the late 1990s a local authority director of social services established a small-scale farm in an urban area to help socialise at-risk teenagers. He managed to secure a major part of the funding to support the work from a European Commission Farming Grant, but he also enlisted service inputs from local mental health and contributions from other NHS service providers (personal communication).

Interpreters and facilitators

Effective boundary spanners develop strong interpersonal relationships, using listening and empathising skills. They seek to explore, discover and understand people, communities and/or organisations other than their own, and to develop a strong understanding of the diversity of roles, responsibilities and cultures. They invest time in obtaining this information, which they then interpret to identify potential common areas for collaboration. They use facilitative skills to draw people into a dialogue and into shared plans of action, helping people from different backgrounds to make sense of each other and position themselves within a common framework. They are good at building trust. Community development practitioners often have particularly strong interpretive and facilitative skills.

 Which parts of these roles are similar to the skills you use in your work?

While these three roles are described in strategic terms, practitioners at many levels inside and outside public health are likely to enact parts of these roles. Understanding how other groups or organisations work, finding imaginative ways through systems and structures, and negotiating and building trust can all be seen as useful skills for a range of people-focused jobs. In much public health work, it might be argued, they are not only useful but also essential. Wenger (2000, p. 235) uses the term 'brokers' for people who introduce ideas from one community to another and comments that 'certain individuals seem to thrive on being brokers; they love to create connections and engage in import–export, and would rather stay at the boundaries.'

Developing trust

Trust is pivotal to successful relationships between individuals, groups and organisations. It is an important aspect of moral leadership and depends on self-esteem. People (or teams or organisations) with poor self-confidence find it difficult to trust others. But trust can be difficult to pinpoint. It is a worthwhile exercise in any group or team to define together what is meant by trust. Box 3.5 sets out the outcome of one team's discussion (Griffiths, 1998).

Box 3.5 Dimensions of trust

If I trust you …

I can give you responsibility for things that are dear to me.

I believe that you will deliver on your promises.

I believe in your good intentions: I will give you the benefit of the doubt.

I forgive you readily when you make mistakes.

I know that you will present my point of view fairly.

Trust is developed over time and may result in a high degree of mutual understanding, knowledge and confidence in the competence of the other person, group or organisation. After a systematic survey of the research literature on trust, Vangen and Huxham (2003) developed a 'cyclical trust-building loop' (see Figure 3.2, page 88). It conceptualises trust as a cyclical process which is triggered when parties are willing 'to take a risk and become vulnerable to the actions of the other partner (s)'. If only modest outcomes are expected, the risk may remain low. If initial outcomes are met, trust will be enhanced and enable more risky initiatives. They suggest this virtuous loop of trust can be maintained if outcomes are realistic 'relative to the level of trust between the participating organisations' (p. 12).

It is relatively easy to commence a programme of working across boundaries, but much more difficult to sustain effective progress over lengthy periods of time. The literature on the effectiveness of cross-boundary working is modest, not least because of its methodological complexities (Williams, 2002). Nonetheless, what research there is suggests that it relies on the skills of individuals who can forge alliances with flair and commitment. So, for example, the Audit Commission (2009) found that gatekeepers to local strategic partnerships between local authorities, the NHS, the third sector and the private sector were very important in keeping the partnership relevant and responsive to local needs. The ability to work collaboratively with people from other agencies and communities, demonstrate awareness of personal impact on others and build constructive relationships with a range of people is integral to public health practitioner standards and competencies.

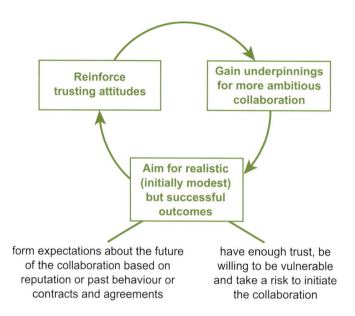

Figure 3.2 The cyclical trust-building loop
(Source: Vangen and Huxham, 2003, p. 12)

3.4 Organisational change and development

The nature of organisational development

Organisational development focuses on creating new ways of working to enable organisations to realise their strategic ambitions and recent definitions have emphasised the importance of workforce engagement and cultural change as keys to success (Local Government Improvement and Development Agency [IDEA], 2011). Organisational development has its origins in behavioural science and Lewin's studies (1946, 1958) on group dynamics, but it now draws on research and insights from systems theory, organisational learning theory and leadership studies. Its theories are highly relevant to public health, which operates in a complex, indeterminate environment within and across organisations with different cultures.

Organisational development and change management are obviously part of everyday life in organisations where leaders are seeking to improve effectiveness and performance. Depending on the desired impact, change initiatives and development may be targeted directly at individuals, groups or at the organisation as a whole. Organisations often focus more on their structures (how they are divided up into units, departments and teams) than on the way in which people work within those structures. This happens in spite of evidence – not least from repeated restructuring of the NHS every three or four years since the 1970s – that 'moving the deckchairs' does not usually or necessarily result in improvements in organisational performance. Indeed, in general there is limited evidence of successful business change, with estimates of the success rate of change programmes ranging between 10 and 30 per cent (Higgs and Rowland, 2000).

Organisations may engage in planned change that is deliberate and organised, but change can also be emergent, unplanned and more spontaneous (Dooris and Hunter, 2007). The change may be continuous or episodic and its purpose more or less ambitious. Examples of emergent change are frequently found when small groups of people get together in communities. For example, the Transition Movement, which aims to promote community self-sufficiency in areas like food in the face of environmental challenges, deliberately avoids organised top-down change. A recent investigation of 28 private and public sector companies, however, indicated that all of them were reacting to shifts in their external environment and most were playing 'catch-up' to deal with existing threats (Oakland and Turner, 2006). The changes they made were planned, with identified goals and resources.

Engaging in organisational change

Detailed and highly structured formal strategic planning, which was at one time seen as essential for organisational change, has given way to a focus on 'strategic thinking', linked to systematic appraisal of the changing external environment (Mintzberg, 1983; Mintzberg et al., 2005). Clearly, the value of this latter approach will depend considerably on the sector in which an organisation is operating. Public health in general and the healthcare sector are both comparatively rapidly changing environments. A wide range of factors influence population health, from economic growth, employment and education to transport and technology. Work to influence these wider determinants is unlikely to be successful unless public health practitioners think strategically about changing themselves and find innovative ways of working with other organisations.

Drivers of successful change include shared vision, leadership, effective project management and organisational learning, and these are closely related to key features of what has been termed the 'learning organisation' (Senge et al., 1994). The concept of a learning organisation emphasises the likely need for continuous change and adaptation, which at times will be radical and dramatic. It focuses on the conditions needed to ensure that an organisation is capable of such development. Key features of such an organisation are:

- personal mastery, building individual skills, knowledge and attitudes, particular openness, without which genuine self-criticism is not possible

- mental models, used to evaluate preconceptions and shed new light on the organisation

- building shared vision, to ensure that teams are clear regarding objectives and means of delivery

- team learning, to ensure that collaborative behaviour is developed as well as specific, technical skill

- systems thinking, which ensures that processes can be improved in sustainable ways.

Which features of Senge's learning organisation seem relevant to public health?

These ideas are highly relevant to public health, which is not a tightly knit organisation with a clearly defined focus but a complex, dynamic system of linkages which aims to transform other organisations and persuade them to take health more seriously. The skill-set which Senge delineates is one which public health practitioners need: for example, to work with GPs on planning for local population health, to support a health initiative in a voluntary sector agency, or to work with local authorities on early interventions with vulnerable groups. It has features in common with 'communities of practice' (Wenger, 2000), which emphasise that flexibility, reflexivity and clarity can facilitate innovation and that team learning must be sustained to drive through change.

Indeed, leadership and organisational development research indicates that the approaches that will probably be most effective in enabling change at any level are the development of trust and effective working methods within teams, as we have discussed in the previous sections. Oakland and Turner (2006), in their review of literature on private and public sector business change, identify 'open communication, participation and cross-training' as key ingredients whereas 'failed efforts were characterised by vague goals and poor communication' (p. 3). Moreover, they argue that 'while support from the top is critical, actual implementation should be carried out from the bottom-up. The idea of empowerment is to push decisions down to where the work is actually done' (p. 5). Their empirical research findings support and extend this view, indicating that the reasons for failure were often bound up with inadequate process management at the operational level. Vision and strategy were in place, but too little attention was paid to the structure, roles, competencies and resources needed to carry through changes in people's behaviour and organisational culture. Learning from past change initiatives was not always evident and less than half of the organisations ran pilot studies or feasibility tests.

> If there is a need to become more competitive or react to a government initiative, the strategic need (must) be translated into quantifiable efficiency and effectiveness improvements that are understood at an operational level ... If this link is broken between the strategic and the operational team there is a risk of misdirected effort leading to no or limited bottom-line benefits or the change will never get off the ground.
>
> (Oakland and Turner, 2006, pp. 23–4)

As a result of this research, Oakland and Turner devised an organisational change framework which identifies readiness for change (not just the need to change, but adequate direction and planning) and processes to achieve change and implementation requirements (see Figure 3.3, page 92). Unless readiness features are in place, organisation can go round and round the implementation loop without success. Unless processes are adequately supported, behaviour will not change and change will not endure. The 'figure of eight' revisits processes at the end to close the loop of change.

While it is important to have a sound logical argument for change, and to make its path as straightforward as possible, the key determinant is likely to lie in the motivation of those who are being encouraged to embark on the journey (Heath and Heath, 2010). Even the most unassailable logical argument in favour of change can fail if the context, particularly the human relationships, is not conducive. The less concrete aspects of change management, encapsulated in 'soft systems' methodology (Checkland and Poulter, 2006), are a further reminder of the need to take fully into account the human aspects of change.

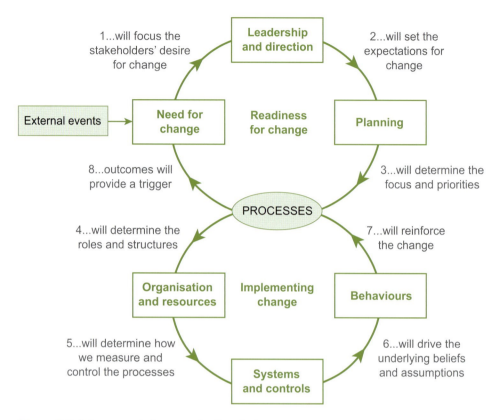

Figure 3.3 A framework for organisational change

(Source: Oakland and Turner, 2006, p. 26)

Influencing others

The organisational change framework is very useful for public health, given its focus on influencing change and development in other organisations and agencies. It suggests that the first stage in persuading a GP, voluntary sector agency or local authority to give a higher priority to health would be to link the proposed change to an external event and need for change within their own local environment (not yours). Finding a trigger to persuade the stakeholders to think about change, set priorities for change and plan a change is a crucial starting point. The next stage is advising on and supporting the processes they (not you) devise. To close the implementation loop and sustain the change it is important to influence actions. Box 3.6 describes the 100,000 Lives Campaign in the USA which used appeals to professionalism, publicity and an engineered deadline to persuade clinicians and managers to act on avoidable deaths.

Box 3.6 The 100,000 Lives Campaign

Don Berwick, as leader of the Institute for Healthcare Improvement, instituted the 100,000 Lives Campaign in December 2004 (now the 5 Million Lives Campaign) to reduce avoidable deaths in hospital. He began with motivation, using the testimony of the mother of a child whose death should have been avoided. He made it a professional duty to take the issue seriously, thereby appealing to the identity of hospital managers and clinicians alike. He used published evidence to show that the astonishing target set (to avoid 100,000 deaths by 9 am on 14 June 2006) was realistic. He publicised the participation of some of the USA's most prestigious hospitals to demonstrate that this was a goal that required the right culture of concern and professionalism. He encapsulated it in a slogan, 'Some is not a number, soon is not a time.' The result: an estimated 122,000 lives saved, on time.

This approach has been replicated with some success in Wales, as the 1000 Lives Plus Campaign.

(NHS Wales, 2011)

The example in Box 3.6 illustrates two key points. First, that an awareness of the potential obstacles and threats to change can help the individual acting as change agent to anticipate and prevent them. In other words, some understanding of the priorities and barriers within the organisations you need to work with is very important to enable you to influence them positively. This understanding might be personal or derived from other people. Second, by using the right incentives, other people can be empowered to react, adapt and devise their own solutions while remaining connected to a very clear and potent objective.

Dooris and Hunter (2007) ask what successful change would look like in public health and suggest some indirect measures of success. These include written roles/job descriptions in an organisation that include health responsibilities, evidence of health-related infrastructures, the setting up of formal health committees and changes in values. These may seem indeterminate compared with more conventional public health 'products', such as measurable engagement and health improvement achieved through a project. The key point, however, as Box 3.6 demonstrates, is that such project successes are more likely to be multiplied if partner organisations – such as hospitals, housing agencies or bus companies – can be mobilised to act themselves (see Chapter 13).

Distributed leadership

Oakland and Turner (2006), among others, make the point that people at the operational level must be actively engaged and take ownership of any change for it to work. This suggests that leadership qualities are required at every level of an organisation and that the range of styles and behavioural flexibility outlined in Section 3.4 are equally relevant to organisational change. Thinking about organisational development from the bottom up is instructive here, especially for public health which needs to galvanise other people, in other organisations and at a range of levels to take action to improve population health. The concept of 'distributed leadership' focuses attention on some of the skills needed for such work: fluidity, sharing roles, opening up boundaries and collegiality (Jones, 2008). Such skills link back to the boundary-spanning roles discussed in Section 3.3. Letting go of overall control and blurring the boundaries between leaders and followers enables the building of leaders at every level (Bennett et al., 2003). Three characteristics of distributed leadership relevant to public health are:

- joint or concerted action through working together to pool initiative and expertise
- open boundaries by widening the leadership group to include people at all organisational levels
- distributed expertise harnessing different varieties of experience to forge a joint dynamic.

In public health, as in other complex management situations, leaders must be open to constructive criticism if real and lasting success is to be achieved. In this context, the concept of 'followership' (Follett, 1949; Grint and Holt, 2011) is useful, not least because without followers leaders cannot deliver. Followers need to have some independence and be willing to question their leaders. If leaders can adopt an open and flexible style they are more likely to empower followers and consequently enrich the group or organisation they are leading. The alignment of situation, leadership style and the nature of the followership is therefore important (for example, Bjungstad et al., 2006).

Conclusion

Change can be chaotic and challenging to drive forward, especially if you are trying to influence it in other organisations or groups. The following questions provide a useful checklist for any practitioner embarking on organisational development and change.

- Culture – does the proposed change match the culture of those required to change?

- Identity – does the proposed change clash with critical aspects of professional identity? How could these be better aligned?

- Achievability – can you 'shrink the change' to make it less daunting, by breaking it into smaller steps?

- Motivation – can those concerned be brought to *care* about the change? Do they *feel* they have the organisational and personal resources to achieve it?

The approaches outlined in this chapter – such as, creative strategic thinking derived from being reflective about the context and community in which you are working, developing the idea of the learning organisation, embracing the need for continuous change and adaptation, and thinking about the whole system in which you work – can help you surf the wave of change positively to deliver improved outcomes. Public health itself is a very good example of all the complexity outlined in this chapter. Organisational development and change management theory and practice are vital to its success, because health needs to be promoted in a range of organisational settings (work, school, home, community and more) and by tackling some of the wider social, economic and environmental determinants of health, such as education and housing. Developing your management and leadership skills is therefore an essential investment.

References

Adobor, H. (2006) 'The role of personal relationships in inter-firm alliances: benefits, dysfunctions, and some suggestions', *Business Horizons*, vol. 49, pp. 473–86.

Alvesson, M. (2000) 'Social identity and the problem of loyalty in knowledge-intensive companies', *Journal of Management Studies*, vol. 37, no. 6, pp. 1102–23.

Audit Commission (2009) *Working Better Together? Managing Local Strategic Partnerships*, London, Audit Commission. Available at: www.audit-commission. gov.uk/SiteCollectionDocuments/AuditCommissionReports/NationalStudies/ 20042009workingbettertogetherREP.pdf (accessed 13 September 2011).

Bar-On (2006) 'The Bar-On model of emotional-social intelligence', *Psicothema*, vol. 18, pp. 13–25.

Belbin, M. (2010) 'Belbin Team Role Theory'. Available at: www.belbin.com/ rte.asp?id=8 (accessed 13 September 2011).

Belbin, M. (1981) *Management Teams – Why They Succeed or Fail*, Oxford, Heinemann.

Bennett, N., Wise, C. and Woods, P. (2003) *Review of Distributed Leadership*, Nottingham, National College for School Leadership.

Bjungsad, K., Thach, E.C., Thompson, K.J. and Morris, A. (2006) 'A fresh look at followership: a model for matching followership and leadership styles', Sonoma, Institute of Behavioral and Applied Management. Available at: www. ibam.com/pubs/jbam/articles/vol7/no3/JBAM_7_3_5_Followership.pdf (accessed 13 September 2011).

Checkland, P. and Poulter, J. (2006) *Learning for Action: A Short Definitive Account of Soft Systems Methodology*, London, Wiley.

Coulson, A. (2005) *Trust and Contracts: Relationships in Local Government, Health and Public Services*, Bristol, Policy Press.

Department of Health (DoH) (2001) *Report of the Chief Medical Officer's Project to Strengthen the Public Health Function*, London, Department of Health. Available at: www.dh.gov.uk/en/Publicationsandstatistics/Publications/ PublicationsPolicyAndGuidance/DH_4062358 (accessed 13 September 2011).

Dooris, M. and Hunter, D.J. (2007) 'Organisations and settings for promoting public health' in Lloyd, C.E., Handsley, S., Douglas, J., Earle, S. and Spurr, S. (eds) *Policy and Practice in Promoting Public Health*, London/Maidenhead, Sage/ Open University Press, pp. 95–112.

Follett, M.P. (1949) *The Essentials of Leadership*, London, Management Publications Trust Ltd.

Friend, J.K., Power, J.M. and Jewlett, C.J.L. (1974) *Public Planning: In Inter-corporate Dimension*, London, Tavistock.

Goleman, D. (1998) *Working with Emotional Intelligence*, New York, Bantam Books.

Griffiths, J. (1998) *What Is Trust?*, on behalf of the West Surrey Health Authority Executive Team (unpublished).

Grint, K., and Holt, C. (2011) *Followership in the NHS: A report for The King's Fund Commission on Leadership and Management in the NHS*, London, The King's Fund. Available at: www.kingsfund.org.uk/leadershipcommission (accessed 20 June 2011).

Handy, C.B. (1985) *Understanding Organizations* (3rd edition), Harmondsworth, Penguin Books.

Handy, C. (1990) *Inside Organisations*, London, BBC Books.

Heath, C. and Heath, D. (2010) *Switch – How to Change Things When Change is Hard*, London, Random House.

Hersey, P. and Blanchard, K.H. (1977) *Management of Organizational Behavior: Utilizing Human Resources* (3rd edition), New Jersey, Prentice Hall.

Higgs, M. and Rowland, D. (2000) 'Building change leadership capability', *Henley Working Paper Series 22*, Henley, Henley Management College.

Hutt, M.D., Stafford, E.R., Walker, B.A. and Reingen, P.H. (2000) 'Defining the social network of a strategic alliance', *Sloan Management Review*, Winter, pp. 51–62.

Janis, I.L. (1972) *Victims of Groupthink*, Boston, Houghton Mifflin Company.

Jones, L.J. (2008) 'Leadership in the "new" NHS', *Nursing Management*, vol. 15, no. 6, pp. 32–35.

Landy, F.J. (2005) 'Some historical and scientific issues related to research on emotional intelligence', *Journal of Organizational Behaviour*, vol. 26, pp. 411–24.

Lewin, K. (1946) 'Action research and minority problems', *Journal of Social Issues*, vol. 2, pp. 34–46.

Lewin, K. (1958) *Group Decision and Social Change*, New York, Holt, Rinehart and Winston.

Local Government Improvement and Development Agency (IDEA) (2011) 'Organisational development'. Available at: www.idea.gov.uk/idk/core/page.do?pageId=9110479 (accessed 15 August 2011).

Mannion, R., Davies, H.T. and Marshall, M.N. (2005) *Cultures for Performance in Health Care*, Buckingham, Open University Press.

Mintzberg, H. (1983) *Power In and Around Organizations*, Englewood Cliffs, New Jersey, Prentice-Hall.

Mintzberg, H. (1989) *Mintzberg on Management*, New York, The Free Press.

Mintzberg, H., Ahlstrand, B. and Lampel, J. (2005) *Strategy Bites Back*, New York, Pearson.

NHS Wales (2011) '1000 lives plus'. Available at: www.wales.nhs.uk/sites3/home.cfm?orgid=781 (accessed 13 September 2011).

Oakland, J.S. and Turner, S.J. (2006) 'Quality management in the 21st century – implementing successful change', *International Journal of Productivity and Quality Management*, vol. 1, no. 1–2, pp. 69–87.

Roberts, N.C. and King, P.J. (1996) *Transforming Public Policy: Dynamics of Policy Entrepreneurship and Innovation*, San Francisco, Jossey-Bass.

Schein, E. (2004) 'The levels of culture' in *Organisational Culture and Leadership*, San Francisco, Jossey-Bass.

Senge, P., Kleiner, A., Roberts, C., Ross, R.B. and Smith, B.J. (1994) *The Fifth Discipline Fieldbook: Strategies and Tools for Building a Learning Organisation*, New York, Doubleday.

Tuckman, B.W. (1965) 'Developmental sequence in small groups', *Psychological Bulletin*, vol. 6, pp. 384–99.

Tuckman, B.W. and Jensen, M.A. (1977) 'Stages of small-group development revisited', *Group Organisation Studies*, vol. 2, pp. 419–27.

Vangen, S. and Huxham, C. (2003) 'Nurturing collaborative relationships', *Journal of Applied Behavioural Sciences*, vol. 39, no. 1, pp. 5–31.

Wanless, Sir D. (2004) *Securing Health for the Whole Population*, London, HMSO.

Webb, A. (1991) 'Co-ordination: a problem in public sector management', *Policy and Politics*, vol. 19, no. 4, pp. 229–41.

Wenger, E. (2000) 'Communities of practice and social learning systems', *Organization*, vol. 7, no. 2, pp. 225–46.

Williams, P. (2002) 'The competent boundary spanner', *Public Administration*, vol. 80, no. 1, pp. 103–24.

Williams, P. (2010) *Special Agents: The Nature and Role of Boundary Spanners*, paper to the ESRC Research Seminar Services: Collaborative Futures: New Insights from Intra and Inter-sectoral Collaboration, University of Birmingham, February 2010. Available at: www.download.bham.ac.uk/govsoc/pdfs/special-agents-paper.pdf (accessed 14 August 2011).

Chapter 4: Developing as a reflective practitioner

Jenny Griffiths

Introduction

Reflective practice has long been a key dimension of professions such as teaching and nursing (Johns, 1995; Brookfield, 1995; Moon, 2004; Rolfe, 2006), but it has not until recently been of major importance to public health. However, the diversity of public health work, the increasing pressure for robust evaluation and the development of professional regulation for the wider public health workforce are combining to highlight the relevance of reflection to public health practice.

This chapter explores the meaning of reflective practice, its place in adult learning and ways in which practitioners can reflect on themselves as learners. It asks why it is important to be a reflective practitioner in public health today and discusses some of the approaches and techniques that may be useful to support practitioners in engaging with the processes of reflection. It ends by considering how reflection can be used in action planning and engagement with complex issues in public health practice.

4.1 Reflective thinking

Reflective practice has been seen as integral to professional development. Don Berwick, President of the American Institute for Healthcare Improvement, has argued that human beings have an innate desire to develop and improve what they do.

> Improvement is, I believe, an inborn human endeavour. My belief arises mostly from watching children. You cannot find a healthy child who does not try to jump higher or run faster. It takes no outside incentive. Children smile when they succeed; they smile to themselves ... Improvement is not forcing something: it is releasing something.
>
> (Berwick, 2004, p. 1124)

If 'releasing' the learning from practice is an essential ingredient in driving forward improvement, it seems important to explore how that might happen. This leads us to consider reflective practice and understand how it might unlock past experience to enhance future practice.

What is reflection?

In professional development, reflection refers to a purposeful way of thinking about experience in order to learn from it. Reflective thought has been viewed as central to education for at least a century. Dewey (1933, p. 9) defined reflective thought as 'active, persistent and careful consideration of any belief or supposed form of knowledge in the light of the grounds that support it and the further conclusions to which it tends.' He noted that people who are reflective tend to be open-minded, responsible and wholehearted.

Dewey's 'active, persistent and careful consideration' is at the heart of effective reflection. The mental processing and structured analysis brought to bear on an experience through reflection deepens the learning from it. To obtain maximum benefit, reflective thought needs to be undertaken with some rigour and stay focused on action.

Why do you think reflection is seen as being important in professional practice?

In the context of adult learning and professional practice, reflection relates to a conscious process of thinking about and interpreting experience in order to learn from it. It is a personal journey with the goal of changing perspectives and influencing future action, arising perhaps from surprise or uncertainty about what is happening. It leads to systematic review, analysis, testing of new ideas and assimilation of these new ideas (Boud et al., 1985; Schön, 1992). This is especially important for experienced practitioners, who have moved beyond initial learning and growing competence into a stage of 'unconscious competence', where skills and expertise may be taken for granted and not interrogated or reviewed. Being reflective is about being continually self-aware and self-critical so that review and learning becomes integral to practice.

Learning from experience

It is sometimes assumed that learning from personal, direct experience at work – as opposed to learning through others in an academic or other developmental setting – is especially effective for practitioners. However, people do not necessarily learn from work experience unless it is followed by a cycle of reflective thought, theorising and planning new learning (Kolb, 1984; Boud et al., 1985; Schön, 1992).

Several educational theorists have drawn attention to key aspects or 'stages' of such a cycle, although in reality they are unlikely to take place in such a discrete way (Atkins and Murphy, 1993). Kolb's experiential learning cycle (1984) is one of the most influential theories (Figure 4.1).

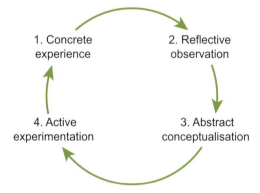

Figure 4.1 Kolb's experiential learning cycle
(Source: Kolb, 1984)

1 **Concrete experience** is 'learning by doing', from direct experience of practice. The experience may be current or may have occurred in the past.

2 **Reflective observation** or analysis focuses on what the experience means for the learner.

3 **Abstract conceptualisation** is the stage of making sense of the experience, applying some theory to its understanding and making generalisations that can be used in the future.

4 **Active experimentation** is putting into practice what has been learned.

Kolb's work has underpinned the development of subsequent models of learning in general and reflection as a particularly important aspect of learning. He highlights the notion of a continuing cycle from experience to learning, informing future experience, and so on, as lying at the heart of reflective practice.

Kolb's learning cycle in Figure 4.1 has been termed a rational model. Why do you think this is?

Kolb's cycle pays most attention to a process of reasoning: gaining experience, analysing and making sense of it, and using the learning extracted to improve practice. But as well as prompting rational analysis, experiences provoke feelings and emotions and these also influence how we experience, reflect on, analyse and use events. Other writers such as Johns (1995) and Gibbs (1988) have emphasised the importance of feelings as an explicit dimension of the reflective process (see Section 4.4).

Reflection in action and reflection on action

A further dimension of reflection relates to when it is undertaken. Schön (1992) made the distinction between 'reflection in action' and 'reflection on action'. Reflection in action takes place in the current, actual situation – it is 'thinking on your feet'. Noting feelings of (perhaps) surprise, confusion or uncertainty, you pause deliberately to reflect on your understanding and previous learning before deciding how to proceed. It is a relatively neglected technique which can enhance skills in behavioural flexibility and help practitioners work with a variety of people in a wide range of settings.

Used much more commonly, reflection on action is a 'cognitive post-mortem' undertaken retrospectively, exploring why you acted as you did, or the dynamics of interaction in the group in which you were participating.

Reflection before or for action uses the understanding gained during reflection to improve performance, building in time for planning and preparation. In a busy work life, adequate preparation before meetings and events can be difficult. It may require real effort and forward-planning to create the time, but the investment will reap considerable rewards in positive outcomes and personal effectiveness (Greenaway, 1995).

4.2 Reflective thinking and public health

It is suggested that health professional development can be aided by systematic regular reflection on the nature of practitioners' responsibilities and their actual and potential impact on people's health (Fleming, 2007; Health Professions Council, 2007). Some key dimensions of the reflective process are shown in Figure 4.2. But why has reflection on practice come to be seen as important in public health? What drivers have created this relatively new agenda and what are the implications for practitioners?

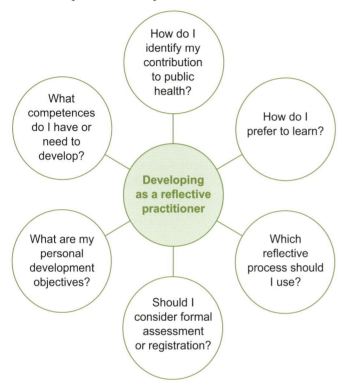

Figure 4.2 Questions relevant to developing as a reflective practitioner

(Source: Griffiths, 2011)

Three features of public health may be seen as influential in moving reflection on practice to centre-stage in public health work: the logic of professional development; the changing conception of the 'public health workforce'; and the increasing variety of the work itself.

Professional development

Reflection has been an integral part of professional development for public health specialists for some years, in particular since the UK Public Health Register (UKPHR) was established in 2003 to enable the regulation of multidisciplinary public health professionals who could demonstrate their specialist competence through creating a reflective portfolio of practice-related learning. As professional development became viewed as important for a wider group than specialists, reflection became more widely relevant. It is worth noting that health promotion and interprofessional health educators also made the case for reflection to have a central role in professional development (Fleming, 2007, 2009).

For those considering a career in the formal public health system, as a practitioner or specialist, reflective thought is regarded as the basis of personal accountability. It is included in public health standards for professional assessment, curricula for training schemes and requirements for continuing professional development. Reflective practice is considered to be fundamental to ethical, safe and effective practice by professional and standard-setting bodies, such as the Faculty of Public Health. The Faculty's code of conduct, *Good Public Health Practice: General Professional Expectations of Public Health Professionals*, states that:

> You must work with colleagues, communities and the public to monitor, maintain and improve the quality of the practice you provide and promote public safety and wellbeing. In particular, you must:
>
> 1 Maintain a portfolio of information and evidence, drawn from your practice
>
> 2 Reflect regularly on your standards of practice in accordance with appropriate guidance on licensing and revalidation ...
>
> (Faculty of Public Health, undated, section 2.3)

For experienced practitioners, reflection underpins the cycle of continuing professional development, which is seen as essential to performance review and development, and therefore to the accountability of staff to the general public. The Faculty of Public Health defines continuing professional development (CPD) as 'purposeful, systematic activity by individuals and their organisations to maintain and develop the knowledge, skills and attributes which are needed for effective professional practice. CPD is a professional obligation for all public health professionals' (Faculty of Public Health, 2009, p. 3).

UKPHR assessment and registration (UKPHR, 2011) guides professional development for public health practitioners. This provides a portfolio-based assessment process for voluntary regulation with the UKPHR, through a devolved process of assessment under way in several parts of the UK. It requires practitioners to demonstrate their competence against 12 standards through a process of critical review and reflection on the public health knowledge and skills they have acquired during their practice (see Box 4.1). It opens up voluntary registration to all autonomous practitioners working at Level 5 or above, as described in the Public Health Skills and Career Framework, whichever sector or type of public health work they engage in.

Box 4.1 Summary of public health practitioner standards

1   Recognise and address ethical issues and dilemmas.

2   Recognise and act within limits of own competence.

3   Act within legal and policy frameworks in ways that respect people's individuality, diversity and autonomy.

4   Continually develop and improve own and others' practice.

5   Promote the value of health and wellbeing and the reduction of health inequalities.

6   Obtain, verify, analyse and interpret data and/or information to improve the health and wellbeing of a population/community/group.

7   Assess the evidence of effective interventions and services to improve health and wellbeing.

8   Identify risks to health and wellbeing, providing advice on how to prevent, ameliorate or control them.

9   Work collaboratively to plan and/or deliver programmes to improve health and wellbeing outcomes for populations/communities/groups.

10 Support the implementation of policies and strategies to improve public health and wellbeing outcomes.

11 Work collaboratively with people from teams and agencies other than one's own.

12 Communicate effectively with a range of different people using different methods.

Practitioners are encouraged to include reflective statements on their learning as part of the commentaries accompanying the evidence of competence against standards (UKPHR, 2011). They are asked for evidence that they have developed and improved their own practice by systematic reflection and by finding opportunities for further development.

The wider public health workforce

Recent workforce reviews in the UK have recognised that the public's health is promoted mainly by what has been termed the 'wider public health workforce' (Department of Health [DoH], 2001), as well as more obviously by the smaller (though considerable) number of public health practitioners and the relatively tiny number of public health specialists. Alongside the specialists and practitioners whose jobs are explicitly focused on promoting public health, most occupational sectors and groups make a very important contribution to public health. It is a paradox that the majority of people who promote 'public health' do not have those two words in their job description. Broadly speaking, three very different workforce groups make up this wider public health workforce (examples of which are given in Box 4.2):

- Those who work directly with individuals and groups, for example, teachers, care workers, including all health and social care professionals, and many paid and voluntary staff in the third sector and private sector. The public health roles of, for example, those in the catering, food and water industries should not be forgotten. The list is very long and roles encompass differing elements of primary, secondary and tertiary prevention.
- Various experts with specialised knowledge of, for example, child health, environmental health, food hygiene, radiation, soil science, virology, and so on.
- Key health influencers, such as chief executives, senior managers and non-executive directors in organisations in all sectors (who have huge influence over workplace health and community leadership for health), local authority councillors, head teachers, and so on, whose remit has a profound impact on population health, particularly on the social, economic and environmental determinants of health.

To enable the best possible outcomes, it was argued, all those who contributed to public health as part of their work, including practitioners, specialists and consultants who worked in the formal public health system, needed to understand, reflect on and develop their knowledge and experience. The Public Health Skills and Career Framework (Public Health Resource Unit and Skills for Health, 2008) reflected this thinking, defining public health as multi-disciplinary, multi-professional and multi-agency. It defined the areas of work within public health, and the competencies they required, enabling anyone anywhere to identify their own contribution and where more knowledge and skills would enable them to develop their practice (see Table 4.1).

Table 4.1 Areas of work in the Public Health Skills and Career Framework, 2008

Core areas of competence for everyone working in public health	Defined areas in which people work
Surveillance and assessment of the population's health and wellbeing	Health improvement
Assessing the evidence of effectiveness of interventions and services to improve population health and wellbeing	Health protection
Policy and strategy development and implementation for population health and wellbeing	Public health intelligence
Leadership and collaborative working for population health and wellbeing	Academic public health
	Health and social care quality

The 2011 NHS Leadership Framework also emphasises 'self awareness', 'managing yourself' and 'continuing professional development' as key competencies (The National Leadership Council, 2011).

This highlights the third driver of reflection noted earlier: the diverse nature of the work itself. The wide range of practitioners making a contribution to contemporary public health is likely to expand further in the future. Few of the people in Box 4.2 (page 108) are likely to have had formal, structured public health training but each one makes a significant contribution to public health. Encouraging a structured approach to reflection on knowledge and skills has the potential to unify and create some sense of shared identity for this disparate workforce.

> ### Box 4.2 The wider public health workforce: some examples
>
> **District council housing officers** contribute to health improvement and health protection by advocating on behalf of families and tenant groups, providing information to people living in social housing and ensuring that action is taken on health risks such as poor drainage and inadequate waste management.
>
> **Community health practitioners** (school nurses, midwives and health visitors) play substantial direct roles in community health improvement and also in surveillance and assessment of population health. Indeed they are active, at different levels, in all the core areas of public health.
>
> **Teachers** are involved in the health improvement and health protection of their students. They have a role in assessing and monitoring risk, including an explicit child protection function, and surveillance and assessment through recording data and submitting reports. They may also informally assess the general health and wellbeing of students and know about health improvement interventions with young people.

 What skills and knowledge do you use in any public health-related work you are involved in?

Practitioners are often able to point to specific public health knowledge but are sometimes less confident about their skills. The core areas set out in Table 4.1 are perhaps more explicit about knowledge than skills, but team working, ethical practice, collaboration and negotiation, leadership, assessing and using evidence, and working across boundaries are implicit to the core areas. They are important for public health but have relevance to a much broader range of occupations. You may be developing these skills outside of a formal system or you may have a personal development plan agreed with you as part of an appraisal process. Whichever route is followed, professional development will involve participating in learning opportunities that use methods of learning you feel comfortable with and a systematic process of reflection to underpin the learning process. It might also be aided by using a competence assessment tool, such as the Public Health Competence Assessment Tool (PHCAT).

4.3 Understanding yourself as a learner

Becoming a reflective practitioner involves understanding yourself as a learner. Learning involves a complex set of processes and there is a long tradition in education of researching and reviewing learning methods to enhance their effectiveness (Schön, 1992). Lectures, seminars, workshops, small group work, individual sessions – and various combinations of these – have moved in and out of fashion through the years and making effective use of them may depend largely on how skilfully they are organised and presented (Hannan and Silver, 2000). Educationalists have developed innovative ways of enhancing the effectiveness of learning by using problem-based learning, decision making problems, case studies and other methods, most of which situate the learner as an active participant. These varied educational methods also raise questions about how people learn and what styles of learning they prefer to engage in.

Learning styles

The observation that people learn in different ways has given rise to theories about 'learning styles'. The notion of learning styles is based on the idea that most people prefer a particular way of taking in information and ideas, and learn most effectively and easily if their learning opportunities and techniques fit this preferred style. In order for learning to be effective, Kolb argued that all four of the stages in his learning cycle (see Figure 4.1) must be followed. But he went on to develop further insights into different types of learning styles based on his learning theory, noting that different people tended to prefer different combinations of concrete experience, active experimentation, reflective observation and abstract experimentation. This Learning Style Inventory was later developed into an assessment method for determining an individual's approach or learning style (Honey and Mumford, 2006).

The four learning styles developed by Honey and Mumford were linked to the four stages of Kolb's learning cycle. Based on observation, these abstracted styles were defined as 'Activist', 'Reflector', 'Theorist' and 'Pragmatist' (see Box 4.3, page 110). The authors argued that they reflected people's different approaches to learning, although they were seen as acquired preferences rather than being fixed in an individual's personality or character. A self-assessment learning styles questionnaire (LSQ) was developed, employing a checklist of work-related behaviours to assess an individual's preferred learning style – and it is still very widely used.

Box 4.3 Preferred learning styles

- **Activists** – have an experience – are people who learn best by doing and by trial and error. They are keen to 'have a go' and get ahead and want to get something done quickly and move on to the next new thing. Activists need particular persuasion of the importance of reflection to review the effectiveness of their actions. This links to Kolb's 'concrete experience'.

- **Reflectors** – learn from it – are people who learn best from observation or listening to the experience of others. Reflectors want to have space and time to process information. They like to review a situation to be sure of 'the facts' (as they see them) before taking any action. This links to Kolb's 'reflective observation'.

- **Theorists** – draw an idea from it – are similar to reflectors, but they need to apply a model, concept or theory to the experience. They learn through logical thinking, questioning assumptions and examples, which enable them to gain abstract understanding of things. They prefer to detach themselves from emotions and personal opinions and may not always be sympathetic to the feelings of others. This links to Kolb's 'abstract conceptualisation'.

- **Pragmatists** – apply a new idea – are similar to activists but like to have an obvious practical application to their activities. They want to put new knowledge and skills into practice and do not like repetition. This links to Kolb's 'active experimentation'.

(Honey and Mumford, 1986)

Learning styles theory accepts that styles are adaptable and can be changed, either because an individual decides they want to change or because circumstances change. Individuals are encouraged to strengthen underutilised styles in order to improve their ability to learn from a wide variety of experiences and opportunities. Kolb argued that those who use all four approaches in his learning cycle are likely to learn more effectively than those who restrict themselves to one or two preferred approaches.

The learning styles approach was subjected to critical review by researchers at the Learning and Skills Research Centre (Coffield et al., 2004). One criticism levelled at the learning styles questionnaire approach related to its reliability and validity – does it actually measure what it is intended to measure? It shifts attention from the learner to abstracted 'learner characteristics' and could obscure the difference between the learning cultures of different subjects. There was also little conclusive evidence of impact. Teaching which used the output from learning styles questionnaires appeared to have no greater success in motivating students or improving their achievements than other teaching.

What strengths and weaknesses do you see in the 'learning styles' approach?

The learning styles approach can enable individuals to reflect on the way they approach learning and, by becoming more self-aware, modify or enhance their ability to learn. Working in a team, it could be very useful to understand and deploy the different styles and strengths that team members may have. However, it does seem rather too simple to reduce the complexity of learning to four styles, especially as studying different types of subject material often requires different skills. Studying the 'art and science' of public health (Acheson, 1998), for example, requires practitioners to learn subjects as diverse as epidemiology, community development, ethics and communication. Arguably, greater attention should be paid to how the learning styles approach is used and how its effects are measured.

Multisource feedback

Multisource feedback is another aid to reflection and self-awareness, which has a long history of use in industrial settings and in organisational psychology and is now widely used in the public sector, particularly for development purposes. It is sometimes entitled '360-degree appraisal', which alludes to the individual being in the middle of a circle of colleagues who provide feedback.

Multisource feedback provides a sample of the attitudes and opinions of colleagues on performance and behaviour. It should be professionally managed and analysed, with a demonstrably valid and reliable questionnaire. Feedback is gathered from a range of sources, such as subordinates, colleagues and peers, and supervisors. Evidence suggests that the most accurate feedback comes from people who have known the subject for between one and three years – long enough to be beyond first impressions, but not so long as to have developed an entrenched view (Seifert et al., 2003). As with preferred learning styles analysis, multisource feedback can be used in team and organisational settings.

Opinions vary as to its value. Smither et al. (2005) undertook a meta-analysis of 24 longitudinal studies and found evidence about its positive benefits in terms of goal setting, feedback and performance, although not its blanket application. The evidence from Seifert et al. (2003) was more equivocal, with doubts about whether it improved employee performance. Smither et al. (2005) suggest that a key question to be asked is: under what circumstances is it useful to use multisource feedback?

Multisource feedback is also, more controversially, being incorporated in appraisal requirements by public health (and other) regulatory and professional bodies, where its focus is more evaluative and should more properly be entitled 'multisource review'. One benefit could be that it provides feedback to the appraiser and the person being appraised from a range of sources, reducing dependence on a single appraiser's or manager's views. Again, it will be important to ask careful questions about how and why it is being used.

4.4 Developing skills in reflective practice

Understanding the potential of reflection and why it is worth engaging in represents the first step in becoming a reflective practitioner. Kolb's experiential learning cycle (see Section 4.1, Figure 4.1) sets out key stages in the reflection process but begs the question: how can busy practitioners factor in reflection on action, let alone reflection in and for action?

Planning in reflection

Educational researchers have argued that reflection should be built into every stage of practice so that practitioners internalise the reflection habit and begin to create a culture of reflection. Research into management learning in the 1990s, for example, identified the value of explicitly undertaking a continuous cycle of planning and reviewing of each experience in preparation for the next (Greenaway, 1995). Although simple, Greenaway's three-stage model in Figure 4.3 is valuable because it gives equal weight to forward planning and to reflecting on previous experience.

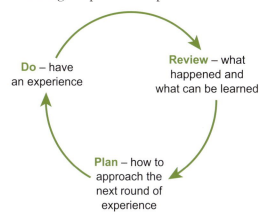

Do – have an experience

Review – what happened and what can be learned

Plan – how to approach the next round of experience

Figure 4.3 The cycle of planning, reviewing and experience

(Source: adapted from Greenaway, 1995)

Rolfe (2006) has developed an alternative formulation of this cycle, which focuses on a sequence comprising: What? So what? Now what? Developed for nursing practice, this draws attention to the importance of developing a full description of what has been experienced before undertaking the scrutiny necessary to interrogate, learn from and make use of it (or avoid repeating it) in future practice.

Reflecting on the quality of one's interaction with others is particularly useful in public health because it is a social activity: practitioners work in teams, across organisations and boundaries and in different organisational cultures. Experience supported by reflection can enable practitioners to learn how to handle the power exercised by others over the outcomes of their work and how to develop relationships with significant others who can help in the achievement of their own aims.

Structuring reflection

Several frameworks of varying complexity have been developed since Kolb's publications on experiential learning and many of the most useful models consciously build on his work, while recognising that effective reflection is not a purely cerebral process. The models described below provide complementary approaches to engagement in systematic reflection. They all include some reflection on feelings as well as thoughts, and acknowledge that an individual's emotions (and those of others involved) at the time and in retrospect will impact enormously on future behaviour. All carry the requirement for practitioners to engage in sensing and feeling as much as knowing and doing. They point towards improving performance by open discussion of fears and how to recognise and disable the triggers that can cause unwanted behaviour, such as becoming angry or upset.

Gibbs' reflective cycle (1988) (Figure 4.4) draws on Kolb's stages of analysis to make sense of the situation, but also explicitly includes feelings as an important aspect of the evaluative stage of reflection. Gibbs' cycle is considerably richer than Kolb's model, especially in encouraging practitioners to reflect from various angles on what happened by using cognition (What did I think?), emotions (What did I feel?), judgement (Was it good or bad?) and analytical ability (What sense does it make?). The model focuses on future action as well by reviewing options (What else might I have done?) and action planning (What would I do if I encountered this situation in future?).

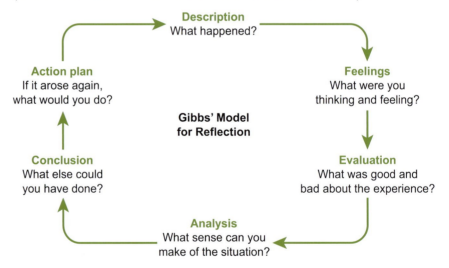

Figure 4.4 Gibbs' reflective cycle

(Source: Gibbs, 1988)

A valuable additional dimension of reflection is captured in the framework for structured reflection developed through work in the Burford Nursing Development Unit in Oxfordshire in the 1990s (Johns, 1995, 2009). Johns guides the analysis of an experience through key questions, but has a particular focus on its context (the factors that influenced it) and on the inclusion of significant others in the analysis. He emphasises the importance of sharing reflections to build a 'community of practice' and enable improved support of others. This emphasis on the context and on the influence of external others is especially useful for public health where, as we have noted, people often work in teams and across boundaries. The Johns framework has five stages.

- **Description** – drawing out the key issues within an experience through a description of thoughts, feelings and contextual background.
- **Reflection** – examining one's motivations and the consequences of actions for all stakeholders, including their possible emotional reactions.
- **Influencing factors** – determining the internal and external factors that influenced actions by self and others.
- **Alternative strategies** – evaluation of one's actions and consideration of other possible choices and their possible consequences.
- **Learning** – thinking about future practice and providing support to others.

In what ways do you think these two frameworks might help you process and learn from an experience you have had?

Below is a case study using the main elements in Gibbs' reflective cycle and in Johns' model. Compare it with your own reflection on how these frameworks might help you learn from an experience.

Stage 1: description (of the experience)

Why were you there – what are the significant background factors? What happened? Who else was there? What was your part in this? What were you trying to achieve? What parts did other people play? What was the result and for whom?

I was involved in a group developing a local mental health promotion and wellbeing strategy. I was responsible for pulling together the evidence base for the strategy. I particularly wanted to ensure that the group recognised the impact of the wider determinants on mental health (e.g. living, work and school environments, and support networks). There were a wide range of professionals in the group from local authority, health and voluntary sector backgrounds. There were three psychiatrists on the group who tried to talk down the arguments about the wider determinants of health. Many of the others accepted the arguments but were not prepared to stand up for them. After a particularly difficult meeting, I said I would not participate again, but my manager suggested that I should ask a couple of other people on the group to help me put my arguments forward. I identified a psychologist and a social worker who restated the arguments using examples from their own experience. The group as a whole decided at the next meeting that it was important to include the need for action in the workplace and in educational settings.

Stage 2: feelings

How were you feeling when the event started? How did other people make you feel? How did your feelings change? How did you feel about the outcome of the event? How do you think other people involved feel about it?

At the first meeting, I was angry and upset and did not handle myself well. I felt I was unprofessional, both at the time and particularly in retrospect. With the benefit of hindsight I can see that I did not present the evidence about the wider determinants of mental health very coherently. I think other people probably felt embarrassed and did not know how to help me because I did not give them the opportunity.

Stage 3: evaluation

Make your own judgement about what happened. What do you think went well or did not go so well? What are the views of others who were involved? Are they the same as or different from your views?

For me, the first meeting was a disaster. I was fortunate that my manager was prepared to coach me in how to identify in advance like-minded people in the group and present the evidence in a way which spans health improvement for individuals with health improvement for populations and does not sound 'political'. I realise now that the clinicians thought I was advocating political action and that I did not value their therapeutic skills.

Stage 4: analysis

Ask yourself more detailed questions about the answers to Stage 3. What preconceptions or personal beliefs have an impact on your understanding of the situation and your reaction to it? What sources of knowledge and/or skills did or should have influenced your decision making?

I was pleased that I stayed focused on evidence throughout. But I allowed my personal views about the contribution of psychiatrists to mental health to influence the way I presented and discussed it. Also, I didn't seek out my natural allies, including the two user representatives on the group who agreed with me, but were too nervous to say so at the first meeting. I was blind to their presence – this is a big learning point for me.

Stage 5: conclusion

You have now explored the issue from different angles and have developed more insight into your own and other people's behaviour. Now ask yourself what you could have done differently. What other choices did you have? How do you now feel about this experience?

I would have been more effective if I had spent some time before the meeting thinking about the likely attitudes of the different players in the group, particularly the doctors to whom others may be deferential. With the benefit of hindsight, I could have presented the evidence base differently, by focusing on the outcomes the whole group wanted to achieve and then identifying the evidence that would support those outcomes. This would have been a much more inclusive way of working and would probably have led to a better-quality strategy as well. Also, I should have asked for contributions from others, or asked the chair of the group to elicit these contributions, including the user representatives who needed to be given an opportunity to speak.

Stage 6: action plan

Think yourself forward into encountering the event or situation again and plan what you would do. What would you do differently and what would you do the same way?

> When a similar situation arises in future, I will think in advance about the membership of the group and find out as much as I can about what individual members want to achieve. I will present my work in a way that is focused on outcomes for individuals and the population as a whole. I will ensure that the link is made between health outcomes for individuals and for populations. I will draw in other members who may be diffident, but support my point of view. Finally, I will refresh and improve my review of the evidence about the impact of the wider determinants, such as working and living conditions on health, and ensure it is relevant to everybody's understanding. My knowledge base was not as up to date as it should have been.

It is important that reflection is not used as a means of over-criticising yourself or 'beating yourself up'. Try to reflect in a balanced way and remind yourself firmly of what has gone well. Reflection is not only for use when a situation has, in your view, not delivered an appropriate outcome or generally gone well. Reflecting on situations where the outcome was good and things went well will also provide much learning for utilisation in the future.

Engaging in professional development

Having considered the process of reflective practice, perhaps the most important requirement is to build in time and space to undertake and record your reflective work. The setting for reflection can influence receptivity and retention. Some people are more likely to reflect productively in a formal setting, such as a seminar room, while others will reflect more productively in an informal setting, such as a café or while out walking. Engaging the senses of vision and hearing can be helpful.

Obtaining feedback from others enhances reflection by encouraging the questioning of taken-for-granted assumptions and enabling practice to be seen through others' eyes. Many people learn most easily, and indeed develop their sense of self, through dialogue with others. A mix of opportunities and methods will offer depth and breadth of learning. Reflection can take place formally or informally, interpersonally (face-to-face, by phone, or video conferencing) or electronically. Formal reflection can be embedded in a variety of personal development processes such as:

- learning sets
- one-on-one, such as appraisal
- coaching or mentoring sessions
- shadowing and secondments.

Informal reflection can happen while chatting with colleagues over a cup of coffee or immediately after a meeting that has gone particularly well (or poorly). Reflection can also take place via e-learning tools, written online materials supplemented with audio, video, or other visual tools.

Like all effective learning methods, reflection enables you to retain control while you change. It also enables you to reconnect with your own deepest aspirations. Some of the questions you ask yourself will concern ethics; for example, how far actions matched beliefs, perhaps what factors made you act in a way not congruent with your beliefs, or how your experience has added to your ethical or moral knowledge (Johns, 1995, and see Chapter 5).

To extract the most learning from your experience you need to respond in writing, at least in note form, to a structured set of questions. This will provide you with a record for future personal reference and, if required, to enable discussion with others. For rapid use when time is short, McKenzie (2010) has suggested that four key questions might structure reflective work.

- What are the most important hard facts?
- Where do I need to dig a bit deeper? (Do I need to read up on something or talk to someone about it?)
- How can I use this in the future? (What are the implications for future policy or practice?)
- How does this make me feel?

The process of reflection will be very personal, unlike most of the report writing undertaken at work. The focus is on your behaviour, so practise being comfortable using the personal pronoun 'I' throughout.

As you develop your reflective skills, your writing will move from a description of the situation and your and others' reactions, to an analysis of context and the roles of others, to an integrated discussion with a focus on learning for the future.

Conclusion

From Dewey onwards, the art of reflection has developed as an important way of turning experience into learning to improve personal practice at work. These processes are valuable in developing your contribution to promoting public health, regardless of whether you are a member of the 'wider public health workforce', a designated public health practitioner or specialist or involved in some other capacity (perhaps as a service user).

The development of voluntary regulation through a public health practitioner assessment process by the UKPHR demonstrates commitment to the value of structured reflection by a public health regulatory body. It lies at the formal end of the spectrum of public health practice. But structured, regular reflection, undertaken in a way that meets the individual's preferences for learning and in a supportive context, can happen in an informal yet systematic way. In doing so, it can make a profound contribution to the development of each and every individual engaged in promoting public health, and to the teams in which they work.

References

Acheson, D. (1998) *Independent Enquiry into Inequalities in Health*, London, HMSO.

Atkins, S. and Murphy, K. (1993) 'Reflection: a review of the literature', *Journal of Advanced Nursing*, vol. 18, pp. 1188–92.

Beard, C. (2007) *Experiential Learning: The Development of a Framework for Effective Practice*, Sheffield, Sheffield Hallam University (unpublished PhD thesis).

Berwick, D.M. (2004) 'Lessons from developing nations on improving health care', *British Medical Journal*, vol. 328, pp. 1124–29.

Boud, D., Keogh, R. and Walker, D. (1985) *Reflection: Turning Experience into Learning*, New York, Kogan Page.

Brookfield, S.D. (1995) *Becoming a Critically Reflective Teacher*, San Francisco, California, Jossey-Bass.

Coffield, F., Mosley, D., Hall, E. and Ecclestone, K. (2004) *Learning Styles and Pedagogy: A Systematic and Critical Review*, London, Learning and Skills Research Centre. Available at: www.lsneducation.org.uk/research/reports (accessed 12 July 2011).

Department of Health (DoH) (2001) *Report of the Chief Medical Officer's Project to Strengthen the Public Health Function*, London, Department of Health. Available at: www.dh.gov.uk/en/Publicationsandstatistics/Publications/PublicationsPolicyAndGuidance/DH_4062358 (accessed 27 August 2011).

Dewey, J.D. (1933) *How We Think*, Lexington, Massachusetts, D.C. Heath.

Faculty of Public Health (undated) *Good Public Health Practice: General Professional Expectations of Public Health Professionals*, London, Faculty of Public Health. Available at: www.fph.org.uk/uploads/B_GPHP.pdf (accessed 27 August 2011).

Faculty of Public Health (2009) *Continuing Professional Development. CPD Policies, Processes and Strategic Direction*, London, Faculty of Public Health. Available at: www.fph.org.uk/uploads/FPH_CPD_Policy_and_Guidance.pdf (accessed 27 August 2011).

Fleming, P. (2007) 'Reflection – a neglected art in health promotion', *Health Education Research*, vol. 22, no. 5, pp. 658–64.

Fleming, P. (2009) 'Facilitating and assessing multidisciplinary reflection', *Connecting Reflective Learning, Teaching and Assessment*, Occasional Paper 10, London, The Higher Education Academy Health Sciences and Practice Subject Centre, pp. 25–34. Available at: http://repos.hsap.kcl.ac.uk/content/m10072/latest/occp10v1.pdf (accessed 27 August 2011).

Gibbs, G. (1988) *Learning by Doing: A Guide to Teaching and Learning Methods*, Oxford, Oxford Further Education Unit.

Greenaway, R. (1995) *Powerful Learning Experiences in Management Learning and Development*, Lancaster, University of Lancaster, Centre for the Study of Management Learning (PhD thesis).

Hannan, A. and Silver, H. (2000) *Innovating in Higher Education: Teaching, Learning and Institutional Cultures*, Buckingham, Society for Research into Higher Education and Open University Press.

Health Professions Council (2007) *Standards of Proficiency: Physiotherapists*, London, Health Professional Council.

Honey, P. and Mumford, A. (1986) *Using Your Learning Styles*, Maidenhead, Peter Honey Publications.

Honey, P. and Mumford, A. (2006) *Learning Styles Questionnaire*, Maidenhead, Peter Honey Publications. Available at: www.peterhoney.com (accessed 26 August 2011).

Johns, C. (2009) *Becoming a Reflective Practitioner* (3rd edition), London, Wiley-Blackwell Publishing.

Johns, C. (1995) 'Framing learning through reflection within Carper's fundamental ways of knowing in nursing', *Journal of Advanced Nursing*, vol. 22, pp. 226–34.

Kolb, D.A. (1984) *Experiential Learning: Experience as the Source of Learning and Development*, Englewood Cliffs, New Jersey, Prentice-Hall.

McKenzie, B. (2010) 'The learner's pool', *pH1 Life in the Middle*, November.

Moon, J.A. (2004) *A Handbook of Reflective and Experiential Learning: Theory and Practice*, London, Routledge Falmer.

The National Leadership Council (2011) 'NHS Leadership Framework' on *NHS Leadership Website*. Available at: http://nhsleadership.org/framework.asp (accessed 30 October 2011).

Public Health Online Resource for Careers, Skills and Training (PHORCAST) 'Public health competence assessment tool'. Available at: www.phorcast.org.uk (accessed 27 August 2011).

Public Health Resource Unit and Skills for Health (2008) *Public Health Skills and Career Framework*, London, Public Health Resource Unit. Available at: www.sph.nhs.uk/sph-files/PHSkills-CareerFramework_Launchdoc_April08.pdf (accessed 27 August 2011).

Rolfe, G. (2006) '"Do not ask who I am" … confession, emancipation and (self) management through reflection', *Journal of Nursing Management*, vol. 14, pp. 593–600.

Schön, D.A. (1992) *The Reflective Practitioner: How Professionals Think in Action* (2nd edition), San Francisco, California, Jossey-Bass.

Seifert, C., Yukl, G. and McDonald, R. (2003) 'Effects of multisource feedback and a feedback facilitator on the influence of behavior of managers toward subordinates', *Journal of Applied Psychology*, vol. 88, no. 3, pp. 561–9.

Smither, J.W., London, M. and Reilly, R.R. (2005) 'Does performance improve following multisource feedback? A theoretical model, meta-analysis and review of empirical findings', *Personnel Psychology*, vol. 58, pp. 33–66.

United Kingdom Public Health Register (2011) *Public Health Practitioner Assessment and Regulation*, London, UKPHR. Available at: www. publichealthregister.org.uk/ (accessed 31 August 2011).

Chapter 5: Ethical issues in public health

Peter Duncan and Alan Cribb

Introduction

Public health practice, like all practice, is inevitably saturated with values and value judgements. This is because public health is aimed at some combination of ends that are deemed desirable (e.g. disease prevention, wellbeing, the reduction of health inequalities) and uses some combination of means that are deemed acceptable (e.g. education, taxation, social engineering). If public health practitioners want to be accountable for their work then they need to be ready to pay attention to, and literally 'offer some account' of, the value judgements embodied in their practice and why and how these judgements can be defended.

In this chapter, we encourage reflection on what we have termed 'practical ethics'; that is, thinking about issues in professional practice in terms of what it is right or good to do. We hope these discussions will motivate practitioners to reflect further on questions of public health ethics, especially as these arise in their contexts of practice. Using a small number of indicative examples, we explore what kinds of values are embodied in public health and begin to tease out some of the tensions between different values. We conclude by making some suggestions about the relationship between this general exploration of values and the particular demands of day-to-day public health practice.

5.1 The relevance of public health ethics

Public health ethics is at least as important as clinical ethics. It would be absurd if society expected high standards of professional accountability from nurses or doctors working in acute healthcare but treated the ethics of public health work (including the work of public health nurses and doctors) as a minor or secondary consideration, when public health practice is designed to significantly affect the lives of large numbers of people.

Nonetheless, it would be understandable if public health practitioners were slightly reluctant to engage with ethics. The field of ethics is often associated with rather abstract, philosophical and unfathomable concerns. Someone who wishes to get on with the practical business of promoting public health may not wish to be 'bogged down' or 'led astray' by questions in philosophical ethics. However, we would suggest that ethics is fundamentally a practical activity and, indeed, one that we cannot really escape from. It is about how we decide what is 'right' or 'good' for us to do, both in general and in particular instances, hence our use of the term 'practical ethics'.

In placing this emphasis on the importance of practical reflection, we are not suggesting that the many complications of ethics can be side-stepped. There are fundamental disagreements about what is or is not justifiable in public health, and about how we can determine what would count as a justification in this area, and the existence of these disagreements needs to be recognised. We are simply suggesting it is better that the complexities and uncertainties associated with ethics are acknowledged explicitly in deliberation about public health policy and practice.

The alternative (which happens too often, partly because of the unfathomable nature of the area) is that these ethical issues are avoided or treated as if they could be managed by purely technical reasoning. It is as if the only real questions were questions about 'what works'.

5.2 Ethics in public health policy and practice

There are two separate, but strongly connected, philosophical understandings of the nature of ethics and the purpose of ethical enquiry. First, ethics attempts to address the question, 'How should we act?' Second, ethics questions what is of value and how it might be possible to produce or increase more of 'the valuable', whatever that happens to be (Lacey, 1976). The connection between these two purposes comes to light when we draw values and action together. If we want to produce more of what we regard as valuable, we need to try to determine what kinds of actions (both generally and in specific instances) are likely to result in more of the value that we are seeking, and are otherwise ethically acceptable. So the central ethical questions for public health promotion are these:

- What are the values that we are trying to produce or increase?
- How should we to go about doing this?

While these are equally important questions – in our view, it is impossible to address one without addressing both – there has sometimes been a tendency for those involved in the application of ethics to healthcare (including public health) to concentrate on the second question. In doing so, they often try to 'develop a kind of philosophical objectivity embodied in rules, principles or ... calculations ... ' (Emmerich, 2010, p. 969). The problem with the relative neglect of questions of values, at least in the field of public health (and in healthcare more generally), is that we run the risk of engaging in the wrong kind of action, however ethically scrupulous we are. This is simply because the values at the heart of the enterprise, including health itself, are so disputed. Consider the example in Box 5.1.

> **Box 5.1 Case study: Joanna Thomas**
>
> Alex Miller is a midwife who has responsibility for the antenatal care of 20-year-old Joanna Thomas. At Joanna's first antenatal appointment it becomes clear that she is a moderate smoker (ten cigarettes per day). Although she recognises the risks that this poses and says she might cut down during her pregnancy, she definitely does not want to give up.

The action that Alex takes in this situation will largely depend on her values as a practitioner promoting public health. Such values may vary considerably. Imagine two different people involved in promoting public health. Person 'A' believes that the best way to promote public health is through preventing disease. Strategies for individual behaviour change should be employed. Expert knowledge and advice should be provided as part of an effort to 'persuade' people to give up health-harming behaviour. On the other hand, person 'B' thinks that the best way to promote public health is by working with individuals or communities to establish what is important to them and helping them develop the skills and capacity to achieve their goals (Green and Tones, 2010).

In summary, we might call the approach of person 'A' the 'medical model' and the approach of person 'B' the 'empowerment model', and either may provide reasonable frameworks for action. However, it is crucial to recognise that both frameworks are laden with values. For person 'A', value lies in professional knowledge, the power of the expert and ultimately in health as disease absence. For person 'B', value exists in people-centred approaches, dialogues as free from hierarchy as possible and health as a process of empowerment. The likelihood is that 'A' and 'B' will, to some extent at least, be unhappy with each other's methods and the values that they represent. The challenge is to work out ways in which we might engage in reasoned appraisal of these (and other) approaches to public health.

How do you think Alex might respond to Joanna on the issue of smoking if she agreed with the values of person 'A' and if she agreed with the values of person 'B'?

If Alex's values are similar to those of person 'A', she will offer strong advice to Joanna about the need to quit smoking, because of the harm that this is doing to herself and her baby. If her values are more akin to those of person 'B', she might engage in a process of exploration with Joanna about why she is smoking. In addition, Alex would encourage Joanna to think about her options with regard to giving up (or not) and support her in being clear about the decision she has reached, why she has made it and its implications. Crucially, Alex would not be trying to *tell* Joanna to give up. We might also imagine that Alex's actions would be determined in some way by the values that Joanna holds. In this and many other examples, how we act as practitioners promoting public health depends on the values that we possess (as well as, hopefully, the values of patients or clients), although our values might rarely be made explicit. The principle adopted in this case ('Alex should actively intervene to stop Joanna smoking' or 'Alex should support Joanna in the decision that she has made') can only reasonably be understood and applied if there is at least some clarity about the values that the professional involved is trying to reproduce. Clarity is also needed with regard to how these relate to the values of the patient or client concerned. This point has wider applicability in promoting public health and returns us to the idea that asking questions about how we should act makes sense only if we have also addressed questions about the values we hold.

While this 'ask about values first' stance may appear reasonable, an important criticism might be that it is also rather unrealistic for practice. In the kind of individual encounter represented by Alex and Joanna, how much time and capacity do healthcare professionals have to analyse their own values, uncover the values of their patient or client and engage in evaluation? Public health practitioners are practical people who often work under pressure. Is it not possible to set out some 'values in general' for public health and then supplement these by establishing a few generalised principles for action?

Principles for public health action

Those involved in healthcare and public health ethics have devoted significant thought to the development of generalised principles, and an example is provided in the following section. With regard to the issue of 'values in general' for public health, one approach to this is to think of the *sources* of public health values. These include those actually working in the field (Tilford et al., 2003) as well as policy makers, politicians and the wider society served by public health work.

This brief indication of the sources of public health values is important because it makes clear that the values underpinning the field are not completely mysterious or ineffable. They emerge (or at least should) from those involved in it. For example, it seems uncontroversial to suggest that all parties in the public health enterprise have 'health' as a value (although there are likely to be significant differences between exactly how the value is interpreted and understood).

We have identified policy makers and politicians as one of the sources of public health values and Box 5.2 contains a statement on health from the UK coalition government. It is an extract from the White Paper *Healthy Lives, Healthy People*, which is the public health strategy for England (2010).

Box 5.2 Healthy Lives, Healthy People

Many premature deaths and illnesses could be avoided by improving lifestyles. It is estimated that a substantial proportion of cancers and over 30% of deaths from circulatory disease could be avoided, mainly through a combination of stopping smoking, improving diet and increasing physical activity ...

(Department of Health [DoH], 2010, p. 19)

 Based on this extract, how do you think the politicians directing the strategy conceive of the value of health? What other values might be underpinning the strategy?

We don't propose to undertake a detailed analysis of the values contained in the White Paper. However, it seems clear that the strategy regards 'health' primarily as the absence of disease and 'public health' as being in large measure about disease prevention. While we need to remind ourselves that others may not agree with this concept of the value of health and the purpose of public health, the White Paper provides us with one, in some ways authoritative, account of the value of health.

Having addressed the question of values, we now consider action and what we should actually do. One way to begin to address action is to think about who and what the promotion of public health is aimed at. Whose health or wellbeing are we trying to promote and improve? Who are we trying to prevent from becoming sick? In general terms, it seems that we are trying to improve the health (in some sense) of both individuals and populations (Naidoo and Wills, 2009). Of course, we would want at some stage to be more careful about exactly who we were aiming our specific efforts at: particular individuals or populations (or aggregations or segments of these such as groups and communities). We would also need to make it clear that promoting public health focuses on individuals and populations. If we add this idea to the concept of health as a value present in *Healthy Lives, Healthy People*, we start to come up with the beginnings of one ethical justification for the field. Promoting public health is valuable because it produces benefit (more health, less disease) for individuals and populations. Translating this into a response to our question about action, we can say that we should act to produce benefit (greater health) for individuals and for populations.

Whose benefit?

The production of benefit does not fully answer the question about how we should act. It is only a start, and indeed some people would say that it does not even approach the crux of ethics. This is because there are many ways in which one person (or group) might act with the intention of benefitting another person (or group), but we would not normally think reference to this intention is sufficient to justify an action. If I come around to your house to tidy up your belongings in your absence, or if I take your money from your wallet and invest it on your behalf in a high-interest account (or perhaps even give it to your favourite charity) then, despite my intention of benefitting you, I may well be judged to be doing the wrong thing. I have intervened in your life without your express permission and I may reasonably be accused of failing to treat you with due respect and of having overstepped the ethical mark.

Arguably, the central challenge for public health ethics is to find ways of differentiating public health work from these kinds of examples. In short, public health work cannot solely rest its legitimacy on the fact that it is designed to produce benefit. It needs to show that it can be ethically warranted overall. That is, as well as being related to benefits or 'goods', ethics, at least on widely recognised interpretations, is concerned about what might be thought of as 'limits' to action – things that we might, as a matter of principle, be required to do or not to do (such as taking money from a wallet without permission). The production of benefit might be called the 'classic' justification for promoting public health. However, the literature sometimes refers to two separate 'classic' justifications and considers the 'individual' justification apart in some way from that of the 'population' justification (see, for example, Wikler, 1978, 1987). Perhaps this is in some measure because the two kinds of public health action that might represent 'individual' work on the one hand, and 'population' work on the other, are often seen as separate. Work with individuals is frequently constructed as 'practice', whereas population-based work is seen as 'policy'. In our view, this dichotomy is unhelpful. It is hard to separate individuals from populations in any ethical justification of public health, simply because we cannot properly understand the former without reference to the latter (and vice versa) (Cribb, 2005; Duncan, 2010).

Take the example of Joanna Thomas again (Box 5.1). Unless we see Joanna's continued smoking as nothing more than wilful behaviour (which seems an incomplete and very unfair view), we have to make reference to wider features of her life. What are her social circumstances? Does she work? What is her level of income? What kind of family and other support does she have? In making these connections beyond the individual consultation, we are helping ourselves frame Joanna's behaviour more appropriately. For example, we know that, for a range of reasons, smoking is a health behaviour associated with inequality; someone is more likely to smoke and to die from smoking-related diseases if they are poor (Marmot, 2010). In seeking a more complete explanation for Joanna's behaviour, we move towards the wider population policy arena. Indeed, the action that Alex Miller, the midwife, might take in relation to that behaviour is only likely to be effective if broader circumstances are explored and understood.

We do not want to separate individual and population justifications for promoting public health, but prefer to see them as strongly connected. Perhaps a helpful general way of understanding this connection in an ethical sense is to regard the justifications as ways of 'seeing' public health that employ different kinds of lenses and therefore examine separate sorts of perspectives. The individual justification operates through a relatively narrow lens to examine a limited number of perspectives and claims. The population justification operates with a wider lens and considers a much larger number of perspectives and claims (Duncan, 2010). If our view is to be complete, we need both of these perspectives.

Of course, there can be tensions between the individual and wider populations in the work of those promoting public health. Indeed, such tensions are a major source of ethical difficulty in the field. Consider the example in Box 5.3.

Box 5.3 The case of Lara Ameen

On Christmas Eve 2010, Lara Ameen, a three-year-old girl from Birmingham, was diagnosed with swine flu (H1N1). She was treated in hospitals in Stockport and Liverpool but died two days later. Previously completely healthy, she would not have been eligible for vaccination against the disease through the National Health Service (NHS) as she was not in a 'high-risk' group, such as older people or those with pre-existing medical conditions, including asthma. Shortly after Lara's death, her mother, Gemma Ameen, criticised the government for not making the vaccine available to all.

(BBC News, 2011)

What do you see as the tensions between individual and population welfare, as set out in the case of Lara Ameen in Box 5.3?

This example provides just one representation from public health of the tension that is often present between the welfare of individuals on the one hand and of wider populations on the other. If Lara had received the vaccine, we can assume that she would not have contracted swine flu and her death would have been avoided. However, the government's decision to restrict vaccination to 'at risk' groups is based on evidence that it is extremely unusual for a previously healthy person to suffer life-threatening consequences as a result of contracting H1N1. In economic and supply terms, the cost of organising a population-wide vaccination programme would be too great to justify the benefits. Of course, in a very important way this kind of argument cannot compare with one inspired by the tragedy of Lara's death and the terrible grief of her parents. As we have suggested, we can see this example through the narrow lens of individual circumstance (Lara's death, the desperate emotional pain of her parents and the belief that it could have been avoided). Initially this perspective might be highly compelling; it would certainly be hard not to feel sympathy for those involved in such a dreadful situation.

Yet the argument developed through the wider lens of overall population benefit is also compelling, although different in tone and nature. As a society, we have limited resources that we are able to devote to healthcare. Generally we know that some people need protection from swine flu more than others, therefore it makes sense to devote resources to those who need it most. Overall, benefit will be maximised because the neediest people will get protection, while the rest of us will find that the health service is better able to help us when we require care in other circumstances, because resources have been more sensibly distributed. Of course, this kind of argument would not apply in other examples related to immunisation, such as measles, mumps and rubella (MMR) immunisation in childhood, where maintaining herd immunity through widespread and effective programmes is crucial to avoid an epidemic (Salisbury et al., 2006).

But in the case of H1N1, which argument should we act on? Should it be according to the compelling personal and individual benefit argument represented by Gemma, Lara's mother, or the equally demanding but different sort of argument for wider population benefit through a more targeted use of scarce resources? Asking these questions is crucial for those engaged in promoting public health because the individual benefit versus population welfare tension emerges so much in their work.

Value conflicts at the local level

There is a third and highly significant level at which those involved in promoting public health often work, alongside an individual level (Joanna Thomas and smoking) and a whole population level (immunisation against H1N1). This is at the level of groups and communities and it provides further exemplification of the tensions related to separate claims and interests that characterise the ethical problem of promoting public health. Consider the issues raised by the hypothetical Barton Heath scenario in Box 5.4.

Box 5.4 Barton Heath housing estate

Barton Heath is a large, sprawling social housing estate on the edge of a small city in the west of England. It fares poorly according to accepted indexes of deprivation and suffers from multiple social problems. Among other indicators of adverse health experience, it has very high levels of coronary heart disease (CHD) and of teenage pregnancies.

Located in the middle of the estate is a comprehensive school attended by the vast majority of local secondary-age children. Next door to this is a family centre, the focus for a small range of community initiatives. The centre is run by a national children's charity and managed by Graham Davies, a community worker. He has recently received funding from the local health service to begin, in cooperation with NHS staff, a young people's sexual health project. This aims to strengthen and develop sexuality and relationships education with local young people, using both the school and other community resources to do so. The project's first activity is a needs assessment, in which young people who have volunteered complete a confidential questionnaire about their relationships. First thing one Monday morning, Graham receives a phone call from a local councillor, Ron Evans, asking why he is going around asking lewd questions and why the NHS is paying for such rubbish when there are much more important things to spend scarce money on.

What issues of values and ethics are highlighted by the Barton Heath case study in Box 5.4?

The Barton Heath scenario raises a cluster of issues to do with values and ethics, some of which we came across in the Joanna Thomas and H1N1 examples. Clearly, Councillor Evans' view of the nature of health and methods for its improvement is quite different from that of Graham Davies, and presumably those who funded the sexual health project. This example raises the issue of resource allocation once again. Exactly how can the decision to spend money on this particular project be justified when there are so many competing possibilities? Of course, we can point to the project's importance in helping to address the 'problem' of local teenage pregnancy rates, but that by itself will not resolve questions of relative priority. For example, why didn't the money being spent on sexual health go towards working on CHD prevention?

This community-based example throws such questions of values dispute and prioritisation of resources into very sharp relief. This is at least partly because this kind of example highlights the complex web of relationships in which many efforts to promote public health are entangled. Disassembling the value disputes contained within this example is also harder because there is sometimes a tendency to regard communities as groups with shared interests and values, whereas delving beneath the surface of Barton Heath will reveal wide diversity with regard to such things. For example, do all the residents, including the young people, uniformly view teenage pregnancy as a problem? (Cribb and Duncan, 2002.)

In the case of Joanna Thomas and Alex Miller, while we argued that Alex had to take account of relationships beyond the individual consultation, what really mattered was her transaction with Joanna and the values espoused by her and Joanna. This relationship might have been based on principles of persuasion, or ones of empowerment. The point is that there was a relatively limited number of ways of conceiving of the relationship and therefore of drawing conclusions about its ethical acceptability.

In Barton Heath, there are many different kinds of relationships going on – between members of the project team and the young people, other local people and their elected representative, and so on – and a range of value positions to take into account. In contrast to the population-based considerations of H1N1, these relationships are relatively close and complex ones, and the diversity of relevant values is obvious. Whether or not the funding is given or withdrawn for the sexual health project will directly affect people who are neighbours or people who share families and friends. Decisions about swine flu vaccination will directly affect some individuals (such as Lara Ameen), but the overall impact will be much less visible because it is spread across the whole population. The impact on wider-value disputes (that is, disputes beyond any controversies about vaccination itself) appears relatively marginal.

Balancing obligations

Ultimately, the differences between the examples are not that clear cut. The framing of the first two examples masks the complex entanglement of relationships, which is manifest in the third example. But this 'framing effect' corresponds in large part with the ways such examples are experienced in real life. That is, sometimes ethical issues are presented and considered as if they had a sharp focus and other times it is more obvious that they are multi-layered.

What is clear from each of the three examples we have considered is that those involved in struggling to promote public health face a range of ethical difficulties in doing so. Furthermore, they cannot simply point to the value of health (however understood) to justify their actions. This is because there are important disagreements about the value of health (and the other values inherent in models of health promotion) as well as serious ethical conflicts and dilemmas to be faced in deciding how they should act.

Public health practitioners need to be able to debate *both* the 'goods' they are promoting *and* the possible 'limits' to their actions, and the tensions within and between these two sets of concerns. The example of fluoridation of water supplies is sufficient to indicate this complexity. The ethics of fluoridation necessarily encompasses debate about the various kinds of harms and benefits that might come about as a result of fluoridation and what other kinds of 'wrongs' might be at stake here. For example, do people have a right to fluoride-free water, or do they, perhaps, have a right to be given the benefits of fluoride? Can the decision about fluoridation be made in a way that somehow respects people's wishes, and so on? In short, how and why might fluoridation be different from the 'taking money from the wallet' kind of example used earlier?

In addition, public health practitioners need to be conscious of the different constituencies that have an ethical claim on them. How can they balance the obligations they believe they have to particular people, to produce individual benefit for example, with a concern for the consequences of their action, which might potentially affect other individuals, wider groups or even whole populations? These are some of the fundamental questions facing those working to improve public health.

5.3 Towards dealing with ethical issues in promoting public health

Those working on the application of ethics to healthcare need to find ways of representing and managing the complexities introduced so far; for example, of dealing with both 'goods and bads' and 'rights and wrongs'. The frequently cited debate in applied philosophy literature between 'consequence-based' (consequentialist) and 'duty-based' (deontological) approaches to ethics is essentially a debate about whether or not questions of right and wrong can be answered wholly by reference to good or bad consequences or whether some other ingredient (which we have signalled here using the shorthand 'limits') is necessary. For the purposes of practical ethics it does not make sense to expect a speedy resolution of this longstanding debate.

Four principles of healthcare ethics

What is necessary are practical ways of acknowledging these different perspectives on, and interpretations of, ethics. The best-known attempt to do this is the 'famous four' principles of healthcare ethics. The four principles were originally proposed and developed by two American philosophers, Tom Beauchamp and Jim Childress (2001). They argued that, everything else being equal, those involved in healthcare should adhere to the following principles:

- beneficence (a concern to do good or produce benefit for patients or clients)
- non-maleficence (a concern to avoid harm)
- respect for autonomy (of patients or clients, in so far as such respect does not impinge on the equal autonomy of others)
- concern for justice (e.g. through the fair distribution of scarce healthcare resources or addressing the natural rights of patients or clients, such as the right to be treated with dignity).

The principles are talked of as being prima facie (Gillon, 1994). This means that each is binding, unless they are in conflict, in which case the principles have to be balanced against one another.

Those working in public health have a responsibility to consider their actions and work out what it would be best to do according to the demands of the principles. An obvious initial worry lies in the idea that they are binding, unless in conflict. What happens in this kind of situation? This worry is an important one. Public health practitioners are busy people and it is understandable that they seek explicit guidance from the principles.

Perhaps the worry can best be addressed by arguing that the four principles allow the establishment of a 'common moral language' (Gillon, 1994, p. 184) through which ethical debate can take place and decisions about action can be reached. They provide a *framework* for decision making, proposing a set of values and obligations that we must (and would surely want to) take into account as we decide what to do. At the same time, the principles do not exclude thought from our decisions because they are prima facie; we should adhere to them if we possibly can, but sometimes we may have to balance them against one another. To the extent that they seek to provide a common moral language and framework, and allow recognition of both consequences and duties, the principles are *pluralist*. That is to say, they attempt to provide an underpinning theory for ethics in healthcare that stands a fair chance of being widely accepted (Jackson, 2006).

Consider again the examples of individual, whole population and community-based public health work that we have discussed in this chapter. If the four principles are to be a useful aid to practitioners, they need to offer reasonable guidance in each of these different kinds of situations.

How helpful are the principles in establishing what we should actually do for each sort of case?

In some respects, the principles appear to offer useful assistance. Consider first Joanna and Alex Miller, her midwife. Alex is perhaps likely to think that giving Joanna advice about the risks of smoking will meet the principle of beneficence. Giving up the habit will, according to Alex, improve Joanna's health. However, awareness of the principle of non-maleficence might prompt Alex to be aware that in any intervention, we stand the chance of not only producing benefit but also creating harm. Alex might be concerned that advice (especially if it is very persuasive) will cause Joanna to be worried about the effects of smoking on her baby to date. She may also be concerned that these worries could be increased because Joanna believes it would be very hard for her actually to give up smoking. These concerns could prompt Alex towards careful consideration of her position in relation to the principle of respect for autonomy. Alex might recognise that her concept of 'health' may not match that held by Joanna, who could view smoking as actually health-enhancing (it is pleasurable for her, allows some relief from a stressful life, and so on). Therefore, Alex's advice must be tempered by recognition of the fundamental importance of Joanna's views and her client's right to decide what she actually wants to do. This relates also to some concepts of the justice principle. For example, Joanna's right to treatment with dignity seems important here, although on other concepts of justice things may appear more complicated. For example, if Joanna continues to smoke, both she and her baby may place a greater burden on scarce healthcare resources than might otherwise have been the case.

Now, consider the case of population-wide availability of the H1N1 vaccine. Here the principle of justice (at least in terms of the fairest use of healthcare resources) is likely to move to the foreground. Can we advocate an intervention that is likely to have limited utility (in terms of avoiding mortality and severe morbidity) within the general population? Wouldn't it be more reasonable to stick to the position of vaccine administration to those groups most at risk? Certainly we might avoid individual tragedies, such as that of Lara Ameen, and this production of individual benefit is clearly important. However, can it outweigh a massive increase in vaccine costs and the effects that this is likely to have on what might be achieved by the overall healthcare budget? Our concerns might be intensified when we think about this example in relation to the principle of non-maleficence. By extending the idea of 'risk' from swine flu to the total population (we are vaccinating everybody because we are all 'at risk'), we may be creating worry and even panic. (Although the panic might exist anyway and is likely to be created and fed by media representations, a sudden change in policy direction may well stoke media 'hype' and public concern.)

Finally, there is the example of the Barton Heath project. Here we can say that the work on sexual health could produce benefit for at least a number of young people who may feel more empowered in their emotional and sexual relationships as a result of the intervention. Against this, there might be reason to believe that the work will raise anxiety among young people and the wider community. (The muddled feelings of adolescence require great sensitivity and it would be very easy for project workers, however well-intentioned, to unwittingly overstep boundaries. And other members of the community, for example parents, might feel that establishment of a sexual health agenda by professionals weakens their own control and authority.) If the project is conducted in a genuinely empowering way, it may meet the principle of respect for autonomy at least in relation to the young people who participate. But, as we have already made clear, there is a range of autonomous interests to be considered in any community and the effects of the work will almost certainly extend beyond those to whom it is directly delivered. Equally, separate conceptions of justice, at least in a distributive sense, will come into play. Councillor Evans is unlikely to be alone in thinking that, in an era of scarce resources and an area with multiple needs, the money for the project could be much better spent elsewhere.

Guidance but not 'answers'

This brief consideration of the three different kinds of examples in the context of the four principles approach indicates their use and potential. For many people they will offer greater clarity in ethical thinking than would come from simply relying on their immediate commonsense reactions. They have certainly prompted thinking and perhaps engendered debate. However, reflecting on the examples also draws out the difficulties with, or limitations of, the principles. We are reminded that they cannot provide us with explicit and definitive guidance. What exactly should be the balance, say, between the production of benefit and respect for autonomy in the case of Joanna Thomas and Alex Miller? Are we right in making a judgement that fair distribution of health resources should trump the avoidance of desperate individual tragedy in the swine flu vaccination example? How exactly can we decide that the potential harms for the wider community are balanced by the benefit for the young people involved in the Barton Heath project? Supporters of the principles quite freely admit that they can't provide definitive answers; their use lies principally in their capacity to support ethical reflection.

Equally, however, there is a striking danger in the idea that the principles might be sufficient for ethical judgement; as if they were equipment that comes up with 'answers' to complex problems in the same way that a sphygmomanometer supplies us with a patient's blood pressure. Ethical deliberation is obviously not like taking a blood pressure reading.

Contained within these two potential criticisms of the four principles, though, lies a possible way forward. While they cannot provide absolute answers, they can help frame debate. They should not be used in a 'machine-like' way, but with sympathy and an awareness of their limitations they may be a useful resource. In our discussion of the examples we have used, much depended on sensitivity, and a preparedness to explore the context and to make connections between separate pieces of information and different judgements.

5.4 The continuing challenge of practical ethics in public health

The discussion so far has concentrated on explaining some of the basic value questions, and the related disputes, underlying public health. Reflecting on these questions forces us to consider (or reconsider) the basic 'value drivers' of public health practice and highlights the need to negotiate ethical 'balancing acts' in the formulation and enactment of practice. The balances we have considered relate, for example, to different concepts of health (including *whose* concepts of health should be in the foreground of policy and practice) and the challenge of paying attention to individual and population level ends, as well as the multiple interests present in any example of community public health.

A further cross-cutting tension, corresponding with two different theoretical traditions but also reflecting a feature of 'commonsense' experience, is the balance between an emphasis on duties and one on consequences. In concrete terms we experience something akin to this tension when we feel 'duty bound' because of questions of principle to take a course of action that might be deemed to have a lower 'cost-benefit' than other options (for example, an intervention that may produce less 'health output' for the same expenditure). As we have noted, the four principles also provide a useful framework for exploring and clarifying some of the key values at stake in these balancing acts and may also be helpful as a springboard for debates or deliberation, although their application is certainly not without difficulty.

In one sense this process of explanation and exploration is an important start. In another sense it might be said that nearly everything still remains to be done. An 'architectural' sketch of some of the structures of public health ethics is useful, but such a sketch not only leaves many more details unidentified but also (and more importantly) leaves all of the 'building' work undone. As we stressed in the introduction, our focus is on practical ethics and practical ethics depends on policy makers and practitioners, as groups or as individuals, taking responsibility for deliberating about, and deciding, what they should do.

Ethics: theory and practice

Practitioners are not entirely alone in this practical ethics enterprise. There is a growing body of theorists engaging with practical challenges in public health ethics (for example, Dawson and Verweij, 2007; and in the journal *Public Health Ethics*; Peckham and Hann, 2009) and policy making agencies and other organisations have offered analyses in the area. In Scotland, an NHS working group report on *Making Difficult Decisions in NHS Boards in Scotland* (NHS Scotland, 2010) recommended that boards developed explicit principles and values for decision making that members could use in individual and population level decision making about treatments and interventions.

In England, the Nuffield Council on Bioethics has produced a much-cited report (Nuffield Council on Bioethics, 2007), which wrestles with, and offers advice about, a range of important and high-profile dilemmas related to infectious disease control, obesity, alcohol and smoking policy, and fluoridation, and considers the question of 'acceptable' kinds and levels of intervention and the possible justifications for such interventions. The report emphasises a concept that it calls 'stewardship': the idea that 'liberal states have a duty to look after the important needs of people individually and collectively' (p. xvi). In relation to public health, this would involve, for example, the state agreeing to and acting on obligations to create conditions for healthy lives and address inequalities in health.

In the light of the discussions in this chapter, how helpful is such ethical direction in public health practice and policy?

Although these are useful places to look for guidance and support, they do not ultimately help with the business of practical ethics. One of the things that is characteristic – one might even argue definitional – of ethics is that we have to make ethical judgements for ourselves. Not only does it seem wrong but also it does not seem to make much sense for someone (simply) to say, 'I am taking ethical responsibility here by doing what X, Y or Z tells me I should do.' There may be cases in which we could provide good reasons for this kind of justification, but these cases certainly could not be the norm if ethics is to retain the sense that we usually give to it. This means, for example, that while we might think a particular approach (like the 'stewardship model') has something to commend it, however much we might wish to endorse it we cannot abdicate or transfer our responsibility to the approach itself. To the extent that we think a model or an analysis is useful for guiding our actions, we are choosing to treat it as such and we remain responsible for those actions.

Reflection on the nature of models as guides and the requirement for action captures one key difference between theoretical ethics and practical ethics. Debating issues in the abstract is quite clearly not the same as being an agent (or one of the agents) responsible for deciding something. The practical agent has an extra layer of 'real world' accountability. There are other equally important, and related, differences. Practical agents (whether practitioners or policy makers) do not 'float above' issues and circumstances, but are entangled in them. We say this for three reasons:

- the ethical issues they face are not neatly separated out into discrete problems, but are all compounded together
- what they can achieve will be partly dependent on their roles and resources and the social and institutional constraints they face
- for the most part, effecting change will not be something they can do on their own, but will depend on them operating in collaboration with, and/or through struggles with, other agents (each with their own resources, constraints and perspectives) (Cribb, 2011).

Conclusion

In an area such as public health, which is so conspicuously bound up with national, local and personal politics, there is inevitably a pragmatic dimension to ethics. This is not to say that the focus should not be on what is right or good. If we are dealing with ethics at all, this much is not negotiable. However, it is to claim that, in addition, we need to be focused on how to do what is right or good.

Public health practitioners and policy makers are accountable for the decisions they make and the influence they have. They cannot hide behind other people, but rather need to be able to provide a reasoned and evidence-based ethical defence of their work. Reflection on, and debate about, values and value tensions can help support this process, but equally important is reflection on, and debate about, the pragmatics of public health work. Public health ethics involves combining values and pragmatism, without losing sight of either. We hope that by drawing out and beginning to explain some of the values and the ethical dilemmas that are deeply embedded in practice, we might help practitioners meet this challenge.

References

BBC News (2011) 'Birmingham girl aged three dies from swine flu'. Available at: www.bbc.co.uk-england-birmingham-12172690 (accessed 14 January 2011).

Beauchamp, T.L. and Childress, J.F. (2001) *Principles of Biomedical Ethics* (5th edition), New York, Oxford University Press.

Cribb, A. (2011) 'Beyond the classroom wall: theorist–practitioner relationships and extra-mural ethics', *Ethical Theory and Moral Practice*, vol. 14, no. 4, pp. 383–96.

Cribb, A. (2005) *Health and the Good Society: Setting Bioethics in Its Social Context*, Oxford, Oxford University Press.

Cribb, A. and Duncan, P. (2002) *Health Promotion and Professional Ethics*, Oxford, Blackwell Science.

Dawson, A. and Verweij, M. (2007) *Ethics, Prevention and Public Health*, Oxford, Oxford University Press.

Department of Health (DoH) (2010) *Healthy Lives, Healthy People: Our Strategy for Public Health in England*, London, The Stationery Office. Available at: www.dh.gov.uk/en/Publicationsandstatistics/Publications/PublicationsPolicyAndGuidance/DH_121941 (accessed 28 August 2011).

Duncan, P. (2010) *Values, Ethics and Healthcare*, London, Sage.

Emmerich, N. (2010) 'Values, ethics and healthcare' (book review), *Sociology of Health and Illness*, vol. 32, pp. 968–69.

Gillon, R. (1994) 'Medical ethics: four principles plus attention to scope', *British Medical Journal*, vol. 309, pp. 184–8.

Green, J. and Tones, K. (2010) *Health Promotion: Planning and Strategies* (2nd edition), London, Sage.

Jackson, J. (2006) *Ethics in Medicine*, Cambridge, Polity Press.

Lacey, A.R. (1976) *A Dictionary of Philosophy*, London, Routledge and Kegan Paul.

Marmot, Sir M. (2010) *Fair Society: Healthy Lives: A Report of the Review of Health Inequalities in England Post-2010*, London, Marmot Review.

Naidoo, J. and Wills, J. (2009) *Foundations for Health Promotion* (3rd edition), Edinburgh, Elsevier.

NHS Scotland (2010) *Making Difficult Decisions in NHS Boards in Scotland: Report of a Short Life Working Group*, Kirkcaldy, NHS Fife. Available at: www.nhsfife.scot.nhs.uk/difficultdecisions/Difficult_Decisions_Mar_2010.pdf (accessed 10 August 2011).

Nuffield Council on Bioethics (2007) *Public Health: Ethical Issues*, London, Nuffield Council on Bioethics.

Peckham, S. and Hann, A. (2009) *Public Health Ethics and Practice*, Bristol, Policy Press.

Salisbury, D., Ramsay, M. and Noakes, K. (2006) *Immunisation Against Infectious Diseases*, London, Department of Health. Available at: www.dh.gov.uk/ prod_consum_dh/groups/dh_digitalassets/@dh/@en/documents/digitalasset/ dh_128827.pdf (accessed 28 August 2011).

Tilford, S.J., Green, J. and Tones, K. (2003) *Values, Health Promotion and the Public Health*, Leeds, Leeds Metropolitan University.

Wikler, D. (1987) 'Who should be blamed for being sick?', *Health Education Quarterly*, vol. 14, no. 1, pp. 11–25.

Wikler, D.I. (1978) 'Persuasion and coercion for health: ethical issues in government efforts to change lifestyles', *Milbank Memorial Fund Quarterly/Health and Society*, vol. 56, no. 3, pp. 303–8.

Chapter 6: Understanding and using theories and models

Jane Wills

Introduction

Any major public health issue that we choose to consider will demand multiple strategies at many levels, from encouraging individuals to change their lifestyle, to engaging with communities for development, to wider social and policy change. So how do practitioners decide what to do? To some extent they use their practice wisdom: what experience has shown them and what they have learned. They will also be sensitive to the context in which they are working, its population's needs and the available resources. These context-specific factors, practitioner insights and client or community needs contribute to an understanding of promoting health that is contingent and contextual. It may be highly developed and practitioners may have a clear understanding of what might work and why. This process of reflection, learning from doing and developing new explanations for phenomena and new situations – 'praxis' as educationalists term it – is central to becoming a 'reflective practitioner'.

However, practice wisdom may not offer sufficient guidance. Practitioners may also use existing theory to guide what they do. This chapter explores the range of theories and models that have been developed in health promotion and public health. It explores why theory is useful to practitioners and examines how theories have been developed at different levels and for a range of different purposes. These include theories at an individual level, for example to explain and predict behaviour change; at group and community level; and at whole-systems level, to situate values and perspectives in health promotion and public health within a wider social framework.

6.1 There is nothing as practical as a good theory

Theories are organised sets of knowledge applicable in a variety of circumstances. They may help to analyse, predict or explain a particular phenomenon or why something happens and the ways in which change takes place in individuals, communities, organisations and societies. In most disciplines the building of theory and progress towards an explanation for phenomena and their relationship is an accepted part of study and research. Theory may consequently help answer different questions. It may be:

- descriptive – what is it?
- explanatory – why is it?
- predictive – what would happen if?
- prescriptive – what should be done?

Health promotion and public health use knowledge and theories derived from research in other disciplines. It is suggested that health promotion in particular is an eclectic discipline or field of study which draws on other disciplines such as sociology, psychology, biomedicine, epidemiology, education, social marketing and communication (Bunton and Macdonald, 2002). Such diversity reflects the fact that health-promotion practice is concerned not only with changing individual health behaviours, but also with the organisation of society and the role of policy and organisational and community structures in promoting health. Traditional public health, on the other hand, draws principally from epidemiology and biomedicine to study the aetiology, incidence and prevalence of diseases and the surveillance and assessment of population health. Within each of these disciplines there are different ways of constructing the knowledge base, different theories and ways of problem solving, with particular methods and tools that are used for investigation and to acquire knowledge.

In Bunton and Macdonald's seminal text on the disciplinary frameworks for health promotion, Thorogood (2002) suggests that sociology, which analyses social class, gender and global issues, can be of use to those promoting health because it looks at the contextual and structural factors that shape and influence health choices. Attention is given not to biological causes of health differences but to the reasons why, for example, working-class people get sick and die earlier. Equally, psychology has been influential in helping us understand how to develop change strategies for individuals through behavioural interventions. It has aided understanding of the role of psychosocial factors, such as social support networks, personal resilience and sense of control, in a wide range of health problems. The ethnographic approach of anthropology has explored the lived experience of diseases and conditions and the socio-cultural conditions which contribute to the communication of diseases. Political science shows how differences in policy can create or limit conditions for diseases; for example, the governance threat posed by HIV/AIDS in southern Africa. Education, social marketing and communication examine how information is structured, disseminated and received in settings such as primary care, where individuals may be given one-to-one advice and counselling on health issues such as smoking, weight reduction and drinking habits.

A theoretical basis for practice pushes practitioners to make explicit their assumptions about why an intervention should work, hence Kurt Lewin's much quoted phrase: 'There is nothing as practical as a good theory' (Lewin, 1951, p. 169). It may be obvious that reducing speed lessens traffic fatalities, or smoke alarms reduce fire fatalities, but what public health practitioners need to know is how to effect change in individuals, communities, organisations and society as a whole.

How do you think theories might help you engage in developing effective practice?

Theories can be used to guide the search for reasons why people are or are not following public health advice, or not caring for themselves in healthy ways. Theories can explain the dynamics of health behaviour, the processes for changing the behaviour, and the effects of external influences on the behaviour. Theories can help pinpoint *what* a practitioner needs to know before developing or organising an intervention, such as how people learn or how messages are communicated. They can provide insight into *how* a practitioner can shape programme strategies to reach individuals, communities and organisations and make an impact on them. Theories also help identify *what* should be monitored, measured, and/or compared in the programme evaluation.

Yet the explicit use of theory in the planning and development of strategy and programmes is not common. Its absence prompted the Royal Society of Public Health (RSPH) to issue a briefing on why theory matters (RSPH, 2009). The US National Cancer Institute (2005) also published a guide to theories appropriate for public health and health-promotion planning entitled *Theory at a Glance: A Guide for Practice*, rather suggesting there is an easy route to theoretical understanding. Guidance on the completion of systematic reviews of evidence also now calls for research studies to include the theoretical principles that guided the investigation (Higgins and Green, 2011).

What accounts for the relative absence of theory in health promotion and public health? While drawing on some modernist theories of change, health promotion can be placed in a post-modern tradition that does not prize rationality in analysing and structuring responses to health concerns and which privileges interpretive methodologies in answering questions. Green (2000, p. 125) asserts that 'For many, theory is equated with a reductionist position, and therefore judged to be incompatible with both holism and empowerment – the central tenets of health promotion.' Public health, on the other hand, has prided itself on its empiricism – relating all knowledge to observed 'facts' – and is often claimed to be devoid of theoretical approaches (Jones and Walker, 1997).

As Chapter 5 highlights, whichever approach we take to promoting health, it is informed by our values – values about what health is, what contributes to its maintenance and what should be done by whom to protect it. A 'medical model' of health, for example, assumes health status and difference to be biological or the result of individual lifestyles, whereas a 'social model' assumes that lifestyle choices are socially shaped and that there are structural variables that determine health and illness (see Table 1.3 in Chapter 1). These models reflect different and divergent philosophical perspectives: a medical focus on the individual and on people's 'agency' or capacity for free will or a social focus on the collective or structural, and on categories such as age, gender, class and social factors. This dichotomy might seem simplistic and not reflective of the complexity involved in promoting health, but it does draw attention to the values that shape public health.

Values determine the way in which the world is seen and, consequently, the selection of activities and priorities and how strategies are implemented. Although rarely articulated explicitly, values inform, shape and guide the direction of public health practice (Wills and Woodhead, 2004), forming the conceptual, emotional and intellectual foreground to individual and collective practice. Jones and Walker (1997, p. 71) noted the need for principles to underpin practice and for an 'internally and externally consistent foundation for fulfilling the public health role.'

6.2 Models of health promotion

In most countries of the world, the principles and action areas of the Ottawa Charter are the guide for practice. In the UK, by contrast, there was a proliferation of models of health promotion in the 1980s as academics and practitioners sought to chart the territory of health promotion in terms of its varied activities and goals across different levels and sectors. Most of these models are what Rawson (2002) calls 'iconic' – in other words, they are exemplars or descriptions of practice. What they do not do is identify the values and conflicts that underpin that practice or provide a guide for how to proceed with an intervention as do, for example, nursing models. Using a model can be helpful, as Naidoo and Wills (2009, p. 76) point out, because it 'encourages the practitioner to think theoretically, and to come up with new strategies and ways of working. It can also help to prioritise and locate more or less desirable types of interventions.'

Models that map activity

Two of the most influential models of health-promotion practice are the models proposed by Ewles and Simnett (1985) and Tannahill (1985). These models depict different approaches and reflect one of the tensions in health promotion and public health practice between approaches that focus on disease prevention and the management of long-term conditions, approaches that seek to promote wellbeing and positive health, and approaches that seek to address the structural determinants of health and ill health through policy interventions. Tannahill's model describes three approaches to health promotion: disease prevention, health education and 'protection', which encompasses environmental and policy interventions. This model, developed by a community physician, sits within a broader medical public health model in which the promotion of health is seen as achieved by medical interventions, such as vaccination and screening, together with the education of patients and individuals to avoid risky behaviours and risks in the environment.

Ewles and Simnett's model (Table 6.1) describes five approaches to health promotion. These range from 'medical' interventions to encourage patient compliance and persuade people to seek early treatment, to a 'societal change' approach which focuses on action to 'change the physical/social environment'. In between lie three different types of health education activity: encouraging behaviour change, informing and educating people about health issues, and empowering clients to set their own agendas in health. Different types of health-promotion activity are seen as important in each approach. In the behavioural approach, for example, the focus of activity is attitude and behaviour change to encourage adoption of 'healthier' lifestyles, whereas in the client-centred approach, it is working with clients' identified health issues, choices and actions.

Table 6.1 Five approaches to health promotion

Approach	Aim	Activity	Values
Medical	Freedom from medically defined disease and disability	Promote medical intervention to prevent or reduce ill health	Patient compliance
Behaviour change	Individual behaviour conducive to freedom from disease	Change client attitudes / behaviour towards adopting healthier lifestyle	Health promoter-led and defined 'healthy lifestyle'
Educational	Individuals with knowledge/ understanding make informed decisions about their health	Educate client about cause/effects of behaviours. Explore values; develop skills	Education as agent to change behaviour
Client-centred	Working with a client on the client's own terms	Respond to client, who identifies health issues, choices, actions	Self-empowerment of client
Societal change	Physical and social environment which enables choice of healthier lifestyle	Political/social action to change physical/social environment	Right and need to make environment health-enhancing

(Source: adapted from Ewles and Simnett, 1985)

How would you characterise the model in Table 6.1 – is it descriptive or analytical?

The model offers a clear and useful account of different ways of thinking about promoting health. It also draws on practice experience as the basis from which to distil the five approaches and, in doing so, attempts to illuminate the dilemmas of health promotion. Yet it still essentially describes how health promotion happens, rather than commenting on the values and conflicts that underpin it. In developing this model the authors commented:

> In our view, there is no 'right' aim for health promotion, and no one 'right' approach or set of activities. We need to work out for ourselves which aim and which activities we use, in accordance with our own professional code of conduct (if there is one), our own carefully considered values and our own assessment of our clients' needs.
>
> (Ewles and Simnett, 2003, p. 43)

Although the different approaches are seen as having distinctive priorities and objectives, and as reflecting very different views of patients/clients, there is an underlying assumption that all approaches are valid depending on the context and that they are interrelated and work most effectively in combination with each other. No one approach is seen to take or should take priority. While this inclusive strategy is reassuring, it may be that recycling descriptions of current practice is ultimately non-productive and does not stimulate practitioners to go much beyond the status quo. Relativism does not encourage clarification of values, whereas the reflective practitioner's task is to go beyond description to analysis (Schön, 1992).

Modelling empowerment

The approaches mapped by these models sit within a paradigm that Collins (1995) calls 'human-developmental'. Within the human-developmental paradigm are those approaches that are about educating individuals to take greater control over their health, variously called 'medical', 'behaviour change', 'educational' or 'empowerment'. All such approaches are concerned with people as individuals and the belief that individuals should change to a defined goal of health behaviour is implicit. Such approaches differ in their views of the ethics and obligations of the practitioner and the basis of the knowledge about what should be changed. Some privilege the view of the health practitioner and others that of the client. The empowerment approach (also known as the self-actualisation model) seeks to develop the individual's ability to control their own health status as far as possible within their environment.

Tones et al.'s empowerment model of health promotion (1990) was also originally developed in the mid-1980s, but places much more emphasis on the role of health education. The model focuses on enhancing an individual's sense of personal identity and self-worth and on the development of 'life skills', including decision making and problem-solving skills, so that the individual will be willing and able to take control of their own life. People are encouraged to engage in critical thinking and critical action at an individual level. The model was developed further over the next two decades, influenced by the focus in the UK on reducing health inequalities. The latest version of the model (see Chapter 10, Figure 10.1) has come to encompass ideas of community empowerment, which require people individually and collectively to acquire the knowledge, understanding, skills and commitment to improve the societal structures that have such a powerful influence on people's health status. It engages people in critical thinking in order to improve their understanding of the factors affecting individual and community wellbeing. It also engages them in critical action that can contribute to positive change at a collective level. Health promotion is seen as deriving from the relationship between education and healthy public policy. The development of policy is not simply to protect populations as conceived in Tannahill's model, but also to create health-promoting environments.

These models of health promotion have stood the test of time and are still widely used because this type of descriptive mapping of health education and promotion activities not only delineates the field but also highlights issues, and even differences, between approaches. What it does not do is provide reliable models of real practice. The development of analytical models or 'analogic' models (Rawson, 2002) of health promotion in the 1980s was an attempt to aid analysis by being explicit about underlying principles or values, not within the models themselves but within the society in which health promotion is undertaken.

The uses of analytical models

Beattie's (1991) analytical model points to the social and political perspectives underlying health promotion approaches. Two axes – mode of intervention (whether authoritative or negotiated) and focus of intervention in a society (whether individual or collective) – generate four different approaches to promoting health (see Figure 6.1, page 154).

In this model social values are seen as driving practice, so that a 'health persuasion' approach to health promotion reflects a paternalist (top–down) and individual-oriented philosophy. Individualism may not necessarily imply paternalism, however, and the model highlights a 'personal counselling' approach based on negotiation. The 'social change' approach assumes a related philosophy of collective action, and Beattie's model demonstrates that collective action could be either participative and community-based or paternalist and state-directed.

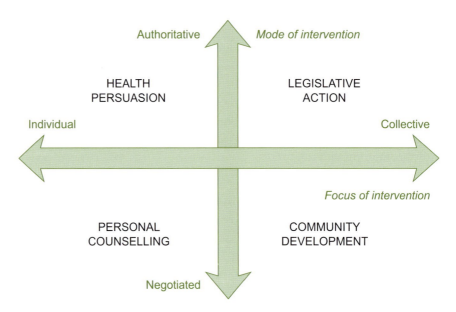

Figure 6.1 Beattie's model of health promotion

(Source: Beattie, 1991, pp. 162–201)

How does Beattie's model differ from the descriptive models you read about earlier?

Beattie's model enables us to reflect on the social and political perspectives underlying health-promotion approaches. Underpinning the conservative model of 'health persuasion', it is suggested, is a bio-pathological model of health that sees health promotion as attempting to repair deficits. Underlying a radical, community-development approach to health promotion are assumptions about empowerment and equity and the mobilisation of communities to effect change (see Freire, 1972). Underlying the libertarian model of 'personal counselling' is an individual non-directive approach in which people are assumed to be free to determine their own lives. Underlying what Beattie terms the 'reformism of legislative action' are assumptions about the role of the state in protecting public health.

Public health and health promotion are fields of activity with specific goals, professions for which individuals can be trained and disciplines that provide different philosophical and epistemological perspectives on an issue. The early attempts to map health promotion showed it as eclectic, drawing from many disciplines, while the analytical models sat within a socio-political paradigm. As we have seen, the models of health promotion were developed in the 1980s as the Ottawa Charter was written and health promotion was emerging as a distinctive area of practice. Its roots in the social science disciplines informed its methods of involvement to access and value the experiences of people themselves (Naidoo and Wills, 2008). Public health, on the other hand, has sat within a biomedical paradigm and its goals have been the recognition and management of risk, identified through epidemiological and statistical analysis of collected data. Tannahill's descriptive model reflects this focus.

In recent years there has been much less interest in providing examples of practice. As the policy emphasis has shifted to a focus on promoting healthier lifestyles, a range of theories and models from social psychology and education have become much more important (Vinck et al., 2004).

6.3 Theories of behaviour and behaviour change

Contemporary public health practice involves behaviour change, whether directed at the individual (for example, smoking or alcohol consumption) or societal level (for example, transport decisions or waste management). Understanding what influences an individual's decisions in relation to their health is a key part of practice. Some of the theories that have been used most frequently in the field of prevention and health promotion include: the Health Belief Model, the Theories of Reasoned Action and Planned Behaviour, Protection Motivation Theory, Health Locus of Control Theory and stage theories such as the Transtheoretical Model of Change (see Conner and Norman, 1996). These theories all imagine a multifaceted dynamic causal structure in which behaviour, personal factors and environmental influences interact.

The focus on rational action

The Health Belief Model (Becker, 1984) was developed to explain why people would or would not participate in programmes to prevent or detect disease. It has been widely applied to explain behaviour, principally in relation to prevention such as screening and immunisation, but also service utilisation. It has also been used to inform programme design.

The Health Belief Model is based on the understanding that a person will take a health-related action (for example, use condoms) if they:

- believe that a negative consequence (e.g. an STI) is likely and will be severe
- have a positive expectation that by taking a recommended action they will avoid a negative consequence (e.g. using condoms will be effective at preventing HIV)
- believe that they can successfully take a recommended health action (e.g. use condoms effectively and with confidence)
- believe that the benefits outweigh the barriers and costs (e.g. reduced risk of infection outweighs embarrassment and potential loss of pleasure).

The model includes four constructs that represent the perceived threat and net benefits: perceived *susceptibility*, perceived *severity*, perceived *benefits*, and perceived *barriers*. An added concept, *cues to action*, could activate the intention to act. A later addition to the model is the concept of *self-efficacy*, or one's confidence in the ability to successfully perform an action. This is particularly important for individuals changing habitual unhealthy behaviours, such as being sedentary, smoking or overeating.

 To what extent do you see this as a convincing account of behaviour change?

The Health Belief Model suggests that behaviour change is a result of a process where information is carefully scrutinised and weighed up before a decision is reached and that individual behaviour will be guided by a rationality of protecting one's health. It is frequently found, however, that people tend to offset long-term benefits, such as health or longer life expectancy, against short-term rewards or costs. Behaviour may instead be guided by other 'rationalities' such as coping or pleasure. The role of smoking in stress relief, for example, makes it a sensible option for many people, even though it is known to be harmful.

Applying the Health Belief Model to programme design might result in health risks being personalised and heightened to encourage an awareness of a threat to health. For example, the campaign to promote the uptake of chlamydia testing framed the issue with the statistic that 1 in 12 people have the disease. This was done in order to try to raise awareness of susceptibility, since higher levels of perceived susceptibility are associated with a greater intention to change behaviour. Numerous theories and models have been derived from research to better understand how to use fear in public information campaigns (for example, Protection Motivation Theory). However, people are unlikely to think of their risk in statistical terms and tend to use the presence of symptoms as a guide (French and Hevey, 2008), which poses difficulties in conditions which are asymptomatic in the early stages, such as chlamydia or hypertension.

Learning and behaviour

In general, attitudes have not been found to be consistently related to behaviour. People may have an intention to change or behave in a particular way (for example, use a condom every time they have sex), but frequently don't actually do this. This failure to demonstrate a consistent relationship between attitudes and behaviour may be because, as we have seen, situational factors also exert a powerful influence on behaviour. These aspects of the behaviour–attitude relationship have been addressed in the Theory of Reasoned Action and its revised version the Theory of Planned Behaviour (Ajzen and Fishbein, 1980). In this model, behaviour is seen as a function of a person's intention, which is comprised of the individual's attitudes towards performing the behaviour and its potential benefits. In deciding to lose weight, for example, the influence of deep-rooted beliefs and values, family and peer opinion and belief in one's ability to manage the change are all important.

There is considerable interest in public health in whether a positive intention can be encouraged by incentives and the National Institute of Health and Clinical Excellence has considered whether there is sufficient evidence to support whether incentives can encourage healthy living (for example, paying people to lose weight). Cash incentives have been found to be a strong motivator in some health behaviours. However, Jochelson's review of incentive programmes (2007) found that when incentives were withdrawn, previous behaviour patterns tended to re-emerge.

The theory of learned behaviour emphasises the influence of perceived social norms concerning the performance of the behaviour. Subjective norms relate to a person's beliefs about what others think they should do (normative beliefs) and by an individual's motivation to comply with the wishes of others. For example, if a smoker feels that most people do not smoke and that most people they value think it would be good for them to quit, then it is more likely they will develop subjective norms that favour quitting. Bandura's social learning theory (1977) asserts that behaviour can be learned or adopted if it is highly conspicuous in public displays even by people who are unacquainted with one another. For example, Sherwin and Parkhurst (2008) have suggested that as numbers of cyclists increase and cyclists become more visible, this will result in more individuals making the decision to cycle.

Self-efficacy is one of the key concepts in most social–psychological models. Self-efficacy refers to a person's confidence in their ability to take action and persist in action. It is seen by Bandura (1977) as perhaps the single most important factor in promoting changes in behaviour. Expectations of self-efficacy have been repeatedly found to be important determinants of the choice of activities in which people engage, how much energy they will expend on such activities and whether they will persist with any behaviour change. When failure is attributed to low personal ability (for example, being physically unfit) and a difficult task (for example, cycling to work), individuals are more likely to give up sooner, select easier alternatives (for example, use personal motorised travel) and lower their goals.

Staged and diffusion models

One of the most widely adopted theories of change is Prochaska and DiClemente's (1984) Transtheoretical Theory of Change (see Figure 6.2), which was developed to explain and predict how individuals move towards adopting and maintaining health behaviour. It uses stages of change as its core construct and integrates processes and principles of change from different theories, hence the name 'transtheoretical'. It is based on the assumption that behaviour change is an ongoing process, rather than a single event, and that individuals have varying levels of motivation or readiness to change.

The theory identifies five stages of change that people will engage in:

- **pre-contemplation** – not considering changing their behaviours or are consciously intending not to change
- **contemplation** – considering making a change to a specific behaviour
- **preparation** – making a serious commitment to change in the next couple of months and beginning to make the necessary preparations to do so
- **action** – explicitly making changes in their behaviour or environment
- **maintenance** – sustaining the change over time
- **relapse** – being unable to sustain the change and exiting from the cycle.

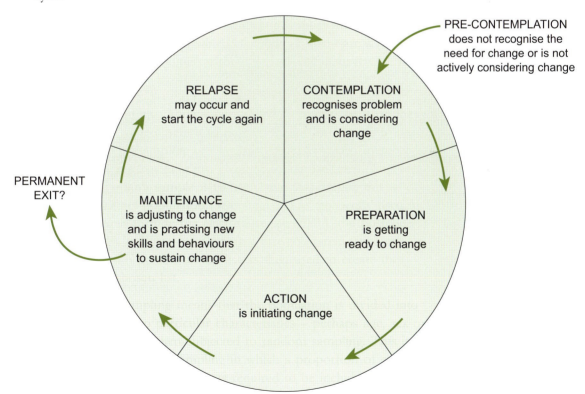

Figure 6.2 Transtheoretical Theory of Change Model

(Source: adapted from Prochaska and DiClemente, 1984)

What advantages and drawbacks do you see in adopting the idea of a cycle of 'stages' to explain behaviour change?

The model is based on observations that people appear to move through these stages in a predictable way, although some move more quickly than others and people may go backwards and forwards around the cycle. In later versions of the model, Prochaska described a final stage of 'termination', where individuals who have changed have no temptation to return to their old behaviour. It applies equally to individuals who 'self-initiate' a change and those responding to advice and encouragement to change. Stages of change theory provides a useful way of tailoring interventions to where people are in the change process. However, there is a decided lack of evidence supporting its practice or the validity of these types of staging algorithms (Riemesma et al., 2003; Brug et al., 2005).

Table 6.2 links the stages of change to the related challenges and actions needed to help an individual who wants to lose weight.

Table 6.2 Use of a stages of change theory to promote weight reduction

Stage of change	Challenge	Suggested action
Precontemplation	Awareness raising	Provide information on the health risks of being overweight
Contemplation	Recognition of the benefits of change	Encourage client to draw up a list of pros and cons of present behaviour. Establish existing harm by taking biochemical measurements (blood pressure, cholesterol) Provide information on the potential benefits of weight loss
Preparation	Support to overcome barriers to weight loss	Assistance with identification of potential barriers and support for overcoming barriers Give information on local support
Action	Programme of change	Work out a plan for weight loss and monitor progress
Maintenance	Follow-up	Organise routine follow-up Work out a plan to prevent relapse

(Source: adapted from Nutbeam and Harris, 2004)

Despite its limited evidence base, stages of change theory has been very popular and applied in motivational interviewing and brief interventions, especially for smoking cessation and alcohol reduction. A recent campaign to encourage greater physical activity among high-risk groups – Let's Get Moving (Department of Health [DoH], 2009) – is based on this model of change and uses an individualised but risk-based approach in general practice. There are ethical concerns that the application of this change model leads to categorising individuals as appropriate for interventions or, conversely, 'not ready'. This may exacerbate existing inequalities, as those who are not ready are likely to be those already least able to access the social, cultural or economic resources and support for making changes.

The process of diffusion of innovation helps to explain the spread of new ideas within a community (Rogers, 1995) and, like the transtheoretical model described above it, suggests that people go through stages before they adopt a new idea:

- initial awareness and increased knowledge
- persuasion and interest in trying out the innovation
- a decision to test out the innovation
- adoption.

The theory is based on observations that the legitimisation of an innovation through a community typically follows an S-shaped trajectory (see Figure 6.3, page 162). It starts with a slow initial uptake by 'early adopters', normally from higher socioeconomic groups, followed by opinion leaders and then the early majority for whom the utility of the innovation must be clear. They are followed eventually by the late majority, who tend to gain information from those around them, and then the laggards, who tend to be more isolated and consequently traditional in behaviour. In this way, change occurs in these groups more as a result of conformity to social norms and compliance to the majority than as an assessment of the costs and benefits of the innovation itself, its ease of adoption or perceptions about its immediate effects.

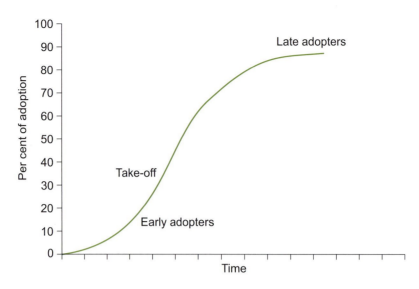

Figure 6.3 The S-shaped curve of the diffusion of innovations theory

(Source: adapted from Rogers and Scott, 1997)

Application of this model would suggest that, although mass media may be influential in raising awareness and the early diffusion of ideas, an opinion leader or a 'change agent' plays an essential role in the communications process by spreading information and stimulating and facilitating change, especially to late adopters. There is a large body of evidence exploring the effectiveness of peers as change agents (e.g. Starkey et al., 2009). What also becomes clear from the model is that different social systems will adopt ideas at different rates, so 'traditional' communities that are homogeneous and isolated are less likely to adopt any innovation.

The complexity of behaviour change

This overview of theories of behaviour change reveals a range of constructs and a diversity of factors at play, which explains why changing behaviours has proven so challenging for policy makers and practitioners. These theories, tested in countless contexts and with different populations, show behaviour to be sometimes rational, but sometimes strongly influenced by emotions, habits and routines. Staged and diffusion models are shown to have serious limitations as intervention methods, but demonstrate that change is a process not an event, as is suggested by social cognition models. An understanding of behavioural models and theories can help in the task of programme or intervention design, but a theory or model does not specify what will work to bring about change. This is an important message for practitioners. Empirical evidence gathered from the evaluation of practice and designated research studies is also needed, identifying which factors are the most significant in determining behaviours.

Behaviour change theories inevitably emphasise the role of the individual in making health choices. When applied to programme planning, such theories tend to disregard the social, environmental and economic forces that shape and constrain individual choices and solely give place to the role of individual factors and social norms.

6.4 Community action and models of development and change

The understanding that there are multiple causes of health problems has shifted the focus of public health and health promotion to broader 'system level' interventions. This is prompted by the recognition that behaviour is influenced by the settings in which people live, work and play and that local values and norms significantly affect attitudes and behaviours of the population (World Health Organization [WHO], 1986). 'Systems' thinking helps to tease out the cycles, interconnections and relationships between different parts of a whole system.

Communities as systems

Communities can be viewed as systems and subsystems which are based on cooperation and consensus on societal goals, norms and values. Community-level models are frameworks for understanding how such social systems function and change, and how communities and organisations can be activated. Bronfenbrenner (1979), for example, describes human development as part of an ecological environment consisting of a set of 'nested structures' or systems which impact on each other, like Russian dolls. He suggests the whole system comprises:

- a microsystem focusing on the individual
- a mesosystem involving linkage with other settings in which the individual participates (e.g. school, workplace and neighbourhood)
- an exosystem concerned with policies that impact on the individual
- a macrosystem of public or government policy.

In public health and health-promotion practice there is an important conceptual difference between those generally small-scale health-promotion activities that are provided in the community for individuals in a specific locality or population subgroup (such as, a breastfeeding support group) and those activities that involve people from the community in defining problems, targets and actions, which are usually defined as 'community development'. Community-based health promotion and public health tends to work around health issues and to a professionally determined agenda, while community development programmes may be large-scale and complex, incorporating many different activities underpinned by explicit values and principles of participation, equity, sustainability and partnership.

Understanding change

Although working with communities is a central feature of public health and health-promotion practice, there is no distinct theory of community change. Theories relate to macro-theories about society and derive from two broad ideological perspectives: a liberal/individualist view privileging consensus reform and a collectivist/socialist view privileging action on the social determinants of health. These reflect different philosophical assumptions about the nature of societal change and the principal sources of health problems as well as degrees of control and top-down or bottom-up approaches. The distinction between these perspectives informs many of the attempts to define and describe health-promotion practice, as in Beattie's model (see Figure 6.1).

Caplan and Holland's model (1990) creates a broad socio-cultural matrix by plotting theories of social change (radical change or social regulation) against theories of the nature of knowledge (subjective or objective). This produces four quadrants, each representing a distinctive approach to health work. The 'traditional' quadrant, for example, aligns with expert-led health education or public health that emphasises social regulation and objectivity. The radical quadrant, where health promotion most comfortably sits, aligns with democratic and inclusive work to achieve radical change that communities themselves identify. The model is explicitly saying that health work is embedded in wider social and cultural practices, ideologies and political struggles. Health promotion is not something apart from the rest of society; indeed, it reflects territory struggles about power, control, autonomy and authority.

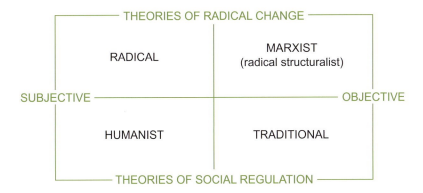

Figure 6.4 Caplan and Holland's approaches to health promotion

(Source: Caplan and Holland, 1990)

What do you think are the strengths of the model developed by Caplan and Holland?

The strength of this model lies in its acknowledgement that tensions exist, for example, between those who claim to be able to provide objective definitions of health, such as the absence of diagnosable disease, and those who would want to provide more subjective, relativist lay-informed accounts. It highlights tensions between those who feel that health can be promoted from within the existing social order through, for example, encouraging lifestyle changes, and those who feel that many problems with health only occur as a result of the existing social order, which therefore needs to be challenged and replaced. This might relate to anti-health industries, such as tobacco or alcohol, or the economic system that produces high levels of unemployment. Equally, we can distinguish public health approaches that privilege fairness, equality and social justice and those values that relate to the effectiveness of public health policy in terms of favouring the least costly option and/or maximising health gains.

Community engagement

Rothman and Tropman (1987) developed a widely used typology that distinguishes between community-level initiatives, drawing attention to how they differ according to levels of community involvement and participation. Other aspects focus on the extent to which the agenda relates directly or indirectly to health and whether they are deficit based (focusing on addressing problems) or asset based (focusing on building strengths). They identify:

- **locality/community development**, when the change strategy is based on capacity building in an effort to get a wide range of community people involved in determining their 'felt' needs and solving their own problems through mutual support, developing skills and sharing activities
- **social planning**, when the change strategy is one in which the practitioner plays a central part in gathering and analysing facts and determining appropriate services and interventions
- **social action**, when the change strategy involves identifying the inequality in society and disadvantaged and oppressed peoples and organising direct action to bring pressure on selected targets, such as a political department, an organisation or an individual.

Guidance on community engagement (NICE, 2008) suggests a theoretical framework that proposes why different levels of community engagement (for example, informing or consulting) could directly and indirectly affect health in both the intermediate and the longer term. For example, consultation with a community over their needs may have an impact on the appropriateness of a service developed, its accessibility and its uptake. Approaches that help communities work as equal partners in what is called co-production may lead to more positive health outcomes and increase social capital and people's sense of belonging to the community and self-efficacy.

While this is proposed as a theory for engagement, and there is plenty of evidence from peer leaders to community champions that supports different approaches to engagement (Swainston and Summerbell, 2007), it is untested as a robust explanatory framework. There are many variables, including the context and timescale for delivery, which will influence its reliability. Critical thinking and reflection on the values and assumptions of such programmes is essential. An understanding of power and control in relation to, for example, the use and ownership of information and resources, the role and agenda of professionals, how leadership is developed and devolved, and the extent of participation and engagement in decision making, informs community development work (Laverack, 2007).

Although community practice does not use a single model of community organisation, several concepts are central to the various approaches. These are shown in Table 6.3.

Table 6.3 Community organisation

Concept	Definition	Application
Empowerment	Process of gaining mastery and power over self/community to produce change	Give individuals and communities confidence, tools and responsibility for making decisions that affect them. Mutual support and action groups build social networks.
Community competence	Community's ability to engage in effective problem solving	Work with community to identify problems, create consensus and reach goals. Develop local leaders, building networks and knowledge and skills
Participation and relevance	Learners should be active participants and work should 'start where the people are'	Help community set goals within the context of pre-existing goals and encourage active participation
Issue selection	Identify winnable, simple, specific concerns as focus of action	Assist community in examining how they can communicate their concerns and whether success is likely
Critical consciousness	Developing understanding of root causes of problems	Guide consideration of health concerns in broad perspective of social problems

(Source: adapted from Nutbeam and Harris, 2004; National Cancer Institute, 2005)

Theory, power and politics

The community has come to be seen as a central resource for change, as reflected in many area-based initiatives. Complex community interventions, such as Sure Start, consist of multiple activities such as building 'community competence', with several layers of organisation. The theory underpinning such interventions can be hard to discern and is, in any case, often ignored in evaluations because the focus is on the inputs and the results, not why change may have taken place.

Health action zones and healthy living centres have been evaluated by new strategies known as 'theory of change' and realistic evaluation (Pawson and Tilley, 1997). These strategies focus on the mechanisms of change in the belief that social programmes are based on implicit or explicit assumptions about how and why such programmes work. The task of the evaluation is to help practitioners unpack and surface these theories and their assumptions, in order to examine the extent to which programme theories hold (Hills, 2004). However, in a report based on six international case studies, Coote et al. (2004) found that large community-based initiatives, far from being theory-driven, are often designed on the basis of informed guesswork and expert hunches and are driven by political imperatives.

6.5 Theories and social change

Public health has been described as entailing 'the organised efforts of society' (Acheson, 1988) or the engagement of 'the social machinery' (Winslow, 1920). Both of these require political involvement and political actions – a study of who or what has the power to organise society as well as how that organisational power is processed. Such study provides a theoretical base for wider efforts to promote health (Bambra et al., 2005).

The central feature of actions to promote health clearly draws from the social science disciplines. It owes much to a political economy analysis of how ill health is generated by poverty, poor housing and work environments, pollution, discrimination and unemployment. The politics of public health is the struggle over the assignment of meaning to suspected causes of ill health, especially the role of economics in the production and distribution of disease. Radical approaches will stress the ways in which 'anti-health' forces, such as the tobacco or some pharmaceutical industries, can contribute to disease. Health inequality and health inequity based on race, ethnicity, gender, class and/or sexuality differences will be addressed through scientific enquiry and the representation of specific groups. The women's health movement, the gay and lesbian health movement and sustainability movements are all examples of what have come to be called health social movements. These are defined as 'collective challenges to medical policy, public health policy and politics, belief systems, research and practice which include an array of formal and informal organisations, supporters, networks of cooperation and media' (Brown and Zavestoski, 2004, p. 679).

What social change theories have you already encountered in this chapter?

We saw earlier in the models of Caplan and Holland (1990) and Beattie (1991) that public health and health promotion demonstrate the tension between the slow, gradual change towards disease prevention through prescriptive expert-led health education and the activism and social action through community development and empowerment. A focus on healthy public policy, using legislation and state intervention as a means to promote health, is challenged by libertarians. These tensions expressed in models of health promotion reflect some of the main theories of how societal change is achieved: whether through reform or conflict. Advocacy or actions designed to gain political commitment, policy support, social acceptance and systems support for a particular health goal or programme have been recognised as one of three major strategies for achieving health promotion goals – the others are enablement and mediation (WHO, 1986). Advocacy may be to protect people who are vulnerable or discriminated against or to empower people who need a stronger voice by enabling them to express their needs and make their own decisions. The tendency is to assume that bottom-up types of practice are inherently preferable to top-down initiatives. Such arguments may, as Carlisle states (2000, p. 375), 'unwittingly run counter to advocacy for social change in the interests of social justice and greater equality in health.'

Mapping theories and models

Debates about social change serve to highlight the philosophical differences that underlie theories and models. There are also similarities in the mapping of different approaches to promoting health. Most refer to a preventive approach: termed 'medical' by Ewles and Simnett (1985), 'preventive' by Tones et al. (1990) and 'disease prevention' by Tannahill (1985); an educational and behaviour change approach (termed 'health persuasion' by Beattie, 1991); an empowerment approach (termed 'client centred' by Ewles and Simnett, 1985); and a social change approach (termed 'radical' by Tones et al. 1990) and 'societal change' by Ewles and Simnett (1985). There are, nevertheless, significant differences in their philosophical and epistemological bases, which the analytical models highlight. Table 6.4 (pages 170–171) shows practitioners how they can locate their practice and how they might draw on theories and models to inform their practice, developing a more coherent and well-founded approach.

Table 6.4 Summary of theories: focus and key concepts

Approach	Theory	Focus	Key concepts	Application
Primary care/ disease prevention	Biomedical	Improve physiological risk factors and personal health behaviours	Risk Causation and association	Screening Health checks
Health education and behaviour change	Health Belief Model	Person's perception of the threat of a health problem and the appraisal of recommended behaviour(s) for preventing or managing the problem	Perceived susceptibility Perceived severity Perceived benefits of action Perceived barriers to action Cues to action Self-efficacy	Design of programmes for behaviour change Patient education
	Transtheoretical Model of Change	Individual's readiness to change or attempt to change towards healthy behaviours	Precontemplation, contemplation, decision/ determination, action, maintenance, relapse Motivation	Smoking cessation Let's Get Moving physical activity programme in primary care
Community action	Community action theories Tones' empowerment model Beattie's model of health promotion	Emphasises active participation and development of communities that can better evaluate and solve health and social problems	Empowerment Community engagement Community development Participation Critical consciousness	Health Action Zones Regeneration areas Community development projects
	Organisational Change Theory Systems theory Diffusion of innovation	Concerns processes and strategies for increasing the chances that healthy policies and programmes will be adopted and maintained in formal organisations	Problem definition (awareness stage) Initiation of action (adoption stage) Implementation of change Institutionalisation of change	Healthy settings

Approach	Theory	Focus	Key concepts	Application
Societal level		Change in societies is achieved through gradual reform or conflict and structural change	Conflict Consensus Reform	Public policy

Conclusion

There is no 'right' approach to promoting health – personal and socio-cultural values will influence an individual's view of the causes of health and ill health and this will lead to different approaches to promoting health being privileged or discounted. This chapter has explored how the frameworks that influence practice may be empirical and built from evidence, whereas others are normative and represent different ideological or ethical positions about what should be such as individual responsibility or the pursuit of social justice.

Public health and health promotion are changing fields. In the 1980s the 'new' public health shifted public health practice from environmental and disease management to a focus on the determinants of health. For a decade from 1997, there was a much greater emphasis on models of community action and development, including participatory approaches, but the renewed focus on achieving population lifestyle changes has led to the theories of behaviour deriving from social psychology achieving much greater prominence. Health education has also re-emerged as a 'new critical health education' (Green and Tones, 2010).

Models are different ways of conceptualising this field. Although they clearly show links to different disciplinary frameworks – social theory, political theory, social psychology, and so on – they are not explanatory or predictive. Understanding where public health practice fits into such models helps practitioners go beyond a 'commonsense' account of their activities. It also clarifies why different parties engaged in public health and health promotion may have very different views as to what it is they should be involved in.

References

Acheson, D. (1988) *Public Health in England. Report of the Committee of Inquiry into the Future of the Public Health Function*, Cmnd 289, London, HMSO (Acheson report). Available at: www.york.ac.uk/yhpho/documents/hea/Website/AchesonReport.pdf (accessed 29 August 2011).

Ajzen, I. and Fishbein, M. (1980) *Understanding Attitudes and Predicting Social Behaviour*, Englewood Cliffs, New Jersey, Prentice-Hall.

Bambra, C., Fox, D. and Scott Samuel, A. (2005) 'Towards a politics of health', *Health Promotion International*, vol. 20, no. 2, pp. 187–93.

Bandura, A. (1977) *Social Learning Theory*, Englewood Cliffs, New Jersey, Prentice-Hall.

Beattie, A. (1991) 'Knowledge and control in health promotion: a test case for social theory' in Gabe, J., Calnan, M. and Bury, M. (eds) *The Sociology of the Health Service*, Routledge, London, pp. 162–201.

Becker, M.H. (ed) (1984) *The Health Belief Model and Personal Health Behaviour*, New Jersey, Thorofare.

Bronfenbrenner, U. (1979) *The Ecology of Human Development. Experiments by Nature and Design*, Cambridge, Massachusetts, Harvard University Press.

Brown, P. and Zavestoski, S. (2004) 'Social movements in health: an introduction', *Sociology of Health and Illness*, vol. 26, no. 6, pp. 679–94.

Brug, J., Conner, M., Harre, N., Kremer, S., McKellar, S. and Whitelaw, S. (2005) 'The Transtheoretical Model and stages of change: a critique', *Health Education Research*, vol. 20, no. 2, pp. 244–58.

Bunton, R. and Macdonald, G. (eds) (2002) *Health Promotion: Disciplines, Diversity and Developments* (2nd edition), London, Routledge.

Caplan, R. and Holland, R. (1990) 'Rethinking health education theory', *Health Education Journal*, vol. 49, pp. 10–12.

Carlisle, S. (2000) 'Health promotion, advocacy and health inequalities: a conceptual framework', *Health Promotion International*, vol. 15, no. 4, pp. 369–76.

Collins, T. (1995) 'Models of health: pervasive, persuasive and politically charged', *Health Promotion International*, vol. 10, no. 4, pp. 317–24.

Conner, M. and Norman, P. (eds) (1996) *Predicting Health Behaviour: Research and Practice with Social Cognition Models*, Buckingham, Open University Press.

Coote, A., Allen, J. and Woodhead, D. (2004) *Finding Out What Works: Building Knowledge about Complex Community-based Initiatives*, London, Kings Fund.

Department of Health (DoH) (2009) *Let's Get Moving – A New Physical Activity Care Pathway for the NHS: Commissioning Guidance*, London, Department of Health. Available at: www.dh.gov.uk/en/Publicationsandstatistics/Publications/PublicationsPolicyAndGuidance/DH_105945 (accessed 29 August 2011).

Ewles, L. and Simnett, I. (1985) *Promoting Health*, Chichester, Wiley.

Ewles, L. and Simnett, I. (2003) *Promoting Health* (5th edn), Edinburgh, Baillière Tindall

Freire, P. (1972) Pedagogy of the Oppressed, London, Penguin.

French, D.P. and Hevey, D. (2008) 'What do people think about when answering questionnaires to assess unrealistic optimism about skin cancer? A think aloud study', *Psychology, Health and Medicine*, vol. 13, pp. 63–74.

Green, J. (2000) 'The role of theory in evidence-based health-promotion practice', *Health Education Research*, vol. 15, no. 2, pp. 125–29.

Green, J. and Tones, K. (2010) *Health Promotion: Planning and Strategies* (2nd edition), London, Sage.

Higgins, J.P.T., and Green S. (eds) (2011) *Cochrane Handbook for Systematic Reviews of Interventions* (version 5.1.0), London, The Cochrane Collaboration. Available at: www.cochrane-handbook.org (accessed 29 August 2011).

Hills, D. (2004) *Evaluation of Community-level Interventions for Health Improvement: A Review of Experience in the UK*, London, Health Development Agency.

Jochelson, K. (2007) *Paying the Patient: Improving Health Using Financial Incentives*, London, Kings Fund.

Jones, I. and Walker, D. (1997) 'The role of theory in public health' in Scally, G. (ed.) *Progress in Public Health*, London, FT Healthcare.

Laverack, G. (2007) *Health-promotion Practice: Building Empowered Communities*, Buckingham, Open University Press.

Lewin, K. (1951) *Field Theory in Social Science: Selected Theoretical Papers*, New York, Harper and Bros., p. 169.

Naidoo, J. and Wills, J. (2009) *Foundations for Health Promotion* (3rd edition), London, Baillière Tindall.

Naidoo, J. and Wills, J. (2008) *Health Studies: An Introduction* (2nd edition), Basingstoke, Palgrave Macmillan.

National Cancer Institute (2005) *Theory at a Glance: A Guide for Practice*, Washington DC, US Department of Health and Human Services. Available at: www.cancer.gov/cancertopics/cancerlibrary/theory.pdf (accessed 29 August 2011).

National Institute for Health and Clinical Excellence (NICE) (2008) *Community Engagement to Improve Health. Public Health Guidance PH 9*, London, National Institute for Health and Clinical Excellence. Available at: www.nice.org.uk/nicemedia/live/11929/39562/39562.doc (accessed 29 August 2011).

Nutbeam, D. and Harris, E. (2004) *Theory in a Nutshell: A Practical Guide to Health Promotion Theories* (2nd edition), Sydney, McGraw Hill.

Pawson, R. and Tilley, N. (1997) *Realistic Evaluation*, London, Sage.

Prochaska, J.O. and DiClemente, C.C. (1984) *The Transtheoretical Approach: Crossing Traditional Boundaries of Therapy*, Homewood, Illinois, Dow Jones Irwin.

Rawson, D. (2002) 'The growth of health promotion theory and its rational reconstruction' in Bunton, R. and Macdonald, G. (eds) *Health Promotion: Disciplines and Diversity* (2nd edn), London, Routledge.

Riemesma, R.P., Pattenden, J., Sowden, A.J., Mather, L., Watt, I.S. and Walker, A. (2003) 'Systematic review of the effectiveness of stage-based interventions to promote smoking cessation', *British Medical Journal*, vol. 326, pp. 1175–77.

Rogers, E.M. (1995) *The Diffusion of Innovations* (4th edition), New York, Free Press.

Rogers, E.M. and Scott, K.L. (1997) 'The diffusion of innovations model and outreach for the National Network of Libraries of Medicine to Native American Communities', *National Network of Libraries of Medicine Outreach Evaluation Resource Centre*, 10 December. Available at: http://nnlm.gov/archive/pnr/eval/rogers.html (accessed 8 August 2011).

Rothman, J. and Tropman, J.E. (1987) 'Three models of community organisation practice' in Cox, F., Erlich, J., Rothman, J. and Tropman, J. (eds) *Strategies of Community Organisation*, Itaska, Illinois, Peacock Publishing.

Royal Society of Public Health (2009) *Why Theory Matters for Effective Health Promotion*, London, Royal Society for Public Health. Available at: www.rsph.org.uk/filemanager/root/site_assets/policy_and_projects/shaping_the_future/WhyTheoryMattersdraft23Jan09.pdf (accessed 29 August 2011).

Schön, D.A. (1992) *The Reflective Practitioner: How Professionals Think in Action* (2nd edn), San Francisco, California, Jossey-Bass.

Sherwin, H. and Parkhurst, G. (2008) 'Exploration of the motivations and existing behaviour of bike rail integrators to inform future promotional interventions', *5th Cycling and Society Symposium*, Bristol, University of the West of England. Available at: www.transport.uwe.ac.uk/cycling_and_society/Henrietta%20Sherwin.PDF (accessed 29 August 2011).

Starkey, F., Audrey, S., Holliday, J., Moore, L. and Campbell, R. (2009) 'Identifying influential young people to undertake effective peer-led health promotion: the example of a stop smoking in schools trial (ASSIST)', *Health Education Research*, vol. 24, no. 6, pp. 977–88.

Swainston, K. and Summerbell, C. (2007) *The Effectiveness of Community Engagement Approaches and Methods for Health Promotion Interventions. Rapid Review*, Teesside, University of Teesside. Available at: www.nice.org.uk/nicemedia/live/11678/34712/34712.pdf (accessed 29 August 2011).

Tannahill, A. (1985) 'What is health promotion?', *Health Education Journal*, vol. 44, pp. 167–8.

Thorogood, N. (2002) 'What is the relevance of sociology for health promotion?' in Bunton, R. and Macdonald, G. (eds) *Health Promotion: Disciplines, Diversity and Developments* (2nd edition), Routledge, London.

Tones, K., Tilford, S. and Robinson, Y. (1990) *Health Education: Effectiveness and Efficiency*, London, Chapman and Hall.

Vinck, J., Oldenburg, B. and von Lengerke, T. (2004) 'Editorial: Health psychology and public health. Bridging the gap', *Journal of Health Psychology*, vol. 9, no. 1, pp. 5–12.

Wills, J. and Woodhead, D. (2004) 'The glue that binds – articulating values in multidisciplinary public health', *Critical Public Health*, vol. 14, no. 1, pp. 7–15.

Winslow, C. (1920) 'The untilled fields of public health', *Science*, vol. 51, no. 1306, pp. 23–33.

World Health Organization (WHO) (1986) *Ottawa Charter for Health Promotion*, Copenhagen, World Health Organization.

Chapter 7: Building evidence-based practice: statistics and epidemiology

Moyra Sidell and Cathy Lloyd

Introduction

This chapter focuses on the production of evidence that can inform public health policy and practice about the health of populations, using quantitative methods of inquiry from a biomedical and social scientific perspective. The emphasis is therefore on the science more than the art of public health (Acheson, 1998), although the boundaries between science and art, particularly in epidemiology, are not clear cut. The evidence considered in this chapter is mainly concerned with preventing disease and prolonging life. It starts by considering the major disciplines involved in collecting information about the public's health, those of demography (the statistical surveillance of the population) and epidemiology, which is concerned with the causes and distribution of diseases. The last section examines attempts, using social scientific methods such as surveys, to explore wider aspects of promoting health and explores the limitations of quantitative statistical evidence in informing public health practice.

7.1 Sources of evidence: demography

Demography provides a framework for studying different aspects of a population, for instance, education and crime, as well as health. Since 1801 a census has been conducted to determine the number of people of different types, groups or categories residing in the UK. Demographers count people according to certain social characteristics, such as age, gender, marital status, housing conditions and, more recently, ethnicity. Demography can identify how many people live and/ or work in a particular geographical area, what kind of work they do, and the age and gender distribution of that population. It is concerned with change resulting from births, deaths, movement of people and alterations in population characteristics.

Demography can also provide statistics on unemployment, indicating the numbers of long-term unemployed people as well as the temporarily unemployed, such as school leavers. Demographic data can be divided into two discrete forms:

- data gathered through population censuses
- data collected through registration systems.

The UK national census

The UK national census provides a snapshot view of individuals at a particular moment in time. It yields information about the size and structure of a particular population as it was on census night. Some of the questions in a census relate directly or indirectly to people's health and therefore are of interest to public health.

The first modern periodic, direct and complete census took place in the USA in 1790. The first UK census followed shortly after in 1801 and it has been repeated every ten years, except in 1941 during World War II. The Population Act 1840 appointed a registrar general responsible for a complete census of the population.

Questions asked in censuses have changed over time to reflect contemporary concerns and, increasingly since 1891, data providing information about aspects of health and lifestyles has been collected. In the 1891 census, questions were asked about the types of dwelling and the number of rooms each household occupied, reflecting concern about overcrowding. From 1911, details were asked about family size, to be considered alongside mortality and morbidity data. The 1921 census contained questions about place of work and methods of transport to work, reflecting growing concern with traffic density. By this time, questions were included about educational level as well as about the ages and numbers of children in the population (for educational planning purposes).

Between the 1991 and 2001 census, changes in the nature of the UK population prompted questions about ethnicity. Since the 2001 census there has been much debate and controversy about how to categorise ethnicity (Gunaratnam, 2007). The latest census, taken in March 2011, utilised a different set of questions related to ethnicity. As well as questions on country of birth, ethnic group and religion, which were asked on the 2001 census, the 2011 census asked how people described their national identity and what passports they held. It also asked two questions about language: 'What is your main language?' and 'How well can you speak English?' Whatever the political implications of this are in terms of public health, this data could be useful in terms of establishing the need for translations or interpreters.

Social class has long been identified as a major indicator of health (Townsend and Davidson, 1982). The 1921 census redefined occupational classification and introduced five socioeconomic groups. This registrar general's social classification has been the subject of much debate and controversy, culminating in a reclassification known as the National Statistics Socio-economic Classification (NS-SeC). This classification was first used in the census of 2001. The census of 2001 also included, for the first time, a specific question on general health in addition to the question on long-term illness. Respondents were asked to assess their own health over the past 12 months as either 'good', 'fairly good', or 'not good', providing subjective quantitative data on general health. This is valuable for public health practitioners because it can be cross-tabulated with a range of other variables such as employment or social class or even how people travel to work. It also allows for a comparison of regional variations in self-reported health, as shown in the maps of the UK in Figure 7.1.

The questions on health have also added to 'the overall picture of health patterns among ethnic minority groups' (Bradby and Chandola, 2010, p. 33). However, issues have been raised concerning the use of ethnicity data in relation to health (Bhopal, 2001; Gunaratnam, 2007).

Census data form the basis of a great deal of statistical information at the national, regional and district level. Indeed, since contemporary censuses extend over some 100,000 separate districts, accurate statistical information about each and every district is available. For public health practitioners, providing information about, for example, lone parents, employment, housing, education and other health-related issues for small areas of the country, can be invaluable for planning local interventions or community profiling.

Hans Rosling (2011), Professor of International Health and an enthusiastic advocate of the power of statistics, points out that the word 'statistic' derives from the word 'state' and that the original purpose of collecting data about the population, in a format such as the census, was to survey the population in order to better control it. He feels that now that this type of data are available to all, it gives the population the power to hold the state to account and can certainly be used to the benefit of the population.

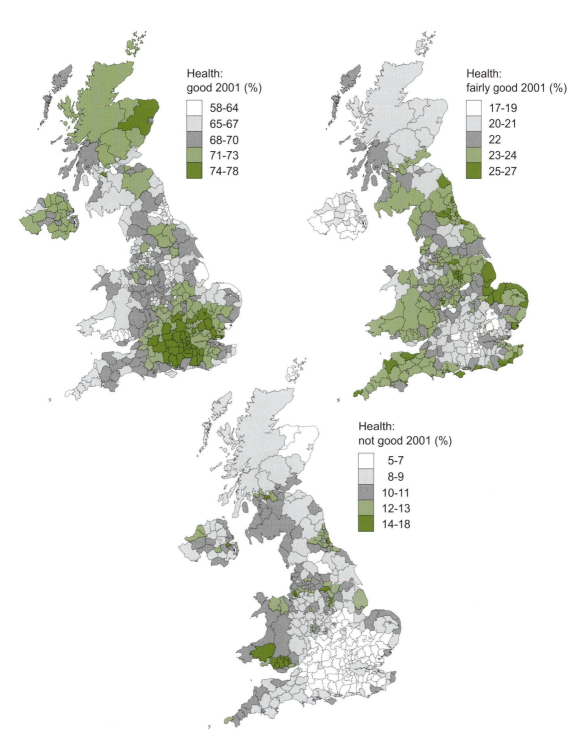

Figure 7.1 Mapping of good and poor health in the UK
(Source: Dorling and Thomas, 2004, pp. 134–35)

Registration systems: counting births and deaths

Demographers count and compare birth and death rates in different places and at different times. These rates are calculated on the basis of returns to the registrar following a birth or death. Since 1836, the registration of births and deaths has been compulsory. Prompt registration was encouraged by instituting a fee payable if the birth was not registered within six weeks. Local registrars were made responsible for registering deaths and births.

Through compulsory recording of deaths (for example, it is illegal to dispose of a body without a death certificate), the Office for National Statistics (ONS) is able to publish detailed mortality statistics. In addition, population data from the census provide information about mortality in relation to cause of death and occupation and this is published every 10 years. This combination of mortality and census data provides valuable information on trends and changes in mortality over time. Mortality statistics are based on death certificates which list the name, age and sex of the deceased as well as the date of death, place of death and cause of death.

What aspects of the death certificate might present problems in recording a death?

The accurate assessment of the cause of death is recognised as being problematic. In fact, the original Death Registration Bill of 1836 did not include provision for cause of death. It was not until the Births and Deaths Registration Act of 1874 that it became a requirement that the cause of death be recorded by the medical practitioner who last attended the deceased, unless there was to be an inquest or a post-mortem. This aspect of the death certificate has provided vital epidemiological information for decades, but its usefulness depends on the accuracy with which death certificates are completed. The procedure is: if the deceased has been seen by a doctor within 14 days before the death and the circumstances of the death are not suspicious, then the doctor fills in the 'cause of death' box. The death certificate asks the certifier to record direct causes of death as well as contributory causes. But it is the 'underlying' cause of death which is most important and that should appear in the lowest completed line of Part 1 of the death certificate.

It is the information on the underlying cause of death that is transformed at the ONS by codifiers into a number that is given to a particular cause of death on a list called the International Classification of Diseases, Injuries and Causes of Death (ICD). For example, cancer of the lung is numbered C34. This is an extremely detailed and wide-ranging classification, which also includes psychiatric conditions including post-traumatic stress disorder (PTSD). Routine mortality statistics are based on this classification of the recorded underlying cause of death, although the ONS now also codes additional causes mentioned on a death certificate.

However, it is not the ICD classification that raises questions about the validity of mortality data, but rather the accuracy and reliability of the certifier of the cause of death. Even when the cause of death is straightforward, there is a wide range of factors that can result in reporting differences. For instance, there are variations in diagnostic decisions between countries and physicians, and over time that can influence mortality statistics. In addition, the cause of death mentioned on the death certificate might mask a serious disease problem that is not identified, either because the person completing the certificate is unaware of it or because the dying person or their family put pressure on the certifying doctor to withhold this information.

Can you think of such a cause?

Causes of death can be underreported when the cause of death is stigmatised, such as suicide, which is unacceptable for some religions. Figure 7.2 (page 182) shows marked international differences in suicide rates.

The Organisation for Economic Co-operation and Development (OECD) admits that:

> The international comparability of death rates from suicide can be affected by reporting differences across countries. A stigma is associated with suicide in many countries, and those recording causes of death may come under pressure to record deaths from suicide as 'unknown' or due to other causes. Caution is required therefore in interpreting variations across countries.
>
> (OECD, 2003, p. 28)

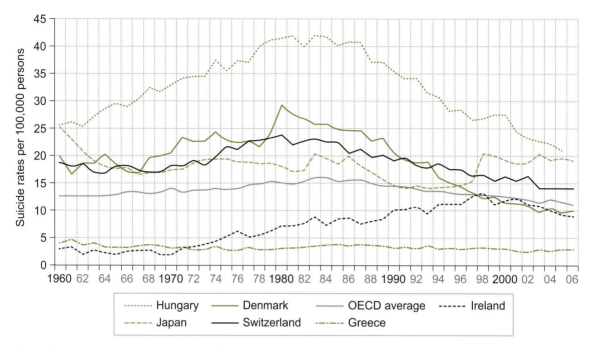

Figure 7.2 International suicide rates (1960–2006)

(Source: OECD, 2010, p. 239)

Pneumonia might appear on the death certificates of many older people when the actual underlying cause of death was senile dementia, with pneumonia a co-pathology. In fact, there has been much controversy in the past about 'old age' as an acceptable cause of death. Peto (1994) estimated that there may be inaccuracies in 30–50 per cent of cases and that this is likely to be more common in older people where multiple pathologies are likely. Nevertheless, death certificates are, potentially, a rich source of evidence for epidemiology, which helps to provide valuable data on the patterns of disease within and between countries.

7.2 Sources of evidence: epidemiology

Epidemiology has been defined as 'the study of how often diseases occur in different groups of people and why' (Coggon et al., 2003, p. 1). It is concerned not only with the distribution of disease within a particular group or population, but also with the factors that put people at risk of contracting a disease, known as 'risk factors'. Box 7.1 explains this term.

Box 7.1 Risk factors

Risk factors are variables that contribute to the risk of developing a disease or condition. For example, some risk factors associated with coronary heart disease include smoking, being overweight, high blood pressure and high cholesterol (low density lipoprotein [LDL]). Over time, research has demonstrated that some risk factors confer a high risk (e.g. LDL cholesterol) whereas other factors actually reduce the risk of coronary heart disease (e.g. high density lipoprotein [HDL] cholesterol).

Epidemiological researchers often use a 'relative risk' statistic in order to compare the risk of developing a disease in those exposed to a certain risk factor with those who are unexposed. For example, the risk of developing lung cancer in smokers compared with non-smokers. Relative risks are also used in randomised clinical trials, such as when comparing the risk of developing a disease in people not receiving a new medical treatment (or receiving a placebo) with people who are receiving an established (standard care) treatment.

Relative risk = risk among exposed/risk among unexposed.

A relative risk of 1 means there is no difference in risk between the two groups.

A relative risk of less than 1 means the disease/condition is less likely to occur in the exposed group than in the control group.

A relative risk of more than 1 means the disease/condition is more likely to occur in the exposed group than in the control group.

Although the term 'epidemiology' literally means the 'science of epidemics', it actually has a much broader remit and explains why and how diseases occur and spread and how they can be contained. The types of events that are of interest to epidemiology include morbidity (disease), disability, mortality (death), recovery and the use of health services. There is also a whole area known as 'psychiatric epidemiology' where the distribution of, and risk factors for, mental illness are studied.

Epidemiologists are in many ways disease detectives (Bailey et al., 2005), tracking down disease to discover why it occurs as well as when and where it occurs. It is a very creative activity. In an essay in the *Journal of Epidemiology and Community Health* (2010), John Last, an Emeritus Professor of Epidemiology and Community Medicine, uses the metaphor of 'joining the dots':

> Epidemiology connects the dots, the isolated bits of information that begin to form a coherent pattern when connected in the right way ... The dots can come from anywhere. Identifying them demands a broad perspective, the ability to see the Big Picture ... Sometimes the way the dots are connected is instantly apparent. Sometimes painstaking investigation and analysis are required.

> (Last, 2010, p. 106)

Last goes on to point out that epidemiology is 'the most eclectic science' because it uses evidence from a wide range of sources. He cites the discovery of the cause of toxic shock syndrome in women from using tampons in the mid 1970s:

> The epidemiological evidence (the connected dots) came from gynaecology, microbiology, toxicology, sociology and the fashion and pharmaceutical industries.

> (Last, 2010, p. 106)

In order to 'connect the dots' epidemiology focuses on populations or communities. These can be very large, such as a nation or continent, or groups within larger populations. So a population such as that of the UK might be broken down into the four nations, or specified health districts. But epidemiology is not just concerned with geographical groupings. Often it focuses on such diverse groups as different occupations or residents in nursing homes. The key feature is that it investigates a 'population at risk': 'The population at risk is the group of people, healthy or sick, who would be counted as cases if they had the disease being studied' (Coggon et al., 2003, p. 1). So the population under study must be capable of having the disease or condition. For instance, studies of prostate cancer would exclude women

Epidemiology is the scientific foundation for public health because it assists in identifying the health problems in particular communities, can assess the relevance of prevention and evaluate the effectiveness of preventive interventions (Tannahill, 1994). Public health practitioners rely, to a large extent, on epidemiological data to provide valuable information about the health of their population. The basic statistical measurements are explained in the next section.

7.3 Mortality and morbidity statistics

These represent measures of deaths in a population (mortality) and measures of disease in a population (morbidity).

Mortality statistics

Mortality data from death certificates and from census and population registers are routinely collected. From these the death rate in a population can be calculated. To calculate a death rate, the number of deaths recorded is divided by the number of people in the population, and then multiplied by 100, 1000 or another convenient figure.

The crude death rate shows the number of deaths in the total population and, for the sake of manageability, is usually calculated per 1000. It is calculated as follows:

$$\text{The annual crude death rate per 1000 population} = \frac{\text{Total number of deaths in a calendar year}}{\text{Estimated mid-year population that year}} \times 1000$$

Crude death rates do not show the burden of deaths in particular groups in the population. For example, one might assume that a town such as Bournemouth is an unhealthy place because it has a high crude death rate, but on closer examination this is found to be due to the fact that it is a popular place to retire to and consequently has a high proportion of older people. To counter this problem, age-specific rates can be calculated as follows:

$$\text{The annual age-specific death rate for the age group 25-50 years per 1000 population} = \frac{\text{Total number of deaths among people aged 25-50 during a calendar year}}{\text{Estimated mid-year population aged 25-50 that year}} \times 1000$$

As well as straightforward age-specific rates, certain special age rates can be calculated which are of particular importance in public health. The infant mortality rate (IMR) is used as an indicator of the overall health of a nation or community. This is because IMR correlates well with young adult mortality, but is more sensitive to socioeconomic and environmental improvements as well as to improvements in healthcare. The IMR is calculated as follows:

$$\frac{\text{The annual infant mortality}}{\text{rate per 1000 live births}} = \frac{\text{Total number of deaths under the age of one year during a calendar year}}{\text{Total number of live births in that year}} \times 1000$$

Other special rates of deaths in infants under one year of age include the annual stillbirth rate, late foetal deaths after 24 weeks of gestation and the annual perinatal mortality rate (stillbirths plus deaths in the first week of life). These are calculated in the same way as infant mortality. Figure 7.3 shows these rates for the UK in 2008.

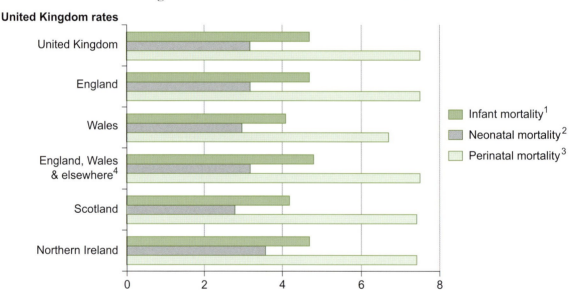

United Kingdom rates

[1] Deaths under 1 year per 1,000 live births

[2] Deaths under 4 weeks per 1,000 live births

[3] Stillbirths and deaths under 1 week per 1,000 live and stillbirths

[4] 'England, Wales and elsewhere' covers both residents and non-residents, comparable with the Scotland and Northern Ireland figures. The separate 'England' and 'Wales' categories cover residents only.

Figure 7.3 Infant, neonatal and perinatal mortality rates (2008)
(Source: Office for National Statistics, 2009, p. 10)

The death rates discussed above are based on all causes of death. The cause-specific death rate is used to calculate how many deaths occurred from specific diseases such as cancer or heart disease. This is calculated as follows:

$$\text{The annual cause-specific death rate per 1000 population} = \frac{\text{Total number of deaths from a particular cause during a calendar year}}{\text{Estimated mid-year population in that year}} \times 1000$$

The calculations made so far can provide the overall crude death rate for a population, the death rate for different age groups and deaths from different causes, but do not allow for a comparison to be made between one part of the country and another.

Why do you think it is important to be able to make comparisons between places?

We noted that Bournemouth has a high proportion of older people and will have a high death rate, whereas a population with a high proportion of young people, in a new town such as Milton Keynes, is likely to have a low death rate. A direct comparison of crude mortality rates for the two localities would obviously produce a distorted picture. So the death rate for a specific condition in a particular area may be higher than the national average simply because the area contains relatively more residents in a susceptible age group than the national population.

Standardised mortality ratios (SMR) can compare mortality rates between different geographical areas, taking age differences into account (see Box 7.2). So, despite the very different age structures of the populations involved, regional comparisons can be made, as Figure 7.4 (page 188) demonstrates for cities in Wales.

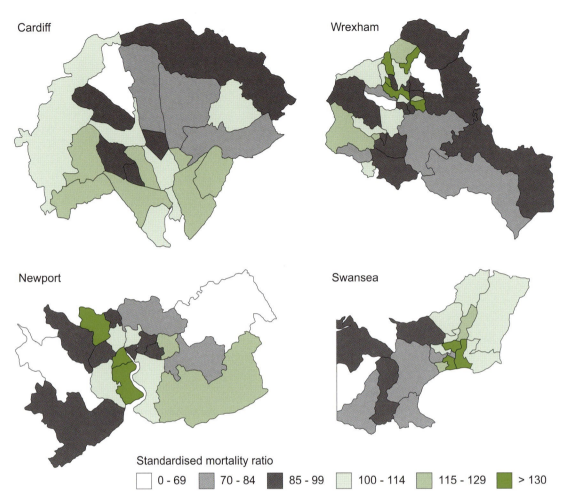

Figure 7.4 Ward-level standardised mortality ratios (all causes, ages 0–74) for four major cities in Wales (1990–1992)
(Source: Williams et al., 1994, Figure 4.4)

Box 7.2 Calculating a standardised mortality ratio

Death rates for age groups (or other groups) in the standard [national] population are multiplied by the population of the same groups in the study population. This produces an 'expected' number of deaths representing what the number of deaths in the study population would have been, if that population had the same death rates as the standard population. The observed (or actual) number of deaths in the study population is then divided by the total expected number and multiplied by 100. This produces an SMR. The standard population always has an SMR of 100, with which the SMR of the study population can be compared. The SMR figure is actually a percentage. This means that if the study population's SMR is 130, its death rate is 30 per cent higher than that of the standard population. If the study population's SMR is 86, then its death rate is 14 per cent lower than that of the standard population.

(Stewart, 2002, p. 80)

As well as comparing death rates for different regions, the SMR can be used to compare the death rates in other groupings of the population; for instance, between different occupational groups.

For example, the SMR for male bus drivers between the ages of 25 and 65 in the UK in 2000 would be calculated as:

$$\frac{\text{Observed deaths in male bus drivers in the UK aged 25-65 years}}{\text{Expected deaths of male bus drivers based on male death rates in UK}} \times 100$$

SMRs are used by National Health Service (NHS) Scotland as part of a patient safety programme that aims to reduce unintended harm from adverse events by 30 per cent and mortality by 15 per cent. They use and publish local hospital SMRs to drive quality improvement by pasting up statistical process charts on hospital wards to demonstrate how improvement is being sustained on a reliable basis (Colin Brown, personal communication, 2011).

So far we have been focusing on mortality data, but how is the distribution of morbidity measured?

Morbidity statistics

Epidemiology also involves estimating the frequency and distribution of diseases in populations. Measures of disease frequency are tools to describe how common an illness is in relation to the size of the population (the population at risk). These measures count the number of cases in a population and a measure in time. The two main types of measure of disease frequency are incidence and prevalence.

Incidence

Incidence is the number of new cases of a disease or disorder that arises in a defined population over a defined period of time.

Incidence rates are calculated as follows:

$$\text{The incidence rate per 1000 population} = \frac{\text{The number of new cases of a disease occurring in a population during a specified time period}}{\text{The population at risk during that period of time}} \times 1000$$

(Source: Royal Free Medical School, 2001, p. 83)

The specified time period is usually a calendar year.

For example, to calculate the incidence of prostate cancer in men in Wales in 2010 per 1000 of the population, you would need to divide the number of new cases of prostate cancer in men in Wales by the number of men resident in Wales in 2010 and then multiply by 1000.

In order to calculate the incidence of chlamydia in a given area – for example Scotland – you would need the actual numbers of men and women in Scotland. If you wanted to calculate the age-specific incidence rate for men and women, because chlamydia infection is higher in younger adults, then you would need the new cases of chlamydia broken down by age as well as by sex. You would then need the numbers of men and women in different age groups in Scotland. Incidence, of course, only applies to reported and diagnosed cases of chlamydia. The actual size of the problem is likely to be higher.

Figure 7.5 shows the incidence rates of syphilis and gonorrhoea for men and women between 2000 and 2009.

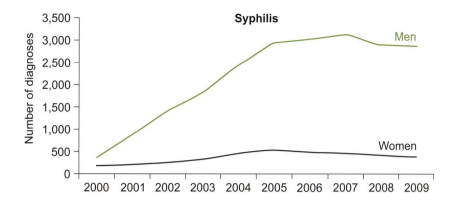

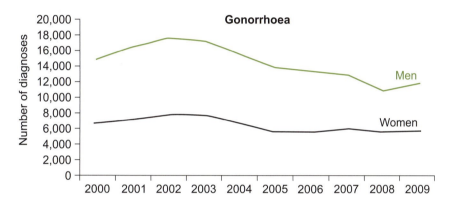

Figure 7.5 New diagnoses of syphilis and gonorrhoea at genito-urinary medicine clinics in the UK by gender (2000–2009)

(Source: Health Protection Agency, 2010, p. 8)

Incidence rates record new cases of a specific disease in a specified timescale, which is useful for comparing trends over time but it does not give you a picture of the total size of the disease or problem. To find this out, prevalence rates are used.

Prevalence

Prevalence is the total number of people suffering from a specific disease at a certain point in time, including old as well as new cases. Prevalence studies are commonly used to survey characteristics such as smoking habits or alcohol use.

Prevalence rates are calculated as follows:

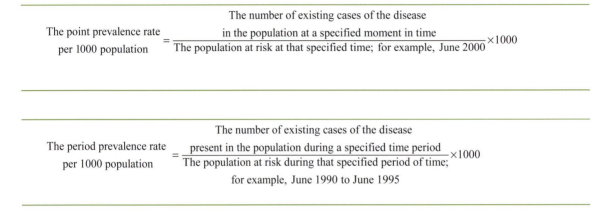

$$\text{The point prevalence rate per 1000 population} = \frac{\text{The number of existing cases of the disease in the population at a specified moment in time}}{\text{The population at risk at that specified time; for example, June 2000}} \times 1000$$

$$\text{The period prevalence rate per 1000 population} = \frac{\text{The number of existing cases of the disease present in the population during a specified time period}}{\text{The population at risk during that specified period of time; for example, June 1990 to June 1995}} \times 1000$$

(Source: Royal Free Medical School, 2001, p. 83)

Incidence and prevalence rates can be calculated separately for men and women as well as other groupings, such as ethnicity.

7.4 Applying epidemiology

There are two broad types of epidemiological inquiry:

- descriptive epidemiology – identifies who gets sick
- analytic epidemiology – tries to go further into finding out why people get sick.

Descriptive epidemiology

A large part of the epidemiological task is concerned with surveillance. Public health departments and agencies, such as the Health Protection Agency, quite literally keep watch on the incidence and prevalence of disease in the population. Data on these are collected regularly and routinely from a range of sources throughout the UK. Sources of morbidity data in the community include those listed in Box 7.3.

Box 7.3 Sources of morbidity data in the community

Public Health Observatory

The Association of Public Health Observatories (APHO) represents a network of 12 public health observatories (PHO) working across the five nations of England, Scotland, Wales, Northern Ireland and the Republic of Ireland. They produce information, data and intelligence on people's health and healthcare for practitioners, policy makers and the wider community. Their expertise lies in turning information and data into meaningful health intelligence. English observatories will be merged into Public Health England from 2013.

Clinical and Health Outcomes Knowledge Base

The Clinical and Health Outcomes Knowledge Base is a one-stop source of all information on health outcomes generated by the National Centre for Health Outcomes Development. Alongside advice on how to measure health and the impact of healthcare, it includes the Compendium of Clinical and Health Indicators. The Compendium contains a wide range of indicators about population health in all areas and enables comparison of figures between areas and the England averages. It includes data around 700 health and local government organisations in England and is now being updated by the NHS Information Centre for Health and Social Care.

The Cochrane Collaboration

The Cochrane Collaboration, established in 1993, is an international network of people helping healthcare providers, policy makers, patients, their advocates and carers make well-informed decisions about human healthcare by preparing, updating and promoting the accessibility of Cochrane Reviews, which are systematic reviews of primary research on a wide range of healthcare and health-policy topics. So far, there are over 4500 published online in the Cochrane Library.

Hospital Episode Statistics (HES)

HES is a collection of NHS hospitals' data, including admissions, main operations and diagnoses. It is a records-based system covering all acute hospitals, primary care trusts and mental health trusts in England. HES records include care provided to NHS patients by the independent sector, including care taking place in treatment centres and care given to private patients in NHS hospitals. HES records are also available for Scotland, Wales and Northern Ireland.

HES information is stored as a large collection of separate records – one for each period of care – in a secure data warehouse. Each HES record contains a wide range of information about an individual patient admitted to an NHS hospital. For example:

- clinical information about diagnoses and operations
- information about the patient, such as age group, gender and ethnic category
- administrative information, such as time waited and date of admission
- geographical information on where the patient was treated and the area in which they lived.

In England HES has transferred to the Health and Social Care Information Centre.

Neighbourhood Statistics

Neighbourhood Statistics provides information on many issues, including health and care, community wellbeing and the social environment. Statistics can be obtained at ward, local authority, health authority, parish and parliamentary constituency level.

General Practice Research Database (GPRD)

GPRD holds anonymised patient-based clinical data submitted regularly by general practices.

Mental health and illness

A wide range of surveys are available on such topics as:

- people with psychotic disorders living in the community
- residents of institutions for people with mental disorders
- homeless people
- prisoners
- children looked after by local authorities
- people providing informal care.

Analytic epidemiology

As well as the basic data on incidence and prevalence of disease, epidemiology is particularly interested in the patterns of disease distribution in human populations.

In order to contribute to causal understanding, to address the question of why people get sick, Bhopal suggests that three main questions need to be asked:

1   How does the pattern of disease vary over time in this population?

2   How does the place in which the population lives affect the disease pattern?

3   How do the personal characteristics of the people in the population affect the disease pattern?

(Bhopal, 2002, p. 18)

Time: when do health problems occur?

The question of when (in time) diseases occur or peak is of considerable interest in epidemiology. For example, it is well established that a range of well-known infectious diseases (e.g. measles, influenza and whooping cough) show cyclical variations in occurrence, which result in epidemics every few years.

Look at Figure 7.6 (page 196) and identify the years in which notifications about pertussis (whooping cough) cases peaked.

In 1978, over 60,000 cases were reported and this fell dramatically in 1981, only to rise again in 1982. The rises may be explained by media coverage of the dangers of the vaccine in the mid 1970s and then again in the early 1980s.

Time can be measured in a variety of ways: secular time (referring to centuries); cyclical time or time intervals such as decades; seasonal time (i.e. summer, autumn, winter and spring); specifying particular times of the week or times of the day.

For example, in relation to secular time in the UK and elsewhere, infectious diseases constituted a major health problem throughout the nineteenth century. Fortunately, most of these diseases have declined and some, such as smallpox, have almost been eliminated. By the end of the twentieth century, however, heart disease and cancer had become the major health problems.

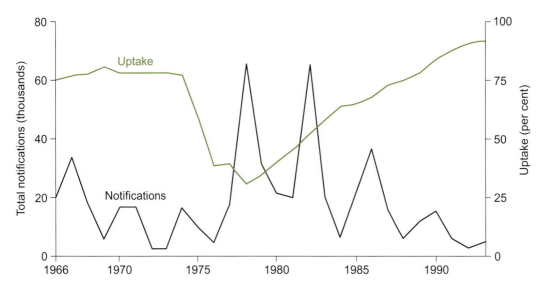

Figure 7.6 Pertussis notifications and immunisation uptake in England and Wales (1966–1993) (Source: Health Education Authority, 1995)

Seasonal variations in the incidence of disease are most common for respiratory tract infections (during winter months). Salmonella food poisoning also frequently shows seasonal variations, with peaks during the summer and over the Christmas period. Hay fever and other allergies occur primarily in the early summer.

Outbreaks of diseases can also be related to specific points in time, locations or events. For example, the exposure of guests at a wedding reception to a certain micro-organism can result in the sudden and simultaneous (or near simultaneous) occurrence of infection, such as typhoid or salmonella food poisoning.

Place: where do health problems occur?

The cholera epidemic of the 1850s demonstrates the influence of geographical and environmental factors on the occurrence of disease. Disease patterns also vary internationally; for example, the global pandemic of HIV infection is not uniformly geographically distributed (United Nations, 2010), as Figure 7.7 shows.

Within countries, regional variations in the occurrence of diseases are not uncommon. In addition, differences in disease patterns between urban and rural communities are frequently observed. Even within one

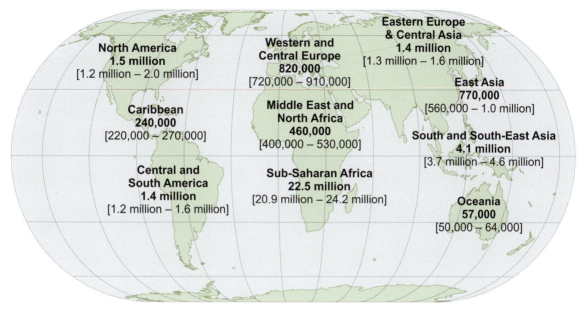

Total: 33.3 million [31.4 million – 35.3 million]

Figure 7.7 Estimated number* of people living with HIV, selected world regions (2009) *Numbers in square brackets refer to range.

(Source: United Nations, 2010, p. 5)

health district, mortality rates due to particular diseases may vary from one electoral ward to another.

However, international comparisons of ill health are not straightforward. In developing countries, access to biomedical treatment and the availability of facilities for investigation can be restricted. This means that there may be problems with the accuracy and completeness of diagnosis. The age structure of the population in developing countries, with a greater proportion of young people than in the industrialised world, also makes comparisons of disease frequency difficult.

Persons: which groups in the population have health problems?

In order to discover the patterns of disease distribution, data are needed on the personal characteristics of the population: the age groups, proportions of men and women, and occupational groups. Other population variables that are important are the social circumstances and conditions in which people live, as well as their religion, culture and ethnic origin.

Figure 7.8 illustrates the prevalence of hazardous drinking by age and sex. It demonstrates that men have higher rates than women, although the rates for both men and women have been decreasing for a number of years. However, women are at particular risk because physiologically they are less tolerant of alcohol than men.

Great Britain
Percentages

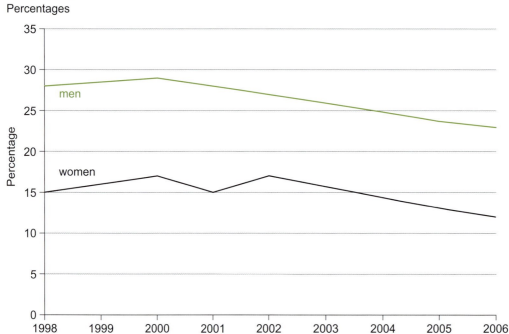

Figure 7.8 Percentage of men drinking more than 21 units a week, and women drinking more than 14 units a week

(Source: Office for National Statistics, 2011, p. 48)

Causation of ill health is difficult to determine. Apart from infectious diseases, such as described in the wedding reception example, most evidence relates to the risk associated with particular factors, rather than the direct causes of ill health. Even in the case of infectious diseases, it is not known why certain people succumb to them when other seemingly similar people do not. Only certain types of causative mechanism are amenable to investigation by epidemiological methods and few diseases can be said to have a single cause.

Despite considerable evidence about the influence various risk factors have on people's health, epidemiologists cannot infer that the link between a risk factor and ill health is a causal one. As Aggleton pointed out: 'there must be no hidden or confounding variable (i.e. a variable that could also be a causative factor) causing both of the variables to change' (1990, pp. 77–78).

The evidence generated by most epidemiological studies is correlational. Box 7.4 explains this term.

Box 7.4 Correlation

Correlation is the term used for an association between two variables. A variable can be anything being measured, for instance height or weight. When an association between two variables is found, it means that when one changes in magnitude, the other one does also. Correlation may be positive or negative. Positive correlation means that if one variable increases so does the other. Negative correlation means that there is still an association but the variables vary inversely; that is, when one increases the other decreases. Finding a correlation does not imply causation. It cannot be said that one variable increasing causes the other to increase. If it is found that weight increases as height increases, this does not mean that getting heavier makes people taller or that getting taller makes people heavier. The apparent association may be caused by a third factor or confounding variable that is influencing both variables simultaneously. For instance, genetic variables will affect the height and weight of someone.

(Adapted from The Open University, 2001, p. 109)

Abramson (2010) puts up a robust defence of the power of correlational evidence by citing many studies that have dramatically changed the public's health. Going back to 1753, he cites the link made between a lack of fresh fruit and vegetables and scurvy as well as the work of Doll and Hill (1950) who found a link between smoking and the increased incidence of lung cancer from their longitudinal study of doctors. But he gives a more recent example of the association found between babies who are put to sleep on their stomachs and sudden infant death syndrome (SIDS). Although the reasons for this finding are still not clear, this correlation has been acted on in the Back to Sleep campaign (Kattwinkel et al., 1992) which has significantly reduced the incidence of SIDS internationally.

However, there is another criticism levelled at epidemiology, which accuses it of not taking enough account of contexts (Baum, 2010). In fact, by trying to isolate risk factors and eliminate confounding variables which might include socioeconomic, cultural and environmental factors, important causal mechanisms can be overlooked. Baum suggests that popular epidemiology presents a way of taking account of context and she cites the example of epidemiologists who have worked in collaboration with local and environmental groups in the Equadorian Amazon to explore the effects of the oil industry on the health of local people (Baum, 2010).

Further limitations of epidemiology and quantitative studies are drawn out after exploring the different types of epidemiological studies.

Types of epidemiological studies

Epidemiological studies generally fall into four broad categories:

- cross-sectional studies
- case–control studies
- cohort studies including longitudinal studies
- intervention studies.

Cross-sectional studies

Cross-sectional studies measure the prevalence of conditions or characteristics of people in a population at a point in time or over a short period. Although they are essentially descriptive studies, their results can often suggest risk factors associated with particular illness or behaviour. They can also be used to find out the prevalence of a health-related behaviour, such as the wearing of seat belts. They are also useful in planning public health interventions, for instance by ascertaining the proportion of a population who exercise.

A population or group can be studied in a variety of ways: questionnaire on physical exercise; taking measurements (such as blood pressure); analysing blood specimens (for example, for blood cholesterol levels); and examining healthcare records.

Case control studies

Case control studies focus on establishing the causes of diseases. The 'cases' are the people with a particular condition, such as high blood pressure or diabetes. The 'controls' are people without the condition. Investigations are then carried out into the previous exposure of the two groups to particular factors that are suspected of causing the symptom or condition. If the two groups differ regarding their exposure to such factors, a causal link between the symptom/condition and the factor is inferred.

Cohort and longitudinal studies

Cohort and longitudinal studies focus on groups of people who show certain attributes or characteristics, such as health behaviours or occupations. The groups are observed over a period of time in order to discover what happens to their individual members and to check whether there are any associations between behaviour and the development of disease. The famous epidemiologist Sir Richard Doll and his colleagues, cited earlier, investigated doctors' smoking habits in this way and followed the sample for over 40 years.

The censuses of 1971 and 1981 saw the introduction of a 'cohort study' on a sample section of the population. This is known as the Office for Population Censuses and Surveys (OPCS) longitudinal study, which also links to a wide range of health and social indicators. Babies born on four days in 1971 were identified and followed up in subsequent censuses. These data are used for medical research as well as demographic purposes. Other examples of cohort studies include the British Birth Cohort studies, the National Study of Health and Growth of School Children, started in 1974 (Stamatakis et al., 2005), and the Millennium baby study which is ongoing (Millennium Cohort Study, 2011).

Intervention studies

These are a type of case–control study where the cases receive an intervention and the controls do not.

The most popular study of this kind is the randomised controlled trial (RCT). RCTs divide the population to be studied into groups on a random basis. One group is then subjected to a treatment, procedure or intervention, while the other is not. If the two groups are matched in terms of their characteristics, any measurable differences between them should be due to the intervention. Ideally, the RCT should be carried out using a double-blind method; that is, neither the researcher nor the subject should know who is in the intervention or control arm of the study.

Drug trials are by far the most common type of intervention study. Their purpose is to discover the effects and effectiveness of new drugs developed by the pharmaceutical industry. Objections to trials such as these are often on ethical grounds. If a study is investigating the effects of a particular treatment on cancer sufferers, for instance, then it could be seen as unethical to withhold the potentially beneficial treatment from the control group who are also cancer sufferers. However, the control group would be receiving the current best conventional treatment. Other ethical problems relate to whether the participants are fully informed about the potential effects of participating. The 1964 Declaration of Helsinki on medical ethics (see World Medical Organisation, 1996) makes it clear that RCT participants must receive adequate information about the aims, methods, expected benefits and possible hazards involved in the intervention. Participants must feel free to withdraw without putting their previous treatment at risk.

Randomised controlled trials use an experimental approach that is largely restricted to single-factor interventions. Interventions are also closed systems, such as schools or health clinics, because these are the contexts in which it is possible to exercise more control and to have more knowledge about the various factors that may influence the outcomes. The experimental approach assumes a greater degree of control over confounding variables than is usually possible or desirable in many of the social settings in which public health interventions take place.

What might be the main problems in trying to use an experimental approach in public health settings?

The random assignment of people in a community setting to intervention and control groups can be problematic given that people are social and cultural beings whose lives cannot become separated from one another. Many public health interventions aim specifically to influence the whole community and in these situations the problem of trying to create experimental conditions is great.

Quasi-experimental design

One response to some of these difficulties has been to use a modified or quasi-experimental design. Instead of using a control group formed by random assignment, the investigator may choose a highly comparable but not randomly selected comparison group. An alternative method is to identify the control group as those individuals who will be exposed to the intervention eventually but who are on a waiting list, and are consequently termed a 'waiting-list control group'.

Even so, the question remains about how useful experimental and quasi-experimental designs are in public health. Here is one view relating to health education that reflects the gap between experimental design and the demands of normal practice settings:

> In practical terms it can be difficult to plan and implement fully controlled experimental studies of health education activities. The use of laboratory type conditions can be both artificial and inappropriate and where interventions have been tested in such artificial situations we have to ask questions about the generalizability of findings to the real world. Even when experimental studies in health education have taken place in normal practice settings the outcomes which result from the extra efforts which typically go into an evaluated study may be an unrealistic guide to what can be achieved in routine practice. Finally, while experiments can establish statistical significance, it may be more important to focus on practical significance.
>
> (Tones and Tilford, 1994, p. 59)

So far this chapter has focused mainly on studying ill health and disease. How can the health of a population be studied in a more positive sense? The next section looks at surveys which address a broad range of factors in relation to health.

7.5 Health surveys

What is a survey?

A survey is a method of researching a population or a sample of that population. The census is a survey which is drawn from the whole population. A survey aims to ask the same questions of all the people in the population or the sample. The items of information gathered are known as variables.

Surveys can focus on factual variables such as age, sex, socioeconomic circumstances and, in the case of health surveys, measurements of health status. They frequently explore attitudes, beliefs and opinions and they can gather information on behaviours, all of which can inform public health.

Scope of health-related surveys

It was noted earlier that the 2001 census included, for the first time, a question on general health, which asked people to rate their health as 'good', 'fairly good' or 'not good', as well as a question about longstanding illness or disability. Before that the only other national large-scale regular survey to ask those two questions was the General Household Survey (GHS). The GHS is an annual survey of around 17,000 people which has been conducted by the ONS since 1971. As well as the two core questions about general health it asks a wide range of questions about socioeconomic conditions. Every alternate year it asks about health-related behaviours, such as smoking and drinking. In 1994 it asked questions on the causes of longstanding illness. In 1998 and 2001 data were collected on the use of the internet, mobile phones and other consumer durables and its 2002 edition, *Living in Britain*, investigated the notion of social capital. This range of variables enables researchers to link health to a much broader social model, so can throw light on and monitor the determinants of health and inequalities in health. Researchers can access the findings and carry out further statistical analysis on variables that interest them. For instance, they may want to draw out the links between those who rate their general health as 'good' with measures of social capital.

In 2008 the GHS changed its name to the General Lifestyle Survey (GLS) and since January 2008 the GLS is part of a new Integrated Household Survey. As well as the GLS the Integrated Household Survey includes:

- Labour Force Survey
- Living Costs and Food Survey
- English Housing Survey
- Life Opportunities Survey.

The Health Survey for England (HSFE) is, as its title suggests, a dedicated health survey. It was started in 1991 and has been carried out annually since then. It combines a health interview with a physical examination carried out by a qualified nurse. It now interviews similar numbers to the GLS. As well as core questions asked annually, it takes a different focus each year. In 2002, it focused on the health of children and young people and on maternal health.

Although covering some behaviours, neither the GLS nor the HSFE is concerned with attitudes and opinions. Other surveys do cover these aspects. At the national level, the British Social Attitudes (BSA) survey is carried out annually and covers England, Wales and Scotland. It monitors the nation's attitudes to a whole range of issues, from religious affiliation to membership of community organisations and participation in voluntary activities, to the impact of transport policies on car use. The BSA and the HSFE are carried out by the National Centre for Social Research.

The King's Fund, an independent foundation that undertakes research and health-policy analysis, carried out a survey in 2004 entitled *Public Attitudes into Public Health Policy* which is mentioned in Chapter 1. They interviewed 1002 members of the public about their 'health expectations', their views on 'individual responsibility and control', the 'role of government' and the 'role of the NHS' (King's Fund, 2004, pp. 4–5). They found a great deal of support for a public smoking ban. With regard to diet and nutrition, they found that government action to ensure that schools provide only healthy meals was very popular. Eighty-two per cent would support laws to limit levels of salt, fat and sugar in foods and 73 per cent would support government action to stop junk foods and sweets being advertised to children. The bar diagram in Figure 7.9 (page 206) shows the percentage of people who agreed with statements about the role of government. This provides useful information on public health.

Characteristics of surveys

Surveys provide quantitative evidence; that is, they aim to quantify the information collected in such a way that the data can be subjected to statistical analysis and that generalisations can be made from them. The quality of surveys is judged in terms of five interrelated criteria (May, 1997).

1 **Standardisation** – each respondent should be asked exactly the same question in exactly the same way so that any difference in their reply is not due to the way that the question is asked.

2 **Replicability** – the survey should be able to be carried out with different but matched respondents and different researchers, and produce the same findings.

3 **Reliability** – it should be possible to obtain the same results using the same questions with the same respondents at different times and with different interviewers.

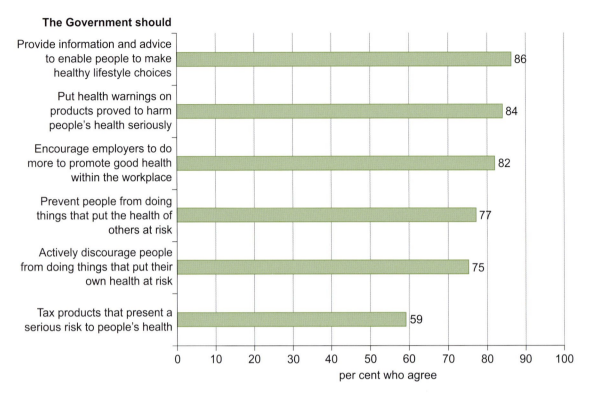

The Government should

Figure 7.9 Percentage of people who agreed with statements about the role of government (Source: King's Fund, 2004, p. 13)

4 **Validity** – the survey should measure what it intended to measure.

5 **Representativeness** – it should be possible to generalise from the survey to the whole population.

Criteria 1, 2 and 3 are closely linked. Standardisation is in many ways an attempt to ensure replicability and reliability. If more than one interviewer is involved in a survey, and in large surveys this is inevitably the case, then they must all be trained in asking the questions. Many surveys give elaborate instructions to the interviewers. Nevertheless, different interviewers can illicit different reactions from respondents merely on the basis of factors such as age or gender.

Certain questions might be more difficult in terms of reliability than others. For instance, the question, 'How do you rate your health?' begs the question, 'What is health?' It might also depend on how a person feels that day or that morning, which might be different from how they feel on another day. Nevertheless, self-assessment of health has been found to be a reliable indicator of future health.

Criterion 4, on validity, is very much dependent on the question asked, which needs to be clear and unambiguous. Criterion 5 is dependent on the sampling procedures. Sampling procedures and the use of questions are addressed next in relation to the characteristics of surveys.

Sampling

The census is the only form of data collection from the population that targets the whole population of the UK. All the other surveys discussed above, out of necessity, focus on a sample of the population. 'Sample' is the technical term for a smaller subset of a larger group, which is the 'population'. This may or may not be the whole population; that is, all UK residents. It may be all students currently at UK universities or any other defined group. Practicalities and issues of manageability govern the need for sampling, but the important issue is that the sample should represent the population from which it is drawn. There are a number of ways to ensure this, depending on the purpose of the survey.

Random sampling

Random samples are also known as probability samples because they enable a statistical generalisation to be made from the sample to the population. Random sampling is a technique whereby each member of the target population has an equal chance of being selected. The usual way to select a random sample is to use a sampling frame; this is a list of those in the target population. Sampling frames frequently used in large health surveys include the electoral register (EL), the postcode address file (PAF) and lists from primary care. A system, such as selecting every tenth person on the list, is then used to create the sample from the chosen list.

Stratified random sampling means that the population is divided into subgroups according to particular characteristics – perhaps age, sex or social class – which are then subjected to random sampling. This is not to be confused with quota sampling in which a proportion of a particular group in the population is required to be included because the research has a particular interest in that group. For instance, a random sample of people in London may fail to include many older women from minority ethnic groups, so the researcher will set a quota of such women to include in the sample in order to be able to elicit their views. A quota sample is actually therefore a non-random sample.

Non-random sampling

A purposive sample is one where people, or organisations, exhibiting particular characteristics are chosen for study; for example, pregnant women over the age of 40 with diabetes. A snowball sample is sometimes used for groups that are hard to reach; for instance, homeless people. In this instance, one interviewee is asked to suggest others who may be willing to be interviewed. Then each of these others will be asked to suggest further people, and so on. These two types of sample are typical of small-scale surveys which, although producing quantitative data, do not claim to be representative. Another type of sample which is becoming increasingly familiar on our streets is the 'next available person' sample, where interviewers try to engage the next available member of the public who passes by.

Asking questions

All surveys ask questions of their respondents in some form or another. This might be in the form of a questionnaire or an interview schedule. Technically, a questionnaire is designed to be filled in by the respondent, whereas an interview schedule is designed to be administered by an interviewer. (This is the way the term is used in this chapter, but the term 'questionnaire' is often used for both ways of asking questions.) In some circumstances, questionnaires and interview schedules are now completed by or with a third party, such as a relative, health/social care assistant or an interpreter; for example, when the population being studied has a high rate of illiteracy in English (Lloyd, 2010).

What do you think are the characteristics of good questionnaires?

Questionnaires are part of everyday life, but you may have noticed how some questionnaires are easier to complete than others. In fact, questionnaires are quite difficult to design. Some general principles exist for the production of good questionnaires. Punch (2003, p. 61) suggests the following:

- keeping questions and items short and as simply worded as possible
- ensuring that each item and question carries only one idea
- avoiding negatives and double negatives
- using language that is clear, unambiguous, relevant and appropriate, and unbiased.

It is often better to use mainly closed questions in questionnaires, because they are easier to codify. Aldridge and Levine (2001) argue that open questions are more difficult to answer in self-completed questionnaires because respondents have to reflect on their answer and this may take time and effort, which they often do not want to invest. However, an argument could be made that open questions allow more attention to be paid to the respondent's point of view, and certainly more use can be made of open questions in an interview schedule where the interviewer records the response. Brevity is a virtue in questionnaires which should not take more than 20–30 minutes of a respondent's time. If there is a need for complex questions then the questionnaire format is probably not appropriate.

The following list includes some common pitfalls in questionnaires (adapted from Aldridge and Levine, 2001).

- The use of insensitive language or language that is class, race or region specific; for instance, it is better to use the term 'midday meal' than 'lunch' which might have class connotations.

- Overlapping categories; for instance, when asking about age it is usual to provide age groups, such as 30–40 and 40–50, but where does a 40-year-old woman place herself? It is better to use the format 30–39, then 40–49, and so on. And when asking about age, always be specific and say 'at your last birthday'.

- Double-barrelled questions, such as 'Do you swim and walk regularly?', with the option to tick just 'yes' or 'no'. This needs to be formulated as two questions with a 'yes' and 'no' reply for each.

Many questionnaires deal with sensitive subjects, so often the anonymity of a questionnaire is useful for gaining information in these circumstances as it avoids the embarrassment of responding to an interviewer (Kelly et al., 1994). Questionnaires can be sent through the post, but this often results in a low response rate. The response rate can be improved if they are given out; for example, at a clinic, with a box for the receipt of the completed ones.

Many of the issues relating to asking questions on a questionnaire also apply to interview schedules but, because the questions in an interview schedule are administered by a trained interviewer, they can be much more complex. Large-scale surveys employ teams of researchers to carry out the interviews, and they are usually trained together. But if the requirements of reliability and replicability are to be satisfied, interview schedules need to contain full instructions for the interviewer in order to try to ensure consistency in the way in which different interviewers carry out the interview. In effect, the instructions are rather like stage directions in a play, which ensure the actor delivers the lines in the way the author intended. Interview schedules are often deemed more attractive for use in any survey that is attempting more than some simple and specific measurements because of the possibility to include many more open questions.

Health surveys can provide a wealth of information on a population – some of it descriptive; some of it analytic – and it should be possible to make generalisations from the survey about the whole population on a wide range of health-related topics. For this to be the case, surveys have to follow specific sampling procedures and ask questions that are meaningful, relevant and unambiguous to the respondent. Surveys have attracted a good deal of criticism, some of which is attributable to poor design, but some criticisms are more fundamental.

Critical views of surveys

Surveys have been criticised for lack of scientific rigour by those who see randomised controlled trials as the only viable form of health research (Aldridge and Levine, 2001).

However, most criticism of surveys is made from a humanistic perspective on the basis that surveys are atomistic: 'they treat society and culture as no more than the sum of the individuals within it' (Aldridge and Levine, 2001, p. 12). In fact, surveys do not pretend to be focusing on individuals per se, but on the aggregate of individuals who make up a population. They describe and analyse populations rather than individual people; that is their strength as well as a limitation. In this way they can identify a great deal about which people adopt a particular health behaviour, but they cannot provide an understanding of the processes involved in why people adopt such behaviour. Chapter 8 looks in detail at the potential of qualitative research in understanding people's behaviour.

A further major criticism of surveys is that they reflect the concerns and presuppositions of the researcher. The questions they ask restrict the respondent's options in answering them. This is particularly the case with closed questions, but even open questions are inviting the respondent to respond to a question which the researcher deems to be important. In addition, in order to ensure replicability and reliability, surveys go to great lengths to ensure that questions are asked in a standardised way. This means that there is very little scope for the respondents to put forward their own point of view if it does not fit into the question asked. This problem is compounded by what Aldridge and Levine term the problem of social desirability:

> Respondents' answers are influenced by their desire to be helpful and to live up to their own self-image or to an ideal which they think will look good to the researcher … They will also try to appear consistent, with the result that their opinions and beliefs will seem more coherent than they really are.
>
> (Aldridge and Levine, 2001, p. 13)

Others have objected to the mythical power of quantitative evidence:

> Quantification has acquired a bogus value – if something can be measured or counted it gains a scientific credibility often not afforded to the unmeasured or unmeasurable. Because of this, a finding or result is more likely to be accepted as a fact if it has been quantified than if it has not. On occasions, our love affair with numbers goes even further: sometimes we may suspect our critical faculties when faced with quantitative information, whether derived from routine or ad hoc sources. As a result, many well known, widely accepted 'facts' of doubtful accuracy have become entrenched in our supposed knowledge of health, disease and health care.
>
> (Black, 1994, p. 425)

Black is not suggesting here that quantitative data do not have their strengths in describing many aspects of populations. Indeed, he believes that quantifying information is so essential that we need constantly to monitor and improve the way it is collected and analysed. He proposes three ways to improve the evidence base for health (Black, 1994): by developing more sophisticated statistical methods to handle this kind of data; by using quantitative methods in combination with qualitative methods; and by acknowledging that some areas of inquiry are simply not amenable to quantitative inquiry, but could be investigated using qualitative methods.

Chapter 8 is devoted to qualitative evidence and discusses further the potential for combining quantitative and qualitative data in the pursuit of public health. Using qualitative methods in combination with quantitative methods can help prevent the problem of ensuring that the questions asked in surveys do not reflect just the concerns of the researcher or those commissioning the research. In-depth qualitative methods, used with a small but purposive sample of people, can help define and refine the research questions and make them relevant to the respondents in a large-scale survey. Qualitative methods can also be useful as a follow-up to a survey that, for example, identifies groups in the population who have been unemployed for over a year. In-depth interviews or focus groups can contribute to the development of understanding of why they have been unemployed and what impact this has had on their health.

Conclusion

Quantitative evidence has its limitations, but it makes a vital contribution to finding out about the population's health. Without such data the extent and nature of inequalities in health would not be exposed. Demography, epidemiology and survey research are powerful and essential tools in efforts to promote public health. Without information on the levels of mortality and morbidity in the population, it is inconceivable that policies and practices to prevent and combat disease could prevail. And without a greater understanding of the distribution of disease within a population, it is difficult to see how policies and practices could be targeted at the appropriate groups in that population. Health surveys can provide much needed information on numerous aspects of a population's health in a much broader sense than disease and death statistics, and they can identify attitudes and behaviours as well as social factors that contribute to the way in which health and ill health is distributed in the population. Nevertheless, the quantitative data that are generated can never be taken at face value and should always be open to critical review and, where appropriate, should be informed and enhanced by qualitative data.

References

Abramson, J.H. (2010) 'Epidemiology: to be taken with care' in Douglas, J., Earle, S., Handsley, S., Jones, L., Lloyd, C.E. and Spurr, S. (eds) *A Reader in Promoting Public Health: Challenge and Controversy*, London/Milton Keynes, Sage/The Open University, pp. 97–106.

Acheson, D. (1998) *Independent Inquiry into Inequalities in Health*, London, HMSO.

Aggleton, P. (1990) *Health*, London, Routledge.

Aldridge, A. and Levine, K. (2001) *Surveying the Social World: Principles and Practice in Survey Research*, Buckingham, Open University Press.

Bailey, L., Vardulaki, K., Langhan, J. and Chandramoha, D. (2005) *Introduction to Epidemiology*, Maidenhead, Open University Press.

Baum, F. (2010) 'Dilemmas in public health research: methodologies and ethical practice', in Douglas, J., Earle, S., Handsley, S., Jones, L., Lloyd, C.E and Spurr, S. (eds) *A Reader in Promoting Public Health: Challenge and Controversy*, London/Milton Keynes, Sage/The Open University, pp. 77–88.

Bhopal, R. (2002) *Concepts of Epidemiology: An Integrated Introduction to the Ideas, Theories, Principles and Methods of Epidemiology*, Oxford, Oxford University Press.

Bhopal, R. (2001) 'Is research into ethnicity and health racist, unsound, or important science?' in Heller, T., Muston, R., Sidell, M. and Lloyd, C. (eds) *Working for Health*, London/Milton Keynes, Sage/The Open University, pp. 168–80.

Black, N. (1994) 'Why we need qualitative research', *Journal of Epidemiology and Community Health*, vol. 48, no. 5, pp. 425–26.

Bradby, H. and Chandola, T. (2010) 'Inequalities and ethnicity: evidence and intervention' in Douglas, J., Earle, S., Handsley, S., Jones, L., Lloyd, C.E. and Spurr, S. (eds) *A Reader in Promoting Public Health: Challenge and Controversy* (2nd edition), London/Milton Keynes, Sage/The Open University, pp. 33–39.

Clinical and Health Outcomes Knowledge Base website. Available at: www.nchod.nhs.uk (accessed 3 October 2011).

Coggon, D., Rose, G. and Barker, D.J.P. (2003) *Epidemiology for the Uninitiated*, London, British Medical Journal Books.

Doll, R. and Hill, A.B. (1950) 'Smoking and carcinoma of the lung', Preliminary Report, *British Medical Journal*, vol. 2, pp. 739–48.

Dorling, D. and Thomas, B. (2004) *People and Places: A 2001 Census Atlas of the UK*, Bristol, Policy Press.

General Practice Research Database website. Available at: www.gprd.com (accessed 3 October 2011).

Gunaratnam, Y. (2007) 'Complexity and complicity in researching ethnicity and health' in Douglas, J., Earle, S., Handsley, S., Lloyd, C.E. and Spurr, S. (eds) *A Reader in Promoting Public Health: Challenge and Controversy*, London/Milton Keynes, Sage/The Open University, pp. 147–56.

Health Education Authority (1995) 'Pertussis notifications and immunisation' (personal communication).

Health Protection Agency (2010) *Health Protection Report*, vol. 4, no. 34, p. 8.

Hospital Episode Statistics [HES] website. Available at: www.hesonline.nhs.uk/ Ease/servlet/ContentServer?siteID=1937 (accessed 3 October 2011). HES statistics are also available through the UK National Statistics and Publication Hub at www.statistics.gov.uk/hub/search/index.html?newquery=hospital +episode+statistics.

Integrated Household Survey website. Available at: www.esds.ac.uk/ government/ihs/ (accessed 30 August 2011).

Kattwinkel, J., Brooks, J. and Myerberg, D. (1992) 'Positionisng and SIDS: AAP task force on infant positioning and SIDS', *Pediatrics*, vol. 89, pp. 1120–26.

Katz, J., Peberdy, A. and Douglas, J. (eds) (2000) *Promoting Health: Knowledge and Practice* (2nd edition), Basingstoke/Milton Keynes, Palgrave Macmillan/The Open University.

Kelly, M. and Charlton, B. (1995) 'The modern and the post-modern in health promotion' in Bunton, R., Nettleton, S. and Burrows, R. (eds) (1995) *The Sociology of Health Promotion: Critical Analyses of Consumption, Lifestyle and Risk*, London, Routledge, pp. 78–90.Kelly, L., Burton, S. and Regan, L. (1994) 'Researching women's lives or studying women's oppression? Reflections on what constitutes feminist research' in Maynard, M. and Purvis, J. (eds) (1994) *Researching Women's Lives from a Feminist Perspective*, London, Taylor and Francis.

King's Fund (2004) *Public Attitudes to Public Health Policy*, London, King's Fund. Available at: www.kingsfund.org.uk (accessed 29 May 2006).

Last, J. (2010) 'Connecting the dots: the power of words and the diversity of epidemiological information', *Journal of Epidemiology and Community Health*, vol. 64, pp. 105–8.

Lloyd, C.E. (2010) 'Researching the views of diabetes service users from south Asian backgrounds: a reflection on some of the issues' in Douglas, J., Earle, S., Handsley, S., Jones, L., Lloyd, C.E. and Spurr, S. (eds) *A Reader in Promoting Public Health: Challenge and Controversy*, (2nd edn), London/Milton Keynes, Sage/ The Open University, pp. 114–20.

May, T. (1997) *Social Research: Issues, Methods and Process*, Buckingham, Open University Press.

Mental Health and Illness website. Available at: www.mentalhealthsurveys.co. uk/index.html (accessed 3 October 2011).

Millennium Cohort Study (2011) Millennium Cohort Study website. Available at: www.esds.ac.uk/ (accessed 12 September 2011).

National Centre for Social Research website. Available at: www.natcen.ac.uk (accessed 30 August 2011).

Neighbourhood Statistics website. Available at: www.neighbourhood.statistics. gov.uk/ (accessed 3 October 2011).

Office for National Statistics (2011) *Smoking and Drinking Among Adults, 2009: A Report on the 2009 General Lifestyle Survey*, London, Office for National Statistics.

Office for National Statistics website. Available at: www.statistics.gov.uk (accessed 30 August 2011).

Organization for Economic Co-operation and Development (OECD) (2003) *Health at a Glance: OECD Indicators 2003*, Paris, Organization for Economic Co-operation and Development. Available at: www.oecd.org/document/11/ 0,3746,en_2649_34631_16502667_1_1_1_1,00.html (accessed 30 August 2011).

Organization for Economic Co-operation and Development (OECD) (2010) OECD Factbook 2010: Economic, Environmental and Social Statistics, Paris, OECD Publishing. Available at: www.oecd-ilibrary.org/economics/oecd-factbook-2010_factbook-2010-en (accessed 30 August 2011).

Peto, R. (1994) 'Smoking and death: the past 40 years and the next 40', *British Medical Journal*, vol. 309, pp. 937–9.

Punch, K.F. (2003) *Survey Research: The Basics*, London, Sage.

Public Health Observatory website. Available at: www.apho.org.uk (accessed 3 October 2011).

Rosling, H. (2011) *The Joy of Stats*, BBC2, 31 March.

Royal Free Medical School (2001) 'Lecture notes' (personal communication).

Stamatakis, E., Primatesta, P., Chinn, S., Rona, R. and Falaschetic, E. (2005) 'Overweight and obesity trends from 1974 to 2005 in English children: what is the role of socio-economic factors?', *Archive of Disease in Childhood*, vol. 90, no. 10, pp. 999–1004.

Stewart, A. (2002) *Basic Statistics and Epidemiology: A Practical Guide*, Oxford, Radcliffe Medical Press.

Tannahill, A. (1994) *Health Education and Health Promotion: From Priorities to Programmes*, Geneva, World Health Organization Regional Office for Europe/ Health Education Board for Scotland.

The Cochrane Collaboration website. Available at: www2.cochrane.org (accessed 3 October 2011).

The Open University (2001) K203 *Working for Health*, Block 1, Unit 4, Milton Keynes, The Open University.

Tones, K. and Tilford, S. (1994) *Health Education: Effectiveness, Efficiency and Equity*, London, Chapman and Hall.

Townsend, P. and Davidson, N. (eds) (1982) *Inequalities in Health: The Black Report*, Harmondsworth, Penguin.

UNAIDS (2010) *Report on the Global AIDS Epidemic 2010*, Geneva, United Nations. Available at: www.unaids.org/documents/20101123_GlobalReport_em.pdf (accessed 14 September 2011).

Williams, H., Dodge, M., Higgs, G., Senior, M. and Moss, N. (1994) *Mortality and Deprivation in Wales*, Cardiff, University of Wales, Department of City and Regional Planning.

World Medical Organisation (1996) 'Declaration of Helsinki', *British Medical Journal*, vol. 313, pp. 1448–9.

Chapter 8: Building evidence-based practice: qualitative approaches and triangulation

Linda Finlay

Introduction

The vast majority of official or statutory public health investigations are based on quantitative methods and approaches. Occasionally, these studies offer a qualitative component: for instance, alongside a survey, a few people may be interviewed in greater depth, adding richness and texture to the quantitative statistics. There is increasing recognition of the value of such evidence, with its sharper focus on both the individual's lived experience and the social context of health/illness. Exciting projects are being developed that combine quantitative and qualitative approaches while, increasingly, new opportunities are opening up for understanding people's health and health needs using qualitative research in its own right.

This chapter focuses on issues surrounding the use of qualitative approaches, and the methods and challenges involved. It begins by considering the evidence base for public health and examines the scope for combining quantitative and qualitative evidence through the example of a health impact assessment (HIA). Following this, the potential contribution of qualitative approaches is investigated using research case studies to raise some critical questions about qualitative methodologies. The chapter ends by examining some of the practical issues and processes involved with data collection, analysis and evaluation.

8.1 Enriching the evidence base: the contribution of mixed methods

Public health workers are urged to provide evidence of the effectiveness of their work, while planners are required to draw on evidence-based practice to improve the quality of services. But evidence comes in various shapes and forms, so the term 'evidence' begs a number of questions. What kind of evidence might best explore health attitudes and explain behaviours? What evidence is needed to show the value of healthcare work? What type of evidence should service users, providers of healthcare and policy makers rely on?

What counts as evidence?

Much depends on how 'evidence' is defined. The prevailing view of the evidence-based practice movement is that evidence should be 'scientific'; that is, utilising measurement and quantification. While results derived from quantitative research have contributed enormously to the public health field, there are gaps and silences. Can the ever-evolving, multi-layered nature of individuals' experiences, healthcare and our social world be measured? Might qualitative measures usefully supplement the evidence base? Qualitative methods are particularly tailored to capturing the opinions, experiences and stories of people. Whereas quantitative data can tell us something about everyone, qualitative data tell us a lot about each one. So it seems logical to explore the ways in which these two types of data can complement each other. Increasingly, a broader range of both quantitative *and* qualitative evidence is being sought and valued. The use of health impact assessments is a case in point.

Health impact assessment as a mixed method

Health impact assessment (HIA) is emerging as an important tool for measuring and delivering healthy public policy (European Centre for Health Policy, 1999). Through *Saving Lives: Our Healthier Nation* (Department of Health [DoH], 1999) and subsequent documents (Social Exclusion Unit, 2000), the British government has identified HIA as a means of ensuring that public policy addresses the wider determinants of health. Box 8.1 sets out the key features of HIAs.

Box 8.1 What is HIA?

Health impact assessment is a technique used to assess the impact of local or national projects (e.g. a new bypass), programmes (such as a community rehabilitation programme for offenders) or policies (such as a local transport strategy) on the health of communities. There are a number of different formal definitions for what people consider HIA to be. The following describes it well:

Health Impact Assessment is a combination of procedures, methods and tools that systematically judges the potential and sometimes unintended, effects of a policy, plan, program or project on the health of a population, and the distribution of those effects within the population. HIA identifies appropriate actions to manage those effects.

(World Health Organization [WHO] and European Centre for Health Policy [ECHP], 1999, p. 4)

HIA is used to help improve health and reduce health inequalities and, more strategically, to inform policy and programme proposals (Health Development Agency, 2004). Its primary output is a set of evidence-based recommendations geared to inform the decision-making process associated with a proposal. These recommendations aim to highlight practical ways to enhance the positive aspects of a proposal, and remove or minimise any negative impacts on health and inequalities (a process known as a prospective HIA).

Although a preferred methodology for HIA is yet to be established, current thinking (see, for example, Association of Public Health Observatories, 2007) suggests that it should be based on a process that takes into consideration:

- both qualitative and quantitative data
- the potential effects and impact on the target population of the proposed policy, programme or project
- the opinions, experience and expectations of the members of the affected community, taking local factors into account
- making practical recommendations to aid decision makers in reaching fully informed decisions and maximising positive impacts and minimising negative ones
- the need for information and recommendations that can be used to continually shape the project or programme in question, providing evidence of both strengths to be developed and weaknesses to be addressed.

(Adapted from The Open University, 2006; Handsley et al., 2007)

Typically, HIA projects are large-scale projects that involve a collection of different research studies, each using a different research design. These multiple studies are designed to take into account the best evidence from both quantitative sources (such as surveys, community profiling and audits) and qualitative sources (such as interviews, participant observation and focus groups). The existing literature and other documentary sources are also reviewed.

However, the available evidence is often limited and/or contradictory and it is important to carefully balance and weigh-up its significance. With HIA, this judgement is usually made through discussion with key stakeholders to ensure any recommendations developed are both relevant and grounded in differing perspectives. For instance, service users and providers will be consulted as well as others in the wider community. The idea of community participation and the need to consult with community stakeholders and informants is central to HIAs.

HIAs are normally carried out prospectively before the implementation of a project, programme or policy in order to inform the initial decision making. However, they can be carried out retrospectively to inform future projects or concurrently with the implementation stage. The aim then is to guide the process and progress of the programme or policy. This was the case in the HIA described below.

An HIA study was carried out by Hirschfield et al. (2001) as part of their Stepping Out project (see Box 8.2). The Stepping Out programme aimed to empower vulnerable young women in the Liverpool area of the UK by encouraging them to participate in social, educational and cultural initiatives. The interventions included the use of groups and one-to-one work to offer support, training and practical skills development. For example, a team of youth workers joined the women on the streets two evenings a week rather than in more formal, centre-based venues. These interventions were evaluated using both quantitative and qualitative methods. The results showed positive impacts on health (such as improved mental health) for the Stepping Out users, particularly resulting from their improved self-esteem. Other health determinants deemed to have been affected included an improvement in social networks and facilitating access to education, training and employment. Box 8.2 illustrates the mix of methods used in the Stepping Out Partnerships HIA in Sefton, Liverpool.

These HIA studies demonstrate the value of using mixed methods and, just as important, show that qualitative approaches can add an important dimension to public health practice. With this in mind, we now explore their contribution in greater depth.

Box 8.2 Multiple methods for a health impact assessment project in Sefton, Liverpool

Multiple methods used in the project focused on:

- a review of the documentary evidence already in existence. This included: monitoring and evaluation reports of the project, the Crime and Disorder Audit ... a full geodemographic profile of the two wards that the project serves and the score on the Index of Local Deprivation.

- interviews with the project manager and a number of the workers in order to ascertain their views about the nature of the intervention, the needs and issues of the client group and the geographical area in which the project operates.

- observation: one of the researchers was invited to accompany two of the detached youth workers in their street work ... enabling the researcher to talk informally with the youth workers and to observe their interactions with the groups of young women that they went up to or who were approached by them.

- finding out the views of the users through a series of face-to-face interviews carried out by the One-to-One workers with their clients using a semi-structured questionnaire and using the results of a user survey (the Self Assessment Questionnaire – SAQ) designed by the research director for another purpose.

- two focus groups at the centre in which the Stepping Out Partnership is based.

- speaking to other key informants and stakeholders who are not directly associated with the project as either employees or users.

(Hirschfield et al., 2001, pp. 17-18)

8.2 The contribution of qualitative approaches

Introducing qualitative approaches

A qualitative investigation aims to explore, describe and/or interpret personal and social experiences, taking into account particular cultural contexts. The approach taken is inductive, exploratory, hypothesis-generating and focused on understanding meanings. This is in contrast to quantitative research, which is deductive and hypothesis-testing, and aims to predict or explain behaviour.

Denzin and Lincoln (1994, p. 2) state that: 'Qualitative researchers study things in their natural settings, attempting to make sense of, or interpret, phenomena in terms of the meanings people bring to them.' They start with open research questions rather than having a hypothesis to test. Rich, textured description is valued, with a focus on the 'hows', 'whys' and 'whats' rather than on questions of 'whether' or 'how many'. In qualitative research, the researcher's role and the research context are viewed with a critical eye. Where possible, the aim is to promote collaborative, empowering, participatory and/or egalitarian relationships.

Qualitative evidence in public health

In the case of public health, qualitative investigation focuses on individuals' everyday meanings, motivations and behaviours related to health. It aims to locate lifestyle risk behaviours within individuals' broader life and cultural contexts to examine how social factors impact on health. In general, qualitative investigation in the field of public health aims to help both practitioners and policy makers ensure that health education and provision are relevant to the needs of service users (see Box 8.3). Some qualitative research will also specifically focus on giving a 'voice' to marginalised, vulnerable or disempowered individuals and groups, with a view to empowering them to take control of their own health. For instance, Choudhry et al. (2002) used a method called participatory action research to examine health issues for a group of south Asian immigrant women. In addition to exploring the women's health needs and understandings, the researchers offered various workshops over a three-year period designed to help the women develop knowledge about their own health.

Box 8.3 Summary of qualitative investigation aims in public health

- To explore individuals' everyday meanings, motivations and behaviours related to health.

- To locate lifestyle risk behaviours within individuals' broader life and social context.

- To examine how social factors (relational, institutional and ideological) impact on health.

- To empower individuals to take control of their own health towards engaging in health-enhancing behaviours.

- To give voice to marginalised, vulnerable or disempowered individuals and groups.

- To better inform service providers and policy makers of users' needs and interests.

Which of the six aims in Box 8.3 would you be most interested in pursuing if you were going to undertake a qualitative investigation?

In addition to the methods outlined in Box 8.2, these different aims are illustrated in action by two further examples from research on public health issues (see Box 8.4).

Box 8.4 Exemplar studies: aims and rationale of public health research

Van Cleemput et al. (2007) examined the health-related beliefs and experiences of gypsies and travellers in England using a mixed-methods study design. The quantitative component demonstrated an excess burden of ill health among gypsies and travellers, which far exceeded that seen in other ethnic minorities and socially disadvantaged groups. The descriptive qualitative strand aimed to put that finding into a cultural context. Policy implications from this study included the acknowledgement that the health needs of gypsies and travellers are not being met by existing policy and that effective healthcare provision requires multi-agency participation and awareness of the specific cultural beliefs/attitudes involved.

Fazil et al. (2004) examined how concepts of empowerment and advocacy impinge on power relationships for service providers working with Pakistani and Bangladeshi families who have children with disabilities. Specifically, they investigated the processes and challenges involved in running an advocacy programme for this group. They argue that there are important cultural and gender factors which need to be taken into account if services for this vulnerable and relatively powerless group are to make a positive impact.

Questioning the value of qualitative evidence

In recent years the qualitative movement has gained growing acceptance in the health and social science arenas. However, in the field of public health the legitimacy of qualitative methods and evidence is still challenged (Green and Thorogood, 2004). Researchers face questions about the validity and generalisability of their findings and are challenged about whether or not their interpretive methods are 'scientific'. Critics claim that qualitative evidence is too anecdotal, subjective, vague, 'soft' and 'airy fairy' (Zyzanski et al., 1992; Labuschagne, 2003). They argue that because qualitative research often involves small numbers of participants, its findings cannot be generalised and are therefore of little value.

However, as noted in Section 8.1, qualitative methods are already being used to enrich HIA work. Green and Thorogood (2004) offer three key arguments about the contribution of qualitative investigations in public health. First, qualitative research fills some gaps that quantitative approaches cannot reach. It has a distinctive role in its search for understanding and context: qualitative methods can therefore address questions about the meaning and purpose of health and interventions, from the perspective of both users and providers.

Second, qualitative approaches are better able to capture complex attitudes and behaviours as they recognise that these are based on people's multiple, ambivalent, ambiguous meanings. Traditional survey research, such as asking people about their health concerns, can result in simplistic, unnuanced answers. In qualitative research it is acknowledged that respondents will be influenced by the context; for example, their relationship with the researcher. If the research is carried out at different times by different people, different 'stories' will be told.

Finally, qualitative investigation is useful in terms of application at both the practice and policy levels. At the level of practice, qualitative evidence can sensitise service providers not only to users' views, but also to how such views might affect health behaviours. Similarly, practitioners' values, beliefs and reactions can be studied to better understand, and so improve, service provision. At the policy level, qualitative studies can provide evidence of population needs. This can inform the implementation of appropriate policies.

With these arguments in mind, advocates of qualitative research are seeking wider acceptance for its specialised contribution. When qualitative research is done as a minor adjunct to quantitative research, there can be a tendency for the qualitative component to be limited to a few superficial, descriptive quotes from participants. For many qualitative researchers this hardly merits the status of 'qualitative research'. In reality, it amounts to little more than the qualitative presentation of quantitative findings. What is needed is a growing commitment to genuine, thorough qualitative evidence involving deeper and more informative results. Such results can only enhance the findings of quantitative studies.

A good example of how qualitative evidence can complement quantitative comes from Winch (1999, cited in Green and Thorogood, 2004), who used a multidisciplinary approach to evaluate an intervention to promote insecticide-treated bed nets in Africa. Significantly, qualitative methods were utilised initially to access local views (and myths) about malaria. This knowledge was fed into various health-promotion interventions, including the use of street theatre emphasising the importance of using nets all year round. To evaluate these interventions, a survey of bed net use was undertaken. When it was discovered that there was still resistance to its use, interviews were used in a further study to investigate the barriers. The results indicated that villagers were concerned about both the cost and the possible toxic effects of the insecticide nets.

In this example, qualitative research was used at the beginning *and* end of the project to answer the 'what' and 'why' questions relating to people's beliefs about malaria and net use. In contrast, the quantitative survey research addressed the question of whether or not the nets were used. In this way, the choice of methodology follows logically from the research question being asked.

8.3 Qualitative methodologies

Qualitative research spans many quite distinct and specialised approaches. This section describes some of these before discussing further the value – and potential problems – of mixing quantitative and qualitative methodologies.

Diverse methodologies

Methodology is the overarching approach to research that encompasses both the underpinning philosophy or theoretical perspective *and* the methods of data collection and analysis used in the research. Researchers have a choice about the different *methods* of data collection (such as interview, participant observation, focus groups and documentary evidence) and analysis.

Underpinning the different methodologies/methods are particular philosophical assumptions or perspectives. Box 8.5 returns to the exemplars introduced in Box 8.4 to demonstrate how the groups of researchers conducted their public health research in different ways – ways that depend fundamentally on which perspective they adopted.

Box 8.5 Exemplar studies: varied methodologies incorporating perspectives and methods

Van Cleemput et al. (2007) engaged their qualitative strand of a broader mixed-methods study by using in-depth non-directive qualitative interviews. Additional data from focus groups offer a measure of 'respondent validation'. In addition, they maintained a scientific, positivist approach by incorporating computer software to manage part of their data analysis.

Hirschfield et al. (2001) describe a fairly complicated and wide-ranging research design for their HIA. They utilised many different methods, including documentary evidence, interviews, surveys, questionnaires, focus groups and fieldwork observation (see their account in Box 8.2 to get a sense of the range of what they evaluated).

Fazil et al. (2004) engaged in an action research project arising from a critical and cultural perspective to evaluate the effectiveness of an advocacy programme offered to Asian families who had children with a disability. Advocate roles were introduced to

---

befriend the families, link them to relevant services and aid communication with services. The researchers interviewed the families on four separate occasions to monitor the progress of the advocacy service. The findings of the research were then fed back to the local service providers and advocates so that they could take on board the issues and problems identified.

The use of multiple methods of enquiry is becoming quite common in public health evidence-based research and this approach is increasingly encouraged by the large funding bodies, such as the DoH, the Economic and Social Research Council (ESRC) and the Medical Research Council (MRC). Public health research is often multidimensional; that is, different aspects of a health intervention project are investigated (as the study by Hirschfield et al. shows). In such cases, it may well be desirable to combine quantitative and qualitative methodologies.

Combining qualitative and quantitative methods and triangulation

Qualitative investigations are often used in tandem with quantitative methods when the researchers aim to address different aspects of the research topic. For example, qualitative methods may be used alongside survey-type research, as in the Van Cleemput et al. (2007) and Hirschfield et al. (2001) examples. Here, the qualitative data can add colour, texture and richness to any demographic data and statistical results and they can also help clarify quantitative findings, particularly where there seems to be a puzzle or contradictions in the findings, as is illustrated in the research by Winch (1999) on bed nets.

Another good example is the work of Kerr et al. (2009), who followed up various large-scale quantitative surveys of the prevalence of gambling. They explored people's experiences of gambling/problem gambling and examined the support available to them. Through the qualitative evidence, the researchers moved beyond simple dichotomies of non-problem versus problem gambling and developed a typology that recognised the complex and malleable nature of gambling behaviour. This importantly shifted the focus from individual pathology to investigations that incorporate contextual factors in explaining problem gambling. When discussing the potential policy impact of the study, the researchers suggest that it will help policy makers set rules for companies that offer gambling establishments so the companies foster an environment that balances freedom to gamble with safeguards.

Sometimes researchers use multiple methods to offset the weaknesses of one method over another. This triangulation (a commonly used term indicating the use of different points to navigate) is used to enhance the validity of findings. For instance, the evidence base could be seen as strengthened if people report similar things when they are being both surveyed and interviewed. Similarly, when the separate analyses of different researchers are triangulated, the results may be seen to have more trustworthiness or credibility.

While studies routinely combine qualitative methods, there is some debate about how easily qualitative and quantitative methods can and should be combined. Problems can specifically arise when these are combined in the same single study. Research by Steward (2006) is a case in point. She studied the nature and impact of teleworking (that is, remote or homeworking), using a survey to identify teleworkers' views of their work and then in-depth qualitative interviews with the same group to follow up the survey and explore how health, illness and sickness were defined and experienced. She found that, far from providing complementary accounts, the two methodologies clashed. Significantly, she discovered that the survey data were often refuted by participants in follow-up interviews and that participants responded differently depending on whether they were writing down their responses or giving them verbally. For instance, Steward found that asking about days 'off sick' produced different answers because the meanings teleworkers ascribed to the terms 'off' and 'sick' varied. She concludes that neither approach can be seen as 'right' (although she gained more information and understanding from the qualitative data): 'A mixed methodological approach', she says, 'served to highlight the complexity and ambivalence [of teleworking] ... It showed how individuals generate information about themselves ... in many ... often irreconcilable ways' (Steward, 2006, p. 105).

Steward argues that it is impossible to produce a consistent version of the object of study because 'truths' are relative; they vary from one person to another and one person's views may vary depending on the context. The object needs to be seen as socially constructed rather than as a fixed reality.

If different methods can produce different results, is this an argument for or against mixing methods?

Care needs to be taken when combining methods as their aims can vary considerably (Yardley and Marks, 2004). Much depends on whether researchers are taking a 'positivist, realist' or 'interpretivist, relativist' approach (i.e. whether they believe there is one reality out there that they are studying and that it needs to be studied scientifically, or whether it is only possible to capture fluid, relative meanings). For instance, Van Cleemput et al. (2007) supported a positivist approach and utilised computer software to ensure the most objective and systematic approach possible to managing data – an approach which suits the research practice preferred by the National Centre for Social Research.

Studies that seek to combine methods that are compatible (in that they draw meaningfully on their different potentials) tend to yield more fruitful results. The practice of combining qualitative and quantitative methods is particularly useful if different questions are being asked. Qualitative methods used in the *planning* stage of a quantitative survey can help to generate survey questions which resonate with people's understandings and meanings and might help avoid the problem identified by Steward (2006). Alternatively, qualitative studies are ideal for *following up* survey results to gain more in-depth information, as shown by Van Cleemput et al. (2007).

8.4 Qualitative methods and processes

The actual process of 'doing' qualitative investigations – be it on its own or in tandem with quantitative studies – requires certain skills. Three particular stages are discussed here: early planning, collecting data and data analysis. Across all these stages, the skill lies in conducting the research or audit appropriately, ethically, systematically and rigorously.

Early planning

There is much to decide in the early stages of planning investigations. What, precisely, is the investigatory focus and question? Who will constitute the participants and how will they be recruited? (In the case of documentary research that does not use participants, how will documents be obtained and how much will be sampled?) Are there particular 'gatekeepers' who need to be approached first (i.e. people who control access to participants: for instance, parents and teachers in the case of research with young people)? What methods of data collection and analysis will be used? What kind of roles will the researcher and participants play? To what extent will participants be involved in the formulation or validation of findings? How will the participants be briefed in order to give their 'informed consent' and how will they be 'de-briefed'? How will the participants' rights and safety be protected?

Given the special relationship found in qualitative studies between the researcher and what is studied, what exactly should the researcher's role be? Beyond seeking to do no harm, qualitative researchers often aim to empower and 'give voice' to their participants. They need to be mindful that their research – which encourages participants to reflect on themselves and the social world around them – has the potential to be transformative, changing both themselves and their participants. In short, there is a power dimension at play – demanding recognition and management. Two key questions here are: 'Whose interests are served by our research?' and 'What wider impact might this research have?' (Finlay, 2006a). Answers to all the questions mentioned here are needed prior to beginning data collection.

After this early planning stage, the investigation is likely to need formal approval; for instance, by the local research ethics committee following the Research Governance Framework (DoH, 2001). The committee's remit includes adjudicating on issues such as informed consent, confidentiality/anonymity, the rights and safety of the participants, the risk to research participants, the legal liability of the researcher and the degree of independent monitoring of the research (e.g. by a supervisor) (Ballinger and Wiles, 2006). The exemplars in Box 8.6 provide some insights into the issue of recruiting participants ethically.

Box 8.6 Exemplar studies: recruiting participants ethically

Van Cleemput et al. (2007) obtained research governance approval (including multicentre research ethics committee ethical review) with secondary approval from primary care trusts and local research ethics committees in each location. The study started with a sampling frame of 269 gypsies and travellers who had consented to participate in the original quantitative study. The group was narrowed down to anyone who had recently accessed health services and then to ensure a maximum variation sample, 27 participants were selected across different age groups, type of accommodation and location. In-depth, non-directive interviews were all conducted by one person (the lead author).While the authors do not specifically discuss any ethical issues arising in their published work, numerous challenges are indicated where they undoubtedly took extra care during data collection and analysis. First, a number of the participants had mental health problems (including depression, schizophrenia, prolonged grief reactions and disabilities associated with drug misuse). Second, participants discussed a range of potentially distressing subjects, including their experience of social hardship arising from both poor environmental conditions and those imposed by a hostile/racist society.

In the HIA study by Hirschfield et al. (2001), considerable care was taken to ensure many different 'voices' were heard. However, gaining access to the women using the Stepping Out service posed problems as some were particularly vulnerable in terms of their mental health and in terms of being excluded by or living on the margins of society. This meant the researchers needed to make special arrangements. It was decided that the researchers should not have direct access to the women who received extra one-to-one support, though they were able to observe the youth workers in interaction with users during their 'street work'. The investigators then designed a semi-structured interview that the one-to-one workers themselves conducted with their clients.

In the research by Fazil et al. (2004), developing trust during the interviews was also a priority. When the researchers asked the participants whether the interviews could be tape-recorded, some participants refused. The researchers therefore recorded the interviews by hand. After each interview, the researcher carefully went through the text with each participant to ensure that they were happy with the recorded information. In addition, throughout the action research process, the advocates and researchers found themselves confronted by a number of sensitive ethical issues. These related to conflicts over ethnicity and gender; for instance, advocates working with just the women in the family found that their interventions had the potential to create family tensions.

In the exemplar studies, what 'risks' did the researcher need to be alert to?

Qualitative research often deals with sensitive, difficult topic areas where risk and safety are germane. However, research risk assessment involves further debate. At what point is a participant deemed to be in danger of harm? For instance, if a participant gets upset during an interview, is that harm? Does this mean that researchers should avoid tackling potentially emotive topics? Some participants welcome the opportunity to talk at a deep and personal level; participants getting upset may therefore not necessarily be a problem. Similarly, precautions taken to minimise risk for the investigators (for example, interviewing in pairs or avoiding going into risky environments) may well be interpreted negatively by participants and be counterproductive. In short, there may be trade-offs between safety and being effective or productive as a researcher.

> Ethical research practice requires a consideration of responsibilities to research participants, professional and academic colleagues, research sponsors and the wider public. Although ethical guidelines exist for most disciplines, qualitative health research often generates ethical dilemmas, which are not easily solved by reference to codes of practice.
>
> (Green and Thorogood, 2004, p. 51)

Probably the best a qualitative researcher can do is to be sensitive to, and critically aware of, the ethical implications of each stage of the research. Attempts should be made to handle these as conscientiously as possible. Care needs to be taken during data collection to regularly review the terms of the research agreement and to check with the participant that they are prepared to continue. The participant may value the opportunity to say something 'off the record' and this needs to be respected.

Collecting data

There are natural affinities between methodology and the methods/ procedures used to collect and analyse data. The choice of methods generally follows from the choice of methodology (Finlay, 2006b). Action research (e.g. Fazil et al., 2004) and mixed methods studies (such as Van Cleemput et al., 2007 and Hirschfield et al., 2001) tend to rely on interview data perhaps in combination with surveys, participant observation and/or focus groups.

Whichever of the many data-collection methods are chosen, the skill lies in being able to carry them off rigorously and sensitively. To illustrate some of the issues and skills involved, consider the case of interviews, focus groups and observation studies – the most frequently employed qualitative methods.

Conducting interviews

Researchers choosing to interview (whether structured or unstructured) need to take care to build a relationship with the participant that ensures the participant feels listened to, safe and respected. Having enabled the participants to share something of themselves, the researcher needs to ensure that they are not being forced to disclose information beyond their choice. Henry and Finlay offer some advice to novice interviewers:

> Talking about thoughts, feelings or one's own present or future plans, can be a threatening and moving experience as well as an enjoyable one. Anyone engaged in a depth interview needs to be aware that new personal understandings might sometimes be disclosed without the participant recognising that this is the case. Your participant needs to be fully informed at the outset, and both of you need to recognize the extent to which personal revelations can be unsettling.
>
> (Henry and Finlay, 2001, p. 6)

Sometimes, as in the study by Hirschfield et al., users may be deemed to be too vulnerable to be interviewed by strangers and other approaches to accessing their views are needed.

Focus groups

Focus groups are a useful way of accessing a range of different interest groups within a community. For example, they may represent the interests of older people, women or people from a minority ethnic group. Focus groups have been used increasingly as a mechanism for assessing health needs and the experiences of service users. Although a good method for accessing a range of different groups of people, the findings of focus groups must be contextualised and not generalised to the wider population.

The role of facilitators is vital – they need to try to promote a relaxed atmosphere initially to enable people to feel comfortable talking in the group. Facilitators might, for example, hand out refreshments as they greet participants or provide some initial warm-up interaction games. Great care needs to be taken when running groups on sensitive topics – particularly if participants have to live or work together after the research. The proceedings of a focus group can be tape-recorded if the group is happy with that. If taping is not possible then the facilitator/researcher will have to make notes at every available opportunity to try to create the most accurate record of the proceedings possible.

Green and Thorogood (2004, p. 128) suggest that the key to recording group interviews is to remember to 'be aware of the context of the data production ... Utterances ... cannot be presented as the essential "views" of the participants.' Group members may say things simply because they are part of the group. For example, perhaps they are feeling some peer pressure and wish to be seen to be going along with what others are saying. Also, sometimes individual members can dominate and influence others in groups. In other words, group dynamics will play a part and need to be taken into account.

Observation studies

Schools, hospital wards and departments, a fitness club and a workplace are typical sites for observation studies, where the researcher observes and records whatever is going on. Negotiating access to the research 'field' requires careful planning as often there are gatekeepers who need to be satisfied. For example, studies attempting to explore service users' views and experiences of their treatment could be derailed by a gatekeeper manager who is defensively reluctant to have user complaints researched by a stranger.

Observation studies are conducted with the researcher taking on varying degrees of participation on a spectrum.

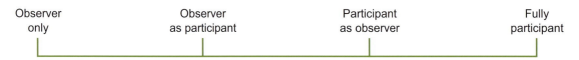

| Observer only | Observer as participant | Participant as observer | Fully participant |

Figure 8.1 Participation spectrum

The middle two points of participation are the most frequently used.

Why might the left and right points on the spectrum present problems?

The right point on the spectrum, where the researcher is fully participant, raises difficult ethical questions because the research role is not known to the people under observation. The other end of the spectrum is also difficult because the researcher can be all too obvious and thereby change the nature of the interactions. The middle two points allow the researcher to become part of the interactions and observe without unduly changing what is being studied. But care needs to be taken to minimise any intrusions to ensure observations are as naturalistic as possible. For instance, the use of video is gaining popularity as a means of recording details of interactions, such as those between healthcare providers and users. Here, having the camera in place before recording can help participants get used to its presence.

With HIA projects and other observational studies, which involve an 'action research' component where health interventions are simultaneously evaluated, additional considerations need to be taken into account. Often the overall goal is to work with community members to implement and research an intervention or social change needed to improve a health problem (Kelly, 2005). This can be time consuming as projects can take several years from the initial discussion stage through to the 'action' being conceived, implemented and evaluated. There is a need to consult and work with community partners at all stages of the research, including the last stage of making public the results of the research. Kelly explores some of the pitfalls:

> To achieve meaningful results, participants must retain a sense of involvement, while the program is simultaneously moving toward its goals. Community members' voices must be heard continuously ... Keeping a diverse group of people together is challenging, and sustaining enthusiasm can be even more difficult, especially as competing needs arise and the group experiences setbacks.
>
> (Kelly, 2005, p. 70)

Data analysis

The analysis of qualitative data is much less concerned with numbers and more concerned with conveying the richness and quality of the data collected. Qualitative investigation can generate large amounts of detailed data. This is a strength as well as a drawback. The strength lies in the richness of the data; the drawback is in the complexity of the analysis required to interpret and present this in such a way that it does justice to that richness. The task of qualitative analysis is to try to derive some order and meaning out of the wealth of data that will probably have been collected. Considering that just one interview transcript can involve many pages of data – qualitative analysis can be time-consuming. But the depth and nuanced subtleties that can be obtained are worth the effort.

Thematic analysis (a method for analysing and describing important patterns within data) is often the analysis method of choice for qualitative public health studies. Braun and Clarke (2006) provide a step-by-step guide to typical phases:

- familiarising yourself with your data
- generating initial codes
- searching for themes
- reviewing themes
- defining and naming themes
- producing the report.

The hope is that themes 'emerge from data'. While it is true that themes need to be grounded in and reflect the data, mostly meanings have to be searched for as they are implicit. They have to be shaped up in successive iterations. Both semantic content and the language itself need to be examined, with key phrases or explanations used by the participants highlighted. These then need to be coded in some way with a word or phrase that captures the essence of the content. To give an example, consider the study described in Box 8.7 by Flowers et al. (1997), which aimed to understand unprotected sex in relationships between gay men.

Box 8.7 An example of interpretive, thematic analysis

Using interpretative phenomenological analysis, Flowers et al. (1997) sought to discover what individual gay men thought and felt about the connection between unprotected anal sex and their relationships. They argued that previous research had not paid sufficient attention to the *quality* of gay men's specific relationships and tended to lump all relationships together. Significantly, their research findings showed that, within romantic relationships, these men often placed more importance on the expression of commitment, trust and love than on their own health.

Applying the thematic analysis method, Flowers et al. came up with such themes as 'casual sex and detachment', 'penetrative sex, relationships and self-involvement' and 'unprotected anal penetration and the romantic rationality'. In their extended analysis and discussion they note how, in the men's accounts of sexual decision making, there seems to be a 'consistent awareness of sexual acts as being communicative ... capturing very powerful expressions ... Semen exchange within a relationship highlights sharing bodies, whilst condom use ... exemplifies keeping bodies separate and isolated' (Flowers et al., 1997, p. 82).

To help with data management, mixed-methods investigators often utilise software packages called computer-aided qualitative data analysis software (CAQDAS), such as *NVivo* or *Atlas-ti*. The use of software prior to further interpretive or explanatory analysis aims to ensure a systematic, scientific approach 'designed for use in applied qualitative research to inform social policy, allowing for rigorous and transparent data management' (Van Cleemput et al., 2007, p. 206).

Van Cleemput et al. (2007) used *Atlas-ti* along with the 'framework' method, where themes/categories are combined with a case-based approach. Iterative analysis through four stages of coding, thematic framework, description and interpretation, focused on four themes they called: the travelling way; low expectations of health; self-reliance and staying in control; and fatalism and fear of death.

Reflexivity

Having analysed their data, qualitative researchers often engage in further analysis to examine the ethics of their research and the central role they have played in the construction and production of the findings. Here, researchers utilise reflective diaries and engage in a process known as reflexivity (Finlay and Gough, 2003). This requires them to self-reflect critically on the ways in which their social background, assumptions, positioning, behaviour, presence and power relations impact on the research process. Reflexivity involves a continuing self-awareness of the research dynamics and claims being made. How this is achieved varies. The reflexive analysis offered by Gunaratnam (2007) on the methodological and ethical dilemmas faced when researching ethnicity provides one good example. Another example is the 'participatory action research' project undertaken by McFadden and McCamley (2003), who investigated young people's sexual health. The authors used reflexivity to explore issues of identity and disempowerment throughout the research project. They tell of their struggle to relinquish their authority as university researchers so that they could share responsibility for the research with younger peer researchers who were taking on the responsibility of interviewing young people:

> At the end of the first phase the peer researchers felt sufficiently equipped to comment critically on the data obtained ... even questioning the supposed expertise of the university researchers ('they should have done it better') and imagining how they (the peer researchers) might improve the study. Listening to such feedback produced initial feelings of annoyance for us – we considered the young people's comments to be overly critical, and quite cheeky! ...

> However, such instances were invaluable in challenging our thinking around what constitutes collaborative research. Despite our aim to diminish the power differentials which dog traditional research approaches, we realised that we had overlooked some central issues within the wider research matrix involving young people as users of power.

> (McFadden and McCamley, 2003, pp. 206–7)

Reflexivity is one of the key ways in which qualitative researchers evaluate the value, integrity and trustworthiness of their research. Subjective elements, which are so much a part of the qualitative research journey, are identified, highlighted and, indeed, actively celebrated (Finlay, 2003). This contrasts with the efforts made in quantitative research to minimise the element of subjectivity in the conduct of the research.

In these ways, the use of reflexivity and critical reflection merges with evaluating the research as a whole – the subject of the next section.

8.5 Evaluation and reflection

The many examples offered throughout this chapter show something of the potential richness, complexity, depth and power of qualitative work. Unlike quantitative research, qualitative research is often less concerned with conceptions of reliability and validity as criteria for judging the quality of research. Reliability (i.e. repeatability and the inner consistency of the means of data collection) is less relevant in the case of qualitative research which, by definition, does not seek to repeat the study; rather, it seeks to elicit a participant's responses within a specific and interpersonal context. Such a situation, therefore, cannot readily be replicated. Qualitative studies are less concerned with generalisability to wider populations and more concerned with looking at underlying meanings and exploring the uniqueness of people's accounts. Validity, then, has a different meaning which should reflect the 'shifting nature of our realities' (Johnson, 2000, p. 82).

If qualitative researchers reject traditional quantitative criteria for evaluation, how can the quality of their research be judged?

New and different criteria, responsive to qualitative research ideals, are necessary to ensure the integrity and value of the research (Finlay, 2006c). Guba and Lincoln (1994) argue for at least two sets of criteria to judge the quality of investigation: trustworthiness and authenticity. Good research also has the power to convince. As Kvale (1996, p. 252) puts it, 'Ideally, the quality of the craftsmanship results in products with knowledge claims that are so powerful and convincing in their own right that they, so to say, carry the validation with them, like a strong piece of art.'

In the light of such criteria, it is suggested that evaluating a given piece of qualitative research is done in terms of five dimensions, called the '5Cs':

1 **Clarity**: Does the research make sense? To what extent is the research systematically worked through, coherent and clearly described?

2 **Credibility**: To what extent do the findings match the evidence and are they convincing? ... Are the researcher's interpretations plausible and justified? ...

3 **Contribution**: To what extent does the research add to debate and knowledge of an issue or aspect of human social life? ... Is it empowering and/or growth-enhancing? ... Does it offer guidance for future action or for changing the social world for the better? ...

4 **Communicative resonance**: Are the findings sufficiently vivid or powerful to draw readers in? Do the findings resonate with readers' own experience or understandings? Alternatively, do the findings unsettle or disturb challenging unthinking complacency? ...

5 **Caring**: Has the researcher shown respect and sensitivity to participants' safety and needs? To what extent is the researcher reflexive about the way in which meanings are elicited in an interpersonal [and cultural] context? Does the research demonstrate ethical integrity and does the researcher show concern for the impact of the research?

(Finlay, 2006c, p. 322)

The examples of studies were selected for this chapter in part because they represent good, clear, trustworthy and convincing examples of research evidence. All have much to offer in terms of being 'caring' as well as making a 'contribution' to knowledge and understanding towards better practice/policy. For instance, the HIA study by Hirschfield et al. (2001) shows a caring concern by engaging with a programme designed to empower vulnerable women and by working hard to hear the voices of diverse stakeholders in order to make recommendations about practice/policy.

The research by Fazil et al. (2004) makes an important contribution to the understanding of empowerment and the cultural and gender issues raised when setting up an ethnically sensitive advocacy service. Specifically, the authors found that empowering individual mothers to negotiate their own lives through advocacy can interfere with family dynamics; mothers would make decisions which were later overturned by husbands. The authors concluded that: 'any process of empowerment will need to demonstrate a high level of cultural sensitivity ... [Further] an advocacy service needs to be very much family orientated to succeed' (Fazil et al., 2004, p. 396).

The study by Van Cleemput et al. (2007) offers an additional layer of credibility because interpretations were 'tested' in a broader community to ensure results could be applied and transferred (i.e. generalised) to the wider population. The researchers describe their procedure in detail:

> We presented the initial thematic findings to volunteer groups of Gypsies and Travellers in each study location. Volunteers attended by open invitation ... A total of 55 attended these five forums. We asked them for their opinions from their own experience and also whether they felt these findings would be true for other groups of Gypsies and Travellers. No concerns were raised about confidentiality, and none of the emerging findings were challenged. Individual themes were confirmed and elaborated. They were recognised as meaningful and important to an understanding of Gypsies and Travellers.

(Van Cleemput, 2007 et al., p. 206)

Does this kind of 'participant validation' lift the credibility of the research for you? Can you think of times when participant validation would not be appropriate?

Participant validation might be used to increase the transparency of the research and foster a sense of collaboration between participants and researchers. However, the process can be problematic: participants may have 'moved on' and it would not be appropriate to pull them back. Ashworth (1993), for instance, supports participant validation on moral-political grounds but warns against taking participants' responses too seriously as it may be in their interests to protect their 'socially presented selves'. Also, there are occasions when participants may feel overly objectified or 'reduced' somehow by an academic representation of their words. So, on ethical grounds, qualitative researchers might also avoid participant validation.

When applying qualitative research methods to public health, researchers are concerned that their research has both value and positive impact. The hope is that research will increase understanding of individuals' health behaviours or change society in some way by informing or changing health practice or policy. Ultimately, the value of qualitative research – whether on its own or as an adjunct to quantitative research – rests on this.

Conclusion

This chapter has looked at using qualitative approaches to build the evidence base in the field of public health. Different examples were provided to highlight the diversity of studies and methods, showing how it is possible to use qualitative approaches on their own as well as in mixed methods projects.

Qualitative researchers often enter uncharted territory that is seemingly beyond the reach of conventional quantitative research. There are specific skills required at every stage, from planning a project to analysing and evaluating its findings. At journey's end, the research may well yield evidence that extends – or sometimes runs counter to – that obtained by quantitative research. What is certain is that much can be learned about people's health-related meanings and motivations by placing them in their broader social context. For the purposes of effective health promotion and a higher profile for public health, such understanding is vital.

The diversity, flexibility and richness of qualitative evidence and its ability to go beneath the surface are beyond dispute. Qualitative evidence is increasingly seen as making a stimulating and humanising contribution to quantitative studies. Is it time that public health practitioners and policy makers emulate professionals in other fields to more regularly embrace qualitative approaches in their own right?

References

Ashworth, (1993) 'Participant agreement in the justification of qualitative findings', *Journal of Phenomenological Psychology*, vol. 24, pp. 3–16.

Association of Public Health Observatories (2007) 'The HIA gateway' in the Association of Public Health Observatories website. Available at: www.apho.org.uk/default.aspx?QN=P_HIA (accessed 1 September 2011).

Braun, V. and Clarke, V. (2006) 'Using thematic analysis in psychology', *Qualitative Research in Psychology*, vol. 3, pp. 77–101.

Choudhry, U.K., Jandu, S., Mahal, J., Singh, R., Sohi-Pabla, H. and Mutta, B. (2002) 'Health promotion and participatory action research with South Asian women', *Journal of Nursing Scholarship*, vol. 34, no. 1, pp. 75–81.

Denzin, N.K. and Lincoln, Y. (1994) 'Introduction: entering the field of qualitative research' in Denzin, N.K. and Lincoln, Y. (eds) *Handbook of Qualitative Research*, Thousand Oaks, California, Sage, pp. 1–17.

Department of Health (DoH) (2001) *Research Governance Framework for England*, London, Department of Health. Available at: http://webarchive.nationalarchives.gov.uk/+/www.dh.gov.uk/en/Publicationsandstatistics/Publications/PublicationsPolicyAndGuidance/DH_4008777 (accessed 1 September 2011).

Department of Health (DoH) (1999) *Saving Lives: Our Healthier Nation*, London, The Stationery Office. Available at: www.archive.official-documents.co.uk/document/cm43/4386/4386-00.htm (accessed 1 September 2011).

European Centre for Health Policy (1999) *Health Impact Assessment: Main Concepts and Suggested Approach. Gothenburg Consensus Paper*, Copenhagen, WHO Regional Office for Europe.

Fazil, Q., Wallace, L.M., Singh, G., Ali, Z. and Bywaters, P. (2004) 'Empowerment and advocacy: reflections on action research with Bangladeshi and Pakistani families who have children with severe disabilities', *Health and Social Care in the Community*, vol. 12, no. 5, pp. 389–97.

Finlay, L. (2006a) 'Going exploring: the nature of qualitative research' in Finlay, L. and Ballinger, C. (eds) *Qualitative Research for Allied Health Professionals: Challenging Choices*, Chichester, Wiley, pp. 3–8.

Finlay, L. (2006b) 'Mapping methodology' in Finlay, L. and Ballinger, C. (eds) *Qualitative Research for Allied Health Professionals: Challenging Choices*, Chichester, Wiley, pp. 9–29.

Finlay, L. (2006c) '"Rigour", "ethical integrity" or "artistry"? Reflexively reviewing criteria for evaluating qualitative research', *British Journal of Occupational Therapy*, vol. 69, no. 7, pp. 319–26.

Finlay, L. (2003) 'The reflexive journey: mapping multiple routes' in Finlay, L. and Gough, B. (eds) *Reflexivity: A Practical Guide for Researchers in Health and Social Sciences*, Oxford, Blackwell Science, pp. 3–20.

Finlay, L. and Ballinger, C. (eds) (2006) *Qualitative Research for Allied Health Professionals: Challenging Choices*, Chichester, Sussex, Wiley.

Finlay, L. and Gough, B. (eds) (2003) *Reflexivity: A Practical Guide for Researchers in Health and Social Sciences*, Oxford, Blackwell Science.

Flowers, P., Smith, J.A., Sheeran, P. and Beail, N. (1997) 'Health and romance: understanding unprotected sex in relationships between gay men', *British Journal of Health Psychology*, vol. 2, no. 1, pp. 73–78.

FrameWork website. Available at: www.framework-natcen.co.uk/ (accessed 1 September 2011).

Green, J. and Thorogood, N. (2004) *Qualitative Methods for Health Research*, London, Sage.

Guba, G.G. and Lincoln, Y.S. (1994) 'Competing paradigms in qualitative research' in Denzin, N.K. and Lincoln, Y. (eds) *Handbook of Qualitative Research*, Thousand Oaks, California, Sage, pp. 105–17.

Gunaratnam, Y. (2007) 'Complexity and complicity in researching ethnicity and health' in Douglas, J., Earle, S., Handsley, S., Lloyd, C.E. and Spurr, S. (eds) *A Reader in Promoting Public Health: Challenge and Controversy*, London, Sage, pp. 147–55.

Handsley, S., Noguera, A. and Beaumont, K. (2007) 'Gauging the effectiveness of community-based public health projects' in Lloyd, C.E., Handsley, S., Douglas, J., Earle, S. and Spurr, S. (eds) *Policy and Practice in Promoting Public Health*, London/Milton Keynes, Sage/The Open University, pp. 321–51.

Health Development Agency (2004) *Clarifying Health Impact Assessment, Integrated Impact Assessment and Health Needs Assessment*, London, Health Development Agency.

Henry, J. and Finlay, L. (2001) 'The interview project: capturing experience and meaning' D317 *Social Psychology: Personal Lives, Social Worlds*, Milton Keynes, The Open University.

Hirschfield, A., Barnes, R., Hendley, J. and Scott-Samuel, A. (2001) *Health Impact Assessment Case Study: The Stepping Out Project*, Liverpool, University of Liverpool. Available at: www.liv.ac.uk/ihia/IMPACT%20Reports/Annex_1-The_Stepping_out_Case_Study.pdf (accessed 1 September 2011).

Johnson, K. (2000) 'Interpreting meanings' in Gomm, R. and Davies, C. (eds) *Using Evidence in Health and Social Care*, London, Sage, pp. 65–85.

Kelly, P.J. (2005) 'Practical suggestions for community interventions using participatory action research', *Public Health Nursing*, vol. 22, no. 1, pp. 65–73.

Kerr, J., Kinsella, R., Turley, C., Legard, R., McNaughton Nicholls, C. and Barnard, M. (2009) 'Qualitative follow-up of the British Gambling Prevalence Survey 2007', London, National Centre for Social Research. Available at: www.gamblingcommission.gov.uk/pdf/Qualitative%20follow-up%20of%20the%20British%20Gambling%20Prevalence%20Survey%202007%20-%20June%202009.pdf (accessed 1 September 2011).

Kvale, S. (1996) *Interviews: An Introduction to Qualitative Research Interviewing*, Thousand Oaks, California, Sage.

Labuschagne, A. (2003) 'Qualitative research – airy fairy or fundamental?', *The Qualitative Report*, vol. 8, no. 1. Available at: www.nova.edu/ssss/QR/QR8-1/index.html (accessed 1 September 2011).

McFadden, M. and McCamley, F.A. (2003) 'Using reflexivity to loosen theoretical and organisational knots within participatory action research' in Finlay, L. and Gough, B. (eds) *Reflexivity: A Practical Guide for Researchers in Health and Social Sciences*, Oxford, Blackwell Science, pp. 200–13.

Social Exclusion Unit (2000) *National Strategy for Neighbourhood Renewal: A Framework for Consultation*, London, The Stationery Office.

Steward, B. (2006) 'Investigating invisible groups using mixed methodologies' in Finlay, L. and Ballinger, C. (eds) *Qualitative Research for Allied Health Professionals: Challenging Choices*, Chichester, Wiley, pp. 93–107.

The Open University (2006) K203 *Working for Health*, Unit 18, Public Health, Milton Keynes, The Open University.

Van Cleemput, P., Parry, G., Thomas, K., Peters, J. and Cooper, C. (2007) 'Health-related beliefs and experiences of gypsies and travellers: a qualitative study', *Journal of Epidemiology and Community Health*, vol. 61, pp. 205–10.

Winch, P. (1999) 'The role of anthropological methods in a community-based mosquito net intervention in Bagamoyo District, Tanzania' in Hahn, R. (ed.) *Anthropology in Public Health: Bridging Differences in Culture and Society*, Oxford, Oxford University Press, pp. 44–62.

World Health Organization (WHO) and European Centre for Health Policy (1999) *Health Impact Assessment, Gothenburg Consensus Paper*, Brussels, World Health Organization Regional Office for Europe and European Centre for Health Policy.

Yardley, L. and Marks, D.F. (eds) (2004) *Research Methods for Clinical and Health Psychology*, London, Sage.

Zyzanski, S.J., McWhinney, I.R., Blake, R., Crabtree, B.F. and Miller, W.L. (1992) 'Qualitative research: perspectives on the future' in Crabtree, B.F. and Miller, W.L. (eds) *Doing Qualitative Research, Research Methods for Primary Care Series*, vol. 3, Newbury Park, California, Sage, pp. 231–48.

Chapter 9: Using evidence to plan and evaluate public health interventions

Moyra Sidell and Jenny Douglas

Introduction

One of the challenges for public health practitioners is to develop effective and appropriate programmes and interventions that meet the needs of their populations and improve health. The success of any public health intervention, however large or small, depends on good planning and evaluation. Effective planning requires information about the needs of the target population as well as evidence about which interventions are likely to work, in what circumstances and with whom. This requires practitioners to utilise existing evidence of the effectiveness of public health practice. Effective public health interventions must also be able to demonstrate their success and, in order to do that, the plan has to include evaluation. All too often evaluation has been something of an afterthought that has been done to satisfy funders or ensure the continuity of the programme. But to be really effective, evaluation needs to be built into the planning process so that it becomes an integral part of the intervention that monitors the progress of the activity, provides feedback and provides sound evidence of the outcomes.

This chapter explores planning and evaluation as a seamless process. It is structured around Nutbeam and Harris's five-stage model of planning and evaluation (2004). But first the broad parameters of planning and evaluation are outlined.

9.1 Why plan and evaluate?

What is planning?

Planning is the vital preliminary stage in a public health intervention where an idea for a project or programme is thought through and translated into action. There are other expressions which are used to describe aspects of planning, and so the terminology can be ambiguous. Box 9.1 sets out some of the words used and their different meanings.

Box 9.1 Terminology used in planning

- Plan: how to get from your starting point to your end point and what you want to achieve.
- Policy: guidelines for practice that set broad goals and the framework for action.
- Programme: overall outline of action; a package of services, or information, in planned sequence that is intended to produce a particular result.
- Strategy: the methods to be used in achieving goals.
- Priority: the first claim for consideration.
- Aim: broad goal.
- Objective: specific goal to be achieved.

(Adapted from Dignan and Carr, 1992; Naidoo and Wills, 2009)

Why plan?

Multidisciplinary public health activity takes place at many levels. Careful and systematic planning of interventions can help ensure that resources are used well and most effectively. It also ensures effective evaluation of public health interventions. Without planning, interventions run the risk of being marginalised and of not being given priority in resource distribution. Perhaps most important of all, planning is a reflective activity: it focuses the mind on the job in hand and forces people to prioritise and justify their activities. Plans can be made for small-scale activities, such as giving a talk to a parent and toddler group, as well as for large events, such as a national no-smoking day or public health intervention to reduce teenage pregnancy and develop appropriate sexual health services. Whatever the scale of the initiative, the planning process is fairly similar. Ewles and Simnett (2003) suggest that all plans should provide answers to three basic questions:

- What am I trying to achieve?
- What am I going to do?
- How will I know whether I have been successful?

Evaluation is the key to answering the third bullet point.

What is evaluation?

How would you define the term 'evaluation'?

Evaluation is basically about judging the worth of an activity, so everyone engages in evaluation when they reflect critically on their actions in order to decide whether to continue or modify what they are doing. Whenever they ask themselves questions such as 'How did that session go?', 'Did I achieve what I set out to do?', or 'Did the service user or colleague really understand what I was explaining to her or was she just being polite when she said she did?', they are engaged in evaluating, albeit informally, their activities. Practitioners are already involved in evaluation, both professionally and in their daily lives – as noted in Chapter 4, it is a fundamental part of reflective practice.

A distinctive characteristic of formal (as distinct from informal) evaluation is its potentially public nature. In principle, the process and findings can be scrutinised and repeated so that it is possible for others to check and confirm or refute them. It is also possible for others to put into action what has been learned and benefit from it. Evaluation is also important in helping to understand why some public health interventions are successful, thus aiding the development of theories about intervention strategies.

The evaluation of public health interventions tends to be more complex and difficult than the evaluation of health services and therapeutic interventions. Although often judged by the same criteria, public health interventions have rather different tasks and goals, which are often hard to measure. The effects of the medical treatment of physically sick individuals are more obvious and immediate than the effects of public health interventions on medically well groups and populations.

All evaluations have two fundamental elements: identifying and ranking the criteria (values and aims), and gathering the kind of information that will make it possible to assess the extent to which these are being met.

Why evaluate?

There are many possible reasons for wanting to evaluate activities aimed at promoting public health. These include questions about effectiveness, the desire to improve practice and a willingness to be self-critical and do the best job possible by consciously learning from experience. In an ideal world, evaluation and planning are inextricably linked as parts of an ongoing cycle. In addition to the desire of individuals to learn lessons that will improve practice, there may also be financial and political pressures that encourage or demand evaluation. Increasingly, projects are required to have an evaluation component in order to be eligible for funding. The World Health Organization (WHO) (1998) recommends that at least 10 per cent of financial resources in any initiative should be set aside for evaluation.

The increased emphasis on evaluation derives generally from the evidence-based approach to policy and practice (see Chapter 7) and the growing awareness of complexity in the health field. Essentially, this means that we should not rely on popular common sense or the received wisdom of the 'experts' when deciding what to do or whether or not something works. It situates evaluation as a required and expected activity that is necessary and valuable. Although the following statements about evaluation were compiled by the Home Office, they apply equally to the public health context.

Evaluation

- provides evidence of a project's success (or failure)
- shows whether resources have been used cost effectively
- helps to avoid mistakes if the project is repeated
- allows improvements to be made to future work
- allows improvements to be made to current projects
- provides information for others who may want to run a similar project
- is an important stage in the process of accountability.

(Home Office Crime Reduction College, 2002, p. 36)

However, before starting to plan and evaluate a public health intervention, the key question to ask is: what evidence is needed to inform this intervention?

9.2 Sources of evidence in planning and evaluation

In order to plan and implement public health interventions, practitioners need to have some idea of the nature of the specific public health issue both locally and nationally. This requires the knowledge, skill and ability to find out, access, appraise critically, synthesise and apply evidence from different disciplines and diverse sources.

In the UK, since the 1990s the accepted orthodoxy has been to base public health practice on the available evidence (McQueen, 2010). Evidence can be obtained from the demographic and epidemiological data sources discussed in Chapter 7 as well as research journals. But evidence can also be found in less formal sources. Davies et al. (2000) noted that critical evidence is held by practitioners and users and that this unpublished critical evidence or 'grey literature' can be accessed via local authority departments or National Health Service (NHS) hospital libraries, which can be valuable sources of knowledge.

There are now many centres aimed at disseminating 'evidence' – for example, the NHS Centre for Reviews and Dissemination and the UK Cochrane Centre (dedicated to providing clinicians with up-to-date information on randomised clinical trials) – as well as national and local initiatives to help make healthcare evidence based. The Evidence for Policy and Practice Information and Co-ordinating Centre (the EPPI-Centre), hosted by the Institute of Education at the University of London, seeks to provide information on evidence-based practice in health promotion. Sources of health information are listed in Box 9.2.

Box 9.2 Sources of health information

Evidence-based resources

The Cochrane Library is an electronic publication designed to supply high-quality evidence to inform people providing and receiving care, and those responsible for research, teaching, funding and administration at all levels.

The Centre for Public Health Excellence at the National Institute for Health and Clinical Excellence (NICE) commissions research to support evidence on how to improve the public's health. Its evidence briefings provide a comprehensive, systematic and up-to-date map of the evidence base for public health and health improvement, with a particular focus on reductions in inequalities in health.

Journals

Key, peer reviewed, journals include:

- *Critical Public Health*
- *Ethnicity and Health*
- *Health Education Research*

- *Journal of Epidemiology and Community Health*
- *Journal of Mental Health Promotion*
- *Health Promotion Practice*
- *International Journal of Health Promotion Education*
- *European Journal of Public Health*
- *Health Education Journal*
- *Social Science and Medicine*

Databases

Although some of the key journals are listed above, public health research is published in a wide array of journals. The following databases should be used to trace relevant articles.

ASSIA contains over 312,000 records from 650 journals in 16 countries.

Global Health contains the Public Health and Tropical Medicine (PHTM) database.

British Nursing Index (BNI) is a UK nursing and midwifery database covering over 240 journals.

Health Management Information Consortium (HMIC) covers UK and overseas health management periodicals, monographs and reports.

CINAHL is an index for 2857 journals from nursing and allied health, from 1982.

Medline is an index for over 3500 journals in medicine, from 1965.

National statistics

The Office for National Statistics (ONS) provides access to key statistics on population trends, mortality, health-related behaviour and indicators of the nation's health via National Statistics Online. The virtual bookshelf provides links to online versions of many statistical publications including *Social Trends, Regional Trends, Health and Personal Social Service Statistics* and *Health Statistics Quarterly.*

International statistics

The WHO provides statistics in both summary format (e.g. World Health Statistics) and in more detail (e.g. levels of mortality, deaths by cause).

The World Bank provides access to a range of health indicators for countries and regions around the world. It includes summary health data.

Regional statistics

The Public Health Observatory is the main source of local statistical information for public health. There are nine public health observatories for England and one in Northern Ireland/ Irish Republic, Wales and Scotland. Links to these are available from the website of the Association of Public Health Observatories, which will continue to be available until the new public health system for England is more fully in place. Local health profiles are available from this website.

Postcode searches can be conducted on the Neighbourhood Statistics area of National Statistics Online, which includes a section on health and social care.

Policy

The Chief Medical Officer's area of the Department of Health (DoH) website has up-to-date information on key public health issues in England.

The NHS Quality Improvement website has information for Scotland.

The Health Evidence Bulletins website has information for Wales.

The Public Health Agency website has information for Northern Ireland.

Other organisations' websites

Many organisational websites provide information on public health topics. The easiest way to trace these is through gateways that list only high-quality websites. Although no longer updated, the Intute website has a 'Nursing, midwifery and allied health' section that includes a range of information on public health.

Researchers have proposed three different levels of practice with regard to the way in which practitioners use evidence when planning health-promotion interventions: planned, responsive and reactive (Nutbeam, 1996; Nutbeam and Bauman, 2006). Nutbeam argued that 'the planned approach to health promotion practice' was based on 'a rational and systematic assessment of the best available evidence concerning population health needs, effective interventions, and the organizational and administrative context for successful intervention' (Nutbeam, 1996, p. 320). In contrast, responsive approaches placed the highest value on the role of the community in defining health needs and solutions, where there may be conflict between the needs identified by the community and priorities identified through more traditional epidemiological analysis. In this approach the use of research evidence is only one of several elements involved in decision making.

Public health interventions are often reactive – that is, rather than being based on a systematic review of the evidence, they are a response to an immediate 'problem' or crisis and a more political agenda. Examples of this in the 1980s were high-profile campaigns about HIV/AIDS, which were funded by central government. A more recent example is obesity, particularly childhood obesity and physical activity, for which public health interventions may be based on epidemiological information about the 'problem', but there is limited evidence of effectiveness of interventions (Roberts et al., 2009). This emphasises the need to evaluate public health interventions.

The evidence needed to evaluate an intervention includes:

- information about an intervention's effectiveness in meeting its goals
- information about how transferable this intervention is thought to be (to other settings and populations)
- information about the intervention's positive and negative effects
- information about the intervention's economic impact
- information about barriers to implementing the interventions.

(Supplement to *American Journal of Preventative Medicine*, 2000, p. 36; cited in McQueen, 2001, p. 264)

There are several measures of effectiveness that attempt to assess health gain and loss. We noted three of these – QALY, PYLL and DALY – in Chapter 1, Box 1.3. The quality-adjusted life year (QALY) was developed within health economics and is used extensively by NICE to assess the cost-effectiveness of treatments and medical interventions. It represents an attempt to add a quality-of-life dimension to the cost-effectiveness equation. Box 9.3 explains its basis and function.

Box 9.3 What is a QALY?

- A quality-adjusted life year (QALY) takes into account both the quantity and quality of life generated by healthcare interventions. It is the arithmetic product of life expectancy and a measure of the quality of the remaining life years.

- A QALY places a weight on time in different health states. A year of perfect health is worth 1 and a year of less than perfect health is worth less than 1. Death is considered to be equivalent to 0; however, some health states may be considered worse than death and have negative scores.

- The QALY provides a common currency to assess the extent of the benefits gained from a variety of interventions in terms of health-related quality of life and survival for the patient. When combined with the costs of providing the interventions, cost–utility ratios result; these indicate the additional costs required to generate a year of perfect health (one QALY). Comparisons can be made between interventions, and priorities can be established based on those interventions that are relatively inexpensive (low cost per QALY) and those that are relatively expensive (high cost per QALY).

(Phillips and Thompson, 2009, p. 1)

The Chief Executive of NICE noted that 'the QALY lies at the heart of every decision NICE has to make' and added that 'it remains the most consistently controversial aspect of its work' (NICE, 2008, p. 5). This is especially true in public health, where its usefulness has been questioned due to its medical focus. Raphael (2001) argues that the increasing emphasis on QALYs (and DALYS) represents a medicalisation of quality of life and a loss of sight of issues of equity in health. Other criticisms have focused on the age bias in QALY evaluations:

They (QALYs) systematically favour interventions targeted at the young who clearly have most to gain in terms of additional years, and are hence fundamentally ageist.

(Green and South, 2006, p. 40)

9.3 Using theory and models in planning and evaluation

Theory can help in the planning and delivery of health-promoting interventions in several ways. Nutbeam and Harris suggest that it can:

- help us understand better the nature of the problem being addressed;
- describe and explain the needs and motivations of the target population;
- explain or make propositions concerning how to change health status, health-related behaviours and their determinants and;
- inform the methods and measures used to monitor the problem and the programme.

(Nutbeam and Harris, 2004, p. vii)

Planning models

All models aim to provide a systematic approach to planning, which not only uses epidemiological evidence in determining priorities for action, but also prioritises the perceived needs of local communities. Table 9.1 (page 256) sets out a planning model for health promotion, which highlights various stages and indicates the potential interconnections between theory and practice. This model suggests that the planning process is complex, but that there are five distinct phases:

- problem definition
- solution generation
- capacity building
- implementation
- process, impact and outcome evaluation.

Table 9.1 The use of theory in programme planning and evaluation

Planning phase	Task	Possible use of theory
Phase 1 Problem identification and prioritisation	Clarify major health issues for a defined population, and prioritise in terms of the potential for effective intervention	Clarify what should be the target elements of an intervention, such as individual beliefs, social norms or organisational practices
Phase 2 Planning a solution	Develop a programme plan which specifies programme objectives, strategies and the sequence of activity	Guidance on how, when and where change can be achieved in the target elements of a programme
Phase 3 Mobilising resources for implementation	Generate public and political support, build the capacity of partner organisations and secure resources	Guidance on how to build partnerships, raise public awareness and foster organisational development
Phase 4 Implementation	Execute the programme as planned, utilising multiple strategies (as appropriate to the programme objectives)	Provide a benchmark against which the actual implementation can be compared with the theoretical ideal
Phase 5 Evaluation	Assess the impact and outcome of the programme according to predefined programme objectives	Define outcomes and measurements which could be used at each level of evaluation

(Source: Nutbeam and Harris, 2004, p. 6)

 Where else in Table 9.1 do you think evaluation might be included, in addition to Phase 5?

Although evaluation is the fifth phase in the model, it needs to be built into the other phases, particularly at phase 2 'planning a solution' where objectives need to be set that can be measured. At phase 3 'mobilising resources and capacity building' the decision needs to be made about who will evaluate and the resource implications need to be built in. Throughout the implementation stage, process evaluation needs to monitor the workings of the intervention before finally assessing the impact of the intervention and evaluating the outcomes. Hawe et al.

(1998) highlighted these issues in their model of health promotion evaluation (Figure 9.1).

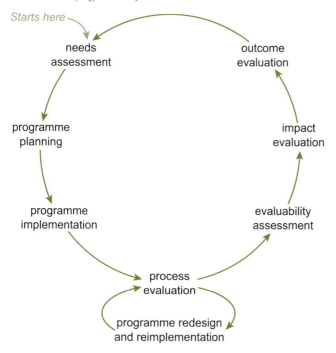

Figure 9.1 Planning and evaluation cycle

(Source: Hawe et al., 1998, p. 78)

As well as impact and outcome, they include process evaluation as the project develops. These three main types of evaluation – process, impact and outcome – can be defined as follows.

Process evaluation assesses the procedures and tasks involved in implementing an intervention (i.e. what is happening?). Components of process evaluation might include: the number and type of people reached by an intervention; what participants thought about the intervention; the quantity and type of activity/service provided; and a description of how services are provided and the quality of services provided (participant satisfaction). Process evaluation should be carried out from the beginning of the implementation stage so it documents the process of implementing the project. Process evaluation usually involves feedback during the course of a project, when things are still taking shape. For this reason it is sometimes called 'formative evaluation'.

Some evaluations are entirely concerned with process. For example, in one-to-one health education encounters, an evaluation might focus solely on the quality and nature of the communication between professionals and service users by asking questions such as: 'Is the communication culturally appropriate?', 'Is the information perceived as credible and relevant?', or 'Is there a good match between the aims of the professional and the needs of the service user?'

Impact evaluation assesses the more immediate effects of a public health intervention. For instance, if the intervention was to introduce an exercise programme for older women who are overweight, the impact evaluation would measure the degree to which the objective of attending the exercise programme had been met.

Outcome evaluation assesses the longer-term goals of the intervention and measures the extent to which an intervention has achieved its intended purpose (i.e. did the desired change take place?). In the example cited above, the overall goal of the exercise programme for the older women might be to help them reduce their weight. In this instance the outcome evaluation would be concerned with measuring any change in the weight of the participants and would require a pre- and post-project measure. The impact evaluation of whether people had taken part in the exercise programme would only require a post-project assessment.

Note that the cycle in Figure 9.1 allows for the project to be redesigned if the process (or formative) evaluation of the project suggests that it is not going to plan. If the project has been running to plan, it will undergo an evaluability assessment followed by impact and outcome evaluation. We will now work through the five stages of Nutbeam and Harris's planning and evaluation model, drawing on Hawe et al.'s cycle to build in these points of evaluation.

9.4 Problem definition and prioritisation

This is the stage where practitioners need to draw on the available evidence using the range of national and local sources identified in Section 9.2. So if, for instance, there seemed to be an unusually high level of teenage pregnancies in a particular area, then a search through the national and local statistics would help establish the actual rate for that area and whether it was markedly different from national rates. If any action was thought necessary, evidence could also be sought on what interventions had been successful in addressing high teenage pregnancy rates either nationally or locally.

It is worth remembering, as evidence is eagerly gathered and plans begin to be devised, that a number of ethical questions should be considered when planning public health interventions (Donnan, 2001, p. 118):

- What should we be doing?
- For whom should we be doing it and at what cost/risk to others?
- Who should decide and how?

This is partly reflected in the increasing concern of public health practitioners to incorporate the ideas and reflect the needs of lay people.

Assessing need

In a classic study, Bradshaw (1972) drew attention to four types of need. The first two – normative and comparative – are defined by experts and reflect professional judgements and standards. Using the medical model, for example, doctors may define some people's health as falling within a 'normal' range, while others may be entitled to (or required to undergo) treatment on the basis of their identified normative health needs. Assessing comparative needs usually involves estimation by professionals of which groups are in greater need of available services or resources. One aspect of national health strategies that many welcomed was that they set out clearer priorities for public health by creating targets for disease reduction and for improving people's quality of life, although some critics have suggested that this unduly restricted the scope of public health activities (Adams, 1994). Whether working to targets or not, it is generally professionals who are assessing people's comparative needs and lay people have, until recently, had little involvement.

Felt needs, the third type of need discussed by Bradshaw, are those that people identify themselves. These may be uncovered by questions addressed to individuals or perhaps by surveys of local residents, but their characteristic feature is that they are perceived by users themselves and generated by their own life experiences. In many cases such needs may be described as hidden or 'latent' because, without knowledge of the services or support that are available or how needs are being defined in the wider world, people may not believe themselves to be 'in need'.

Expressed need is what people say they need; it is the turning of a felt need into a request, call or even demand for action. For example, people may grumble for years about the restricted opening hours of the local health centre without doing anything about it. However, if they are consulted about opening hours, the grumbles may turn into expressed demands for change. Local mothers may feel the need for a safe crossing place on a busy road and find out that on other roads traffic has been better controlled. This may turn their felt but latent need into an expressed need and they will begin to make demands for traffic controls. Expressed needs may reinforce normative needs because the process of channelling the felt need into an expressed need may itself be mediated by professionals and may reflect the realistic options open for action. On the other hand, people's expressed needs may conflict with public health practitioners' priorities.

A central problem in identifying needs is determining what needs themselves are and, in particular, what types of needs should be regarded as legitimate, an issue that is further discussed in Chapter 14. Some policy makers may give more value to needs assessed by large-scale quantitative methodologies, while smaller-scale qualitative studies, which aim to involve consumers, may not be given equal value. This raises ethical issues when determining priorities for action: whose needs count?

An initiative by Coventry Primary Care Trust provides an example of the involvement of consumers in developing sexual health services for teenagers. They set up a local Teenage Pregnancy Partnership Board (TPPB) which decided to commission some research to find out what it was that pregnant teenagers and young parents felt that they needed. This was because, as Lawlor and Shaw (2002) argued, the debate about teenage pregnancy and young parenthood focuses on the negative, largely because young people have remained silent in much of the discussion. The negative focus is produced by people who are not themselves 'young mothers'.

In order to obtain the views of groups of people who may have been socially excluded or marginalised in the past, some attention must be paid to the research methodologies and research methods employed. In the Coventry example, they used qualitative methods, one-to-one in-depth interviews and small focus-group work rather than more quantitative methods. Postal questionnaires may exclude people who have low literacy skills and those whose first language is not English. The response rate for postal questionnaires is known to be much lower than that for face-to-face interviews and they may only be completed by the most motivated people. The issue of language also needs to be considered when undertaking surveys in multilingual and multicultural areas. There is a growing research literature on developing appropriate research methodologies for undertaking research with black and minority ethnic communities (Gunaratnam, 2007; Lloyd, 2010).

Assessing local health needs and listening to local voices is not a straightforward matter. Local people do not speak necessarily with one voice. Although they may share common problems or interests, they may have different agendas and express different needs. Some may speak louder than others, some may find it hard to express themselves, and others may not be interested at all. As well as questionnaires, phone-ins and high-street surveys, practitioners have adopted a number of other strategies in an attempt to overcome the difficulties and tap into the most comprehensive local voice possible. These include using key informants and focus groups and setting up health forums. A range of methods used to find out the needs of local people are reviewed in the next section.

Methods used in health needs assessment

Working with key informants

This resembles the grapevine approach, where key individuals are interviewed because they have particular access to local knowledge. They may be formal or informal leaders, the landlord of the local pub who has 'an ear to the ground', religious or cultural leaders, or the head teacher at a local school.

This approach may provide a distorted or biased view because it may not be possible to disentangle the informant's own interests from the interests of the local population. It may provide only a superficial picture of the local community and not represent the views of minority groups or groups with special concerns.

Health forums

A health forum for a particular locality would comprise a mixture of professionals, members of voluntary organisations, community groups and local residents. It differs from a focus group (see Chapter 8, Section 8.4) in that the forum is a cross-section of the community rather than a special interest group. Once set up, a health forum would meet regularly, deal with health issues as they arise, and have a finger on the pulse of the local community and its health needs.

In assessing the needs of communities, both focus groups and health forums have their relative strengths and weaknesses. Focus groups have special access to the needs of specific groups in the community whose voices may not otherwise be heard, but of necessity they have their own agenda which may conflict with that of other groups. Reconciling those different agendas may be very difficult. A health forum can bring together different interest groups, but runs the risk of becoming elitist and dominated by the professionals.

Community profiling

Community profiling uses social research in a community primarily in order to listen to the voice of (often) marginalised people and then to feed that voice into an assessment of their collective needs, with a view to creating what Moran and Butler (2001, p. 60) refer to as a 'living health profile'. The term 'community profile' is therefore broader than an assessment of needs as it also takes into account the resources available within that community to meet those needs. Hawtin et al. explained a 'community profile' as:

> A comprehensive description of the needs of a population that is defined, or defines itself, as a community, and the resources that exist within that community, carried out with the active involvement of the community itself, for the purpose of developing an action plan or other means of improving the quality of life in the community.
>
> (Hawtin et al., 1994, p. 5)

A community profile, then, is more than a health audit; it produces a database of all the resources in the community. This need not be on a large scale, such as a city-wide profile. Indeed, many general practitioners are being encouraged to adopt a community profiling approach to the services they offer. This community-oriented primary-care approach is very much about planning, rather than responding to patients who present themselves at the surgery. Community profiling has been a longstanding approach in health promotion. For example, in a project in Sandwell in the West Midlands, aimed at assessing the health needs of black and minority ethnic communities in Smethwick, a community profile was developed which included all the voluntary and religious organisations, as well as those statutory organisations that might impact on the determinants of health (Douglas, 1996).

Community profiles are a written snapshot of the community's natural and built environment, together with the social, economic, political, cultural and religious structures of support within this. A health needs assessment can draw on a community profile to inform local plans by looking at unmet needs for services, and provide information that will allow services to be tailored to local populations. The range of information that a community profile draws on is shown in Box 9.4.

Box 9.4 Information for building a community profile

- The demographic and social mix of the people – taking into account such factors as age, class, gender, ethnicity, religion and disability.
- The housing available to them in the area.
- Access to jobs, training and income in, and accessible from, the area.
- Public services and facilities, schools, colleges, health centres, police services, etc., in the area and accessible nearby.
- Shops, entertainment, sport and culture in the area and nearby.
- Voluntary organisations and services, local associations and political parties.
- Family and community networks to which people contribute and on which they can call.
- An audit of local skills to assess the resources available in the community.

What questions about a community would the types of information set out in Box 9.4 help you answer?

In assessing the health needs of a particular community, a profile would be valuable to address the following questions.

- How healthy is the community?
- What does it need to be healthier?
- What does it need to stay healthy?
- What are the best ways to accomplish these goals?
- What resources exist in the community to help it become healthier?

There are several frameworks for developing such profiles (Jack and Holt, 2008; Hill et al., 2010). Public health observatories developed health profiling in the UK and Ireland to cover a range of indicators and domains, including morbidity, mortality, lifestyles, demography and wider determinants of health (Hill et al., 2010).

Rapid appraisal

Rapid appraisal is a methodology that has become popular as a way of collecting information on which priorities can be based. Rapid appraisal does not rely solely on gathering new information but can collect secondary data (from demographers, epidemiologists and large-scale social surveys) as well as information from any source deemed appropriate.

One of the problems identified with the rapid appraisal method is that it relies mainly on key informants who may or may not represent the local population well. It is important that the wider community is involved. Setting priorities with, rather than for, people seems eminently sensible if people are to feel committed to a plan of action (see Chapter 11). But there may also be conflicting interests in the setting of priorities: there are those priorities that are set by others, as well as the practical or real interests on the ground.

Participatory appraisal

Participatory appraisal is another method of involving local communities in assessing and appraising their own needs, identifying problems and determining the priorities for solving those problems. For example, participatory rapid appraisal (PRA) was used in the Ardoyne area of North Belfast to define the health and social needs of women and to formulate joint action plans between the residents and service providers. The PRA team interviewed 20 key informants, including local health and social service professionals, voluntary organisations and representatives from community groups, using two focus-group discussions. Each group was led by a skilled facilitator who used a semi-structured interview schedule covering a broad framework of issues.

> The goal was to elicit the community views and opinions of the locality through a guided questioning route, and for the sub-team to emerge from the focus group with a deeper understanding of the 'community's' priority health and social need issues. The group also discussed how to improve the uptake of existing services and

new ways to meet gaps in services. … In Ardoyne, where health and social services management is largely localized, PRA provided a powerful vehicle for active participation of civil society in planning and evaluating services.

(Lazenbatt et al., 2001, pp. 571–6)

The nature of information on needs is dependent on the research methodology or methodologies chosen. Cross-sectional epidemiological surveys will provide general information about a population – how many people smoke, for example, and their knowledge of the effects of smoking. However, if a greater understanding of when and why people smoke is required, then qualitative methodologies will be more valuable.

9.5 Generating solutions

Having defined the issue or problem, we can move to solution generation, which is stage two of the Nutbeam and Harris (2004) cycle.

Setting aims and objectives

Aims or goals are broad statements that set out what the programme or initiative expects to achieve. In everyday conversation the terms 'aims' and 'objectives' are often used interchangeably. However, aims tend to be broader, and specific objectives often contribute to the aim. Objectives are statements that map out the tasks needed to reach the aims or goals, including a timeframe for the achievement of each task. It is important to set clear aims and objectives, not least because unless there are clear aims and objectives it is not possible to evaluate the programme or project. Effectiveness lies at the heart of evaluation and tends to be what most people have in mind when they hear or use the word 'evaluation'. And effectiveness is concerned with whether an activity has achieved what it set out to do in relation to its aims and objectives.

Identifying aims and objectives is not always straightforward. Certain kinds of aims and objectives are, by their nature, easier to describe than others, but it is important that the various parties involved try to be as explicit and specific as possible about what they are aiming to achieve.

Green and Tones (2010) suggest that objectives should be SMART. This is an acronym for specific, measurable, achievable, realistic and time limited. Objectives have to be measurable and testable for evaluation of effectiveness to take place. This involves identifying smaller-scale objectives that contribute to an aim as well as finding a way of assessing or measuring the extent to which these objectives have been achieved. Objectives should be clearly understood, state what is to be accomplished and be measurable. To be useful in evaluation the objectives should include:

- the outcomes to be achieved or what will change
- the conditions under which the outcome will be observed or when the change will occur
- the criterion for deciding whether the outcome has been achieved or by how much it has changed
- the priority population or who will change.

Deciding what will be an appropriate and feasible measure of effectiveness or change is a crucial step in planning and carrying out an evaluation. Where it is difficult to gather information directly about the outcome of an activity, and where it is not possible to demonstrate a direct link between public health activities and the desired outcome, intermediate and indirect indicators are often used. Measurable objectives and intermediate indicators can be selected even where the main aim of an activity or a project is something as general and seemingly abstract as empowerment. A reviewer of community intervention evaluation suggested this can be done by:

> an interactive dialogue between evaluator and program workers which shows how a common but indistinct objective … 'to empower residents' can be broken down and translated into more practical and recognisable terms … (which) represent specific things happening to specific people. There may, for example, be attitudinal changes across the community as a whole, skills changes within the immediate group involved, changes in the makeup of advisory boards or groups.
>
> (Hawe et al., 1998, p. 205)

Therefore, setting aims and objectives that will facilitate the evaluation can enhance the planning activity by stimulating discussion and debate about the direction of the project or programme.

Mobilising resources: capacity building

Capacity building is intricately linked to the previous stages in the Nutbeam and Harris model. When setting objectives, it is essential that they are realistic and manageable. This means being aware of the resources available and identifying likely constraints. Resources exist in a variety of forms, and may include hard cash, availability of volunteers, political responsiveness or particularly useful skills possessed by colleagues, members of the advisory board or the target group.

Evaluation needs to be built into the resources in terms of time, expertise and personnel. Decisions need to be made about who evaluates – is it to be internal or external? This decision will often depend on the size and scope of the intervention. It will also depend on the requirements of any fundholders involved. A strategy that is often adopted is for those involved in implementing the project to evaluate the process while external evaluation researchers evaluate the outcomes.

For small-scale interventions it is possible that the planning and organisation will be taken on by the public health practitioner. Other programme plans may require an advisory group with the participation of a variety of people: these are the 'stakeholders'. Green and Tones (2010) define primary, secondary and key stakeholders as follows.

- **Primary stakeholders** are the potential beneficiaries – those who are directly affected, either positively or negatively, by the initiative.
- **Secondary stakeholders** are those involved in implementing and evaluating the initiative.
- **Key stakeholders** are those whose support is essential to the continuation of the initiative – for example, fundholders.

(Green and Tones, 2010, p. 159)

Once the group is assembled, it will be necessary to discuss how the process of planning will work and familiarise the members with public health interventions. Ideally, all major stakeholders should be involved in the planning of the intervention. As the group becomes oriented, there will be some role negotiation while each person understands what contribution they can usefully make (see Chapter 3 for some wider discussion of roles in a group). It is essential that each member of the group feels valued and useful, otherwise tensions could set in and undermine the goals being pursued. Responsibility for different tasks will need to be delegated and a group responsibility for the whole undertaking will need to be fostered. Again, it is important to build evaluation tasks into this process. Table 9.2 suggests how the evaluation tasks could be shared.

Table 9.2 Suggested sharing of evaluation tasks in health promotion programme evaluation

Evaluation task	People responsible
Finding out if the programme is reaching the target group	Secondary stakeholders (the programme staff) but with involvement from primary stakeholders
Observing programme operations to see if the programme is being implemented properly	Secondary stakeholders
Assessing participants' satisfaction with the programme	Secondary stakeholders (the programme staff) but with involvement from key stakeholders
Assess programme quality	Key and primary stakeholders
Making a preliminary assessment of programme effects	Secondary stakeholders
Assessing the short-term effects and determining if they are really caused by the programme	(External) Evaluation research staff, possibly with support from primary stakeholders
Assessing longer-term effects and determining if they are really caused by the programme	(External) Evaluation research staff, possibly with support from primary stakeholders

(Source: adapted from Hawe et al., 1998, p. 11)

Developing funding proposals

Practitioners often need to develop proposals for public health interventions, whether they are applying for funding from their own organisation or an outside organisation. However, there is increasing recognition of the need to fund interventions more appropriately, so practitioners may have to bid competitively for funding. This means that developing clear and coherent funding proposals is essential.

In developing a funding proposal, it is important to have very clearly stated aims and objectives and very clear timescales as the success of the initiative will be measured against these. There must be a clear rationale for carrying out an intervention, based on prior epidemiological evidence. Funders are increasingly concerned with the relationship of research to theory and practice and the ways in which users and the public are involved in developing the programme or proposed research project. Having a clear dissemination strategy is equally important. Your own organisation may have guidance on writing and funding proposals and funding bodies themselves usually give very clear guidance as to what is expected of the person writing the proposal in terms of content. One of the important aspects of developing funding proposals is to ensure that they are properly and realistically costed. A realistic assessment of the resources required and the outcomes expected is extremely important, and plans for evaluating the initiative must be built into the funding proposal.

9.6 Putting it into action: implementing the plan

Putting the plan into action is the exciting and nerve-racking part. If some time has passed between planning and implementation, it is always worth making a final check to ensure that no significant changes have occurred. For instance, there may be changes in government or NHS policy that need to be taken into account and plans may need adjusting accordingly. Doggedly implementing a plan when circumstances have changed is a waste of time and resources. This is where process evaluation can be invaluable.

Process evaluation

Process evaluation should go hand in hand with implementation. It involves monitoring the progress of the implementation of the plan; that is, making sure that the plan is being carried out as intended, appropriate people are involved as outlined in the plan, and the plan is actually feasible and manageable in practice. In general, the following four questions should be addressed.

1   Is the programme reaching the target group? Are all parts of the programme reaching all parts of the target group?

2   Are participants satisfied with the programme?

3   Are all the activities of the programme being implemented?

4   Are all the materials and components of the programme of good quality?

(Hawe et al., 1998, p. 61)

The process approach considers that what people learn as a result of becoming involved in a project or programme is no less relevant than reaching pre-set targets. Describing and analysing the process, rather than impacts and outcomes, becomes a key feature of the evaluation. As a result, the evaluation might be more acceptable to community development workers and community activists, who may take a more radical or democratic view of what evaluation should be and have as much interest in less tangible benefits as in reaching targets and statistical 'success'.

Process evaluation should therefore be seen as an opportunity to learn, make adjustments to the programme and respond to feedback from users of the programme. If the programme is really not working in the way that was intended then more radical changes may need to be made (see Figure 9.1). Process evaluation needs to continue throughout the implementation stage until the programme is deemed to have reached the point of evaluability in the planning and evaluation cycle, when it is ready for the impact and outcome evaluation to begin.

9.7 Impact and outcome evaluation

Methods for evaluation

Designing a formal evaluation means choosing methods that are appropriate to the purposes of the evaluation and this choice will be influenced by the kind of public health intervention being pursued and the values and assumptions underlying it. The range and scope of quantitative and qualitative methods are explored in Chapters 7 and 8 and there are three broad (and, in practice, often overlapping) categories from which to choose:

- experimental and quasi-experimental methods concerned with establishing cause and effect
- survey techniques that aim to identify significant patterns
- qualitative methods that focus on description and interpretation.

Although randomised controlled trials have been held up as the gold standard in the evaluation of public health interventions, it has become increasingly clear that this method is not always appropriate (Springett, 2001; Green and South, 2006). Some evaluations will require different quantitative methods, or a mix of both qualitative and quantitative research methodologies.

Reflecting on evaluation

Many evaluations in the field of public health use a mixture of designs and methods and may be described as pluralist (in varying degrees), although, as noted in Chapter 8, combining qualitative and quantitative methodologies is not without its critics. Some researchers have argued that the logic, values and rules underlying experimental and quantitative design, on the one hand, and qualitative, illuminative design, on the other, are so different that the two cannot, with integrity, be added together (Lincoln and Guba, 1985). However, others have accepted the value of mixing methods, while remaining sensitive to their differences. Baum (2010) suggests that mixing methods enables particular public health research questions to be answered and that the use of multiple methods enables triangulation between the methods and allows a more detailed understanding of complex issues. The WHO European Working Group on Health Promotion Evaluation (Rootman et al., 2001) also stressed the importance of using a range of methodologies for public health evaluation and not focusing on randomised controlled trials.

The case study in Box 9.5 provides an example of such methods. It describes a three-year project to promote physical and mental wellbeing in a deprived community. Chances4Change have sponsored a wide range of projects and have encouraged mixed-method evaluation. Another significant driver has been the requirement of funders for increasing amounts of evaluation. Many projects initially did little evaluation and focused mainly on reaching targets for attendance and throughput, but the innovative use of simple tools has enabled useful evaluation work to be done (Lockwood, 2011).

Box 9.5 Naturally Active case study

Naturally Active was a three-year programme within the Chances4 Change project funded by Big Lottery in south-east England. Its aim was to provide and promote physical activity and mental wellbeing for black and minority ethnic communities, older people, children and young people and individuals with mental health problems from the more deprived wards of Dartford and Gravesham. A range of outdoor activities were developed, which included walking and playing golf. Three types of evaluation tools were developed:

- questionnaires to collect socio-demographic data on participants, their physical activity behaviour and likes and dislikes in relation to physical activity

- pre- and post-activity data collection, which recorded levels of health and mental wellbeing

- more detailed qualitative evaluation of each activity to identify the needs of specific client groups, which included conducting focus groups and/or professional medical assessment.

The tools developed utilised a mixture of methods, combining quantitative and qualitative methods aimed at measuring process, during the implementation phase as well as impact and outcome. In developing appropriate evaluation tools, consideration was given to the age of the participants and levels of literacy, since some of the activities of the project were aimed at children and young people. Hence questionnaires required the use of accessible language and symbols. One of the Naturally Active projects, the Sikh Ladies Walking Group, was evaluated by carrying out two group interviews. The first group interview was conducted after the first walk with three women and the second was conducted just before the close of the group with 25 women. The independent evaluation provided information about the *impact* of the walking group on health and wellbeing and the *outcome* of the walking group on changes in lifestyle of the women who participated, longer-term mental health improvements and social and cultural benefits.

Why do you think the Naturally Active case study (Box 9.5) used a range of evaluation methods?

The programme used a range of methods for evaluation to try to capture the complexity, process and outcomes of the various interventions. With such a wide range of activities an evaluation strategy had to be developed which moved beyond merely measuring the volume of activities and the number of participants. With such varied groups of participants in terms of age, ethnic background and health status, the evaluation had to try to capture different views about its value. In approaching evaluation it faced challenges encountered by most projects and interventions which happen in 'real time' and in 'real localities' rather than in laboratory conditions where other variables and confounding factors can be removed.

Conclusion

Planning and evaluation are integral to effective public health practice and should be considered together when developing public health interventions. The planning of any intervention needs to be thorough and yet remain flexible. Above all, planning should be based on sound information and information should include the knowledge and views of those involved, whether individuals or communities.

This chapter has shown how values of participation, empowerment, a focus on the whole person and critical awareness can be built into the processes of planning and evaluation. Although few would argue about the principle that all public health practice should have its basis in sound evidence, there is a continuing and lively debate about what this means exactly and the best ways of achieving it.

References

Adams, L. (1994) 'Health promotion in crisis', *Health Education Journal*, vol. 53, pp. 354–60.

Baum, F. (2010) 'Dilemmas in public health research: methodologies and ethical practice' in Douglas, J., Earle, S., Handsley, S., Lloyd, C.E. and Spurr, S. (eds) *A Reader in Promoting Public Health: Challenge and Controversy*, London/Milton Keynes, Sage/The Open University, pp. 77–88.

Bradshaw, J. (1972) 'The concept of need', *New Society*, vol. 19, pp. 459–68.

Davies, H.T.O., Nutley, S.M. and Smith, P.C. (2000) *What Works? Evidence Based Policy and Practice in Public Services*, Bristol, Policy Press.

Dignan, M. and Carr, P. (1992) *Programme Planning for Health Education and Promotion* (2nd edition), Baltimore, Maryland, Williams and Wilkins.

Donnan, S. (2001) 'Ethics in public health' in Pencheon, D., Guest, C., Melzer, D. and Muir Gray, J.A. (eds) *Oxford Handbook of Public Health Practice*, Oxford, Oxford University Press, pp. 118–25.

Douglas, J. (1996) 'Developing health promotion strategies with black and minority ethnic communities which address social inequalities and their impact on health' in Bywaters, P. and Mcleod, E. (eds) *Working for Equality in Health*, London, Routledge, pp. 179–96.

Douglas, J., Earle, S., Handsley, S., Lloyd, C.E., Jones, L.J. and Spurr, S. (eds) (2010) *A Reader in Promoting Public Health: Challenge and Controversy* (2nd edition), London/Milton Keynes, Sage/The Open University.

Ewles, L. and Simnett, I. (2003) *Promoting Health: A Practical Guide* (5th edition), London, Baillière Tindall.

Green, J. and South, J. (2006) *Evaluation*, Maidenhead, Open University Press.

Green, J. and Tones, K. (2010) *Health Promotion Planning and Strategies* (2nd edition), London, Sage.

Gunaratnam, Y. (2007) 'Complexity and complicity in researching ethnicity and health' in Douglas, J., Earle, S., Handsley, S., Lloyd, C.E. and Spurr, S. (eds) *A Reader in Promoting Public Health: Challenge and Controversy*, London/Milton Keynes, Sage/The Open University, pp. 147–56.

Hawe, P., Degeling, D. and Hall, J. (1998) *Evaluating Health Promotion: A Health Worker's Guide*, Sydney, MacLennan and Petty.

Hawtin, M., Percy-Smith, J. and Hughes, G. (1994) *Community Profiling: Auditing Social Needs*, Buckingham, Open University Press.

Health Evidence Bulletins Wales website. Available at: http://hebw.cf.ac.uk/ (accessed 2 September 2011).

Hill, A., Balanda, K., Galbraith, L., Greenacre, J. and Sinclair, D. (2010) 'Profiling health in the UK and Ireland', *Public Health*, vol. 124, pp. 253–58.

Home Office Crime Reduction College (2002) *Passport to Evaluation*, York, Home Office Crime Reduction College.

Intute website. Available at: www.intute.ac.uk (accessed 2 September 2011).

Jack, K. and Holt, M. (2008) 'Community Profiling as part of health needs assessment', *Nursing Standard*, vol. 22, no. 18, pp. 51–56 .

Lawlor, D.A. and Shaw, M. (2002) Too much too young? Teenage pregnancy is not a public health problem, *International Journal of Epidemiology*, vol. 31, pp. 552–554.

Lazenbatt, A., Lynch, U. and O'Neill, E. (2001) 'Revealing the hidden "troubles" in Northern Ireland: the role of participatory rapid appraisal', *Health Education Research*, vol. 16, no. 5, pp. 567–78.

Lincoln, Y. and Guba, E. (1985) *Naturalistic Inquiry*, Thousand Oaks, California, Sage.

Lloyd, C.E. (2010) 'Researching the views of diabetes service users from south Asian backgrounds: a reflection on some of the issues' in Douglas, J., Earle, S., Handsley, S., Lloyd, C.E., Jones, L.J. and Spurr, S. (eds) *A Reader in Promoting Public Health: Challenge and Controversy* (2nd edition), London/Milton Keynes, Sage/The Open University, pp. 114–20.

Lockwood, A. (August 2011) (personal communication) PhD student, Faculty of Health and Social Care, The Open University.

McQueen, D. (2010) 'The evaluation of health promotion practice: twenty-first century debates on evidence and effectiveness' in Douglas, J., Earle, S., Handsley, S., Lloyd, C.E., Jones, L.J. and Spurr, S. (eds) *A Reader in Promoting Public Health: Challenge and Controversy* (2nd edition), London/Milton Keynes, Sage/The Open University.

McQueen, D. (2001) 'Strengthening the evidence base for health promotion', *Health Promotion International*, vol. 16, no. 3, pp. 261–68.

Moran, R.A. and Butler, D.S. (2001) 'Whose Health Profile?', *Critical Public Health*, vol. 11, no. 1, pp. 59–74.

Naidoo, J. and Wills, J. (2009) *Foundations for Health Promotion* (3rd edition), London, Balliere Tindall.

National Institute for Health and Clinical Excellence (NICE) (2008) *Report on NICE Citizens Council meeting: Quality Adjusted Life Years (QALYs) and the severity of illness*, London, National Institute for Health and Clinical Excellence. Available at: www.nice.org.uk/media/2C3/31/CCReportOnQALYsAndSeverity. pdf (accessed 2 September 2011).

NHS Quality Improvement Scotland website. Available at: www. healthcareimprovementscotland.org/home.aspx (accessed 2 September 2011).

Nutbeam, D. (1996) 'Achieving "best practice" in health promotion: improving the fit between research and practice', *Health Education Research*, vol. 11, no. 3, pp. 317–26.

Nutbeam, D. and Bauman, A. (2006) *Evaluation in a Nutshell: A Practical Guide to the Evaluation of Health Promotion Programs*, Sydney, McGraw-Hill.

Nutbeam, D. and Harris, E. (2004) *Theory in a Nutshell: A Practical Guide to Health Promotion Theories* (2nd edition), Sydney, McGraw-Hill.

Phillips, C. and Thompson, G. (2009) *What is a QALY?*, London, Hayward Medical Communications. Available at: www.medicine.ox.ac.uk/bandolier/painres/download/what?QALY.pdf (accessed 15 September 2011).

Public Health Agency Northern Ireland website. Available at: www.publichealth.hscni.net (accessed 2 September 2011).

Raphael, D. (2001) 'Evaluation of quality-of-life initiatives in health promotion' in Rootman, I., Goodstadt, M., Hyndman, B., McQueen, D., Potvin, L., Springett, J. and Ziglio, E. (eds) *Evaluation in Health Promotion: Principles and Perspectives*, Copenhagen, WHO, pp. 123–47.

Roberts, K., Cavill, N. and Rutter, H. (2009) *Standard Evaluation Framework for Weight Management Interventions*, London, Association of Public Health Observatories/National Obesity Observatory/NHS. Available at: www.noo.org.uk/uploads/doc721_2_noo_SEF%20FINAL300309.pdf (accessed 2 September 2011).

Rootman, I., Goodstadt, M., Potvin, L. and Springett, J. (2001) 'A framework for health promotion evaluation' in Rootman, I., Goodstadt, M., Hyndman, B., McQueen, D., Potvin, L., Springett, J. and Ziglio, E. (eds) *Evaluation in Health Promotion: Principles and Perspectives*, Copenhagen, WHO, pp. 7–38.

Springett, J. (2001) 'Appropriate approaches to the evaluation of health promotion', *Critical Public Health*, vol. 11, no. 2, pp. 139–52.

World Health Organization (WHO) (1998) *Health Promotion Evaluation: Recommendations to Policy Makers, Report of the World Health Organization European Working Group on Health Promotion Evaluation*, Copenhagen, WHO Regional Office for Europe.

Chapter 10: Educating for health

Jackie Green

Introduction

Health education came under fierce critical scrutiny in the last quarter of the twentieth century. It stood accused of failing to respect individual autonomy and blaming individuals if they were unable to change their behaviour. The target of criticism was generally referred to as 'traditional' health education, whereas, to be more precise, it was a particular model of health education – the preventive or medical model. Critics paid little attention to alternative models of health education that existed at the time and were characterised by a set of values more consistent with those of the Ottawa Charter (World Health Organization [WHO], 1986).

This chapter investigates those alternative models and demonstrates that health education has an important role within contemporary public health. It explores how health education can contribute to individual and community empowerment and considers its role in supporting and facilitating changes in health behaviour. The chapter discusses why communication is central to effective health education and how communication strategies might be used by public health practitioners to empower, as well as influence, people. Some of the more controversial approaches to influencing behaviour change, such as nudge theory and social marketing, are also considered.

10.1 The role of health education

The preventive or medical model of health education focuses on medical intervention and patient compliance, using professional authority to persuade people to minimise/avoid risks to their health. It has a role to play but has been justifiably criticised for trying to change individual behaviour without giving due consideration to the social and environmental determinants of that behaviour, which might make change difficult or even impossible. Such an approach can lead to 'victim-blaming', a notion developed by Ryan (1976). Moreover, the persuasive efforts of health professionals to change behaviour have been seen as failing to respect individual autonomy and voluntarism.

This does not mean that health education has been superseded – it remains at the core of much public health practice. But it does shift the focus to alternative models of health education characterised by a commitment to equity, empowerment and voluntarism (Tilford et al., 2003). 'Voluntarism' means without coercion and with the full understanding and acceptance of the purposes of the action (Green and Kreuter, 1999). Such models have more to offer contemporary public health. They are endorsed by the 'stewardship' approach to public health advocated by the Nuffield Council on Bioethics (2007) which states that programmes should:

- aim to ensure that it is easy for people to lead a healthy life
- not attempt to coerce adults to lead healthy lives.

Are there any situations when persuasion or coercion would be ethically acceptable?

Although the principle of voluntarism should generally be upheld, Green and Tones (2010) qualify this with the provision that an individual's right to free choice should not impinge on the rights of others or have a negative effect on the wellbeing of the community. For example, legislation about drink-driving is undoubtedly coercive in denying choice to drivers, but protects others from risk. Similarly, it is important to safeguard vulnerable groups. Persuasive messages directed at parents about protecting children from dangers in the home may therefore be justified. Such tensions between individual and population-level rights and benefits, and their implications for practitioners, are explored in Chapter 5.

Numerous taxonomies of health-education and health-promotion models exist (see Chapter 6) and it is not the intention to revisit them in any detail here. Nonetheless, it is worthwhile noting that the 'educational model' is concerned with enabling informed choice and the voluntary adoption of behaviour. However, it assumes that freedom of choice exists and does not acknowledge the environmental and personal factors that might constrain choice. In contrast, an 'empowerment model' addresses this issue by directly focusing on enabling individuals and communities to achieve control over their health.

10.2 An empowerment model of health education

The contribution of both individual and community empowerment to improving public health has been recognised in the English public health White Paper *Healthy Lives, Healthy People*: 'We need a new approach that empowers individuals to make healthy choices and gives communities the tools to address their own, particular needs' (Department of Health [DoH], 2010, p. 2). The Marmot Review also identified empowerment as the 'centre of action to reduce health inequalities' (Marmot, 2010, p. 34). Before considering the role of health education as the primary means for achieving empowerment, we need to understand what empowerment is.

Self-empowerment has been defined as, 'a state in which an individual possesses a relatively high degree of actual power – that is, a **genuine** potential for making choices' (Tones and Tilford, 2001, p. 40). It is characterised by a number of psychological attributes. Important among these are beliefs about self and the amount of control an individual has. At a general level, the notion of 'locus of control' (Rotter, 1966) refers to an individual's perception about the extent to which events in their life are contingent on their own actions. Those with an external locus of control would see events as unpredictable and due to chance, fate or others in a more powerful position. In contrast, an internal locus of control would be associated with the belief that events are consequent on one's own actions. Clearly, those with an internal locus would be more likely to take action to control their health. More specifically, the concept of 'self efficacy' (Bandura, 1982) refers to an individual's belief about their ability to carry out a particular action successfully (see Chapter 6). Those who believe that they are capable of performing actions are more likely to attempt them than those who do not. According to Bandura, self-efficacy beliefs can be influenced by four main factors:

- **direct experience** – previous success or failure
- **vicarious experience** – observation of other people's experience (so-called modelling)
- **verbal persuasion** – encouragement about likely success
- **physiological state** – the level of fear or stress.

An empowered individual will also have a high level of self-esteem. Although this will, in part, be influenced by beliefs about control, it is more broadly the product of the whole range of beliefs about self – the so-called 'self concept' – and the value attached to its various elements. Skills, including general life skills and specific skills, are also necessary to empowerment. On the one hand, they ensure that actions can be accomplished successfully and, on the other, the possession of skills and the experience of using them successfully can enhance self-esteem and sense of control. Not least among these skills is the ability to access and interpret information about health. While it is accepted that knowledge alone is generally insufficient to change behaviour, having accurate information about the factors that impact on health and about health choices and their consequences is essential to empowerment. The concept of 'health literacy' focuses specifically on this set of skills and has been defined as, 'the cognitive and social skills which determine the motivation and ability of individuals to gain access to, understand and use information in ways that promote and maintain good health' (Nutbeam, 1998, p. 357).

There are undoubtedly similarities between empowerment and health literacy. Indeed, Tones (2002) has argued forcefully that health literacy is merely a rebranding of empowerment. Nonetheless, its particular focus on skill development provides useful pointers to educational opportunities. In contrast, the issue of power is more central to empowerment.

The actual power individuals or communities have is influenced by a constellation of environmental factors. Conversely, active, participating communities may be able to change the environment to reduce exposure to health risks or make it more health enhancing. This two-way effect is known as 'reciprocal determinism' – a notion central to social learning theory (Bandura, 1986). An empowered community will be more likely to have the motivation and capability to influence the environment. It is more than a collection of empowered individuals and would have additional attributes such as:

- a sense of community
- commitment to achieving collective community goals rather than just individual goals
- high levels of social capital – the social resources available within the community.

Although health literacy has its origins in patient education and ensuring compliance with treatment regimens, the notion has been extended to include the capacity to take action at either the individual or the community level. Nutbeam (2000) distinguishes three levels of health literacy:

- functional health literacy – sufficient literary skills to deal with health information
- interactive health literacy – also includes the personal and social skills and motivation and self confidence required to take personal action
- critical health literacy – also includes the skills needed to take social and political action as well as individual action.

How can health education contribute to empowerment? Health education has been defined as 'any planned activity designed to produce health- or illness-related learning' and learning itself as 'a relatively permanent change in capability or disposition' (Tones and Tilford, 2001, p. 30). Health education may therefore achieve changes in:

- awareness, knowledge and understanding
- beliefs, values and attitudes – about self and also specific health issues
- skills
  - information finding and interpretation
  - problem solving and decision making
  - specific psychomotor
  - social interaction
  - social activism
- behaviour.

The scope of health education is very broad and it can potentially contribute to individual and community empowerment at all the various levels outlined above. For example, the development of skills will enable people to take action and also affect their self-efficacy beliefs, sense of control and self-esteem. Raising awareness about the negative effects of the environment on health may motivate people to act collectively.

At its most radical, health education is concerned with addressing the fundamental causes of disadvantage and ill health and achieving political and social change. It involves critical consciousness raising to generate awareness and concern about social injustice along with the development of skills to take appropriate social and political action. The term 'critical consciousness raising' was popularised by Freire (1972) and was central to his educational approach, which sought to empower disadvantaged people and enable their liberation from oppressive social structures. Such health education is very much in tune with critical theory and has been referred to as critical health education (Green and Tones, 2010).

Regardless of whether the primary aim of health education is to achieve change in individual behaviour, empowerment or social and political change, the target of health education is generally assumed to be individual members of the population or communities. The definition offered by Green and Kreuter (below) draws attention to the often overlooked potential for targeting both professional groups and policy makers who are in a position to influence or bring about change:

> health education is aimed primarily at the voluntary actions people can take on their own, individually or collectively, as citizens looking after their own health or as decision-makers looking after the health of others and the common good of the community.
>
> Green and Kreuter (1999), p. 14

The legitimate target of health education can therefore be much broader. The education and training of professional groups is fundamental to the way services are delivered and in particular to enabling people to achieve control of their health through working in ways that are participatory and empowering. Furthermore, tackling the structural factors that impact on health may require professionals to have the skills to work with communities to achieve environmental change or to mediate, lobby and advocate on their behalf.

Health education and healthy public policy are frequently presented as alternative strategic approaches. But it seems impossible to envisage how policy change might be achieved without some form of learning – and hence education as the means for achieving learning – whether it is among policy makers themselves, advocates for change or communities seeking change. Not only can health education be used to influence individual behaviour, it also has a key role in contributing to policy change and tackling the structural determinants of health. Drawing on Tones and Tilford (2001) and Green and Tones (2010), its broader role may be summarised as:

- personal empowerment – to enable individuals to gain control over their health and the voluntary adoption of health actions through developing the necessary skills, knowledge, beliefs, values and attitudes

- community empowerment and critical consciousness raising – to develop the skills and motivation to act collectively to tackle environmental and structural barriers to health

- agenda setting – to develop awareness among key stakeholders about the need for environmental and policy change

- professional education and training – to enable professionals in different sectors to work with communities to address their health needs and become effective advocates for health.

Health education – and particularly an empowerment model of health education – is therefore the major driver for achieving public health goals.

10.3 Supporting and facilitating change

Health education programmes are more likely to be effective if they specify their learning objectives and their target group precisely. Reference to theory can identify which variables to consider – including both intrapersonal and external environmental factors.

As identified in Chapter 6, there are numerous theories and models to draw on in order to identify the determinants of behavioural intentions and actions. A simple example of the importance of identifying the key variables is provided by the West of Scotland Cancer Awareness Project Bowel Cancer Campaign. The campaign aimed to encourage those with signs and symptoms of bowel cancer to present earlier. The Health Belief Model (HBM) (Becker, 1984) indicates that taking such action would be more likely if an individual believes that: they are susceptible; the consequences are serious; the recommended action will reduce susceptibility or consequences; and the benefits will outweigh the cost. Cues to action and positive health motivation more generally will also contribute.

> **Box 10.1 West of Scotland Cancer Awareness Project Bowel Cancer Campaign**
>
> Insight from public research found:
>
> - reasonable levels of awareness of the disease, but poor awareness of signs and symptoms
> - low awareness of incidence levels
> - lack of awareness that disease can be effectively treated if detected early
> - fear of diagnosis of cancer is a major issue but there are also issues about embarrassment and stigma to present
> - focus on 'risk' factors in communications may alienate target audience.
>
> (National Health Service [NHS] Scotland, undated)

How might you overcome the barriers noted in Box 10.1, drawing on insights from the Health Belief Model (HBM)?

The main barriers reported in Box 10.1 relate to lack of awareness and fear. Applying the HBM to the insights derived from research into public perceptions about bowel cancer shows low awareness of the incidence and hence the level of risk of developing the disease. The costs of seeking early advice are perceived to be high in terms of embarrassment and fear of being diagnosed with cancer. There is also little awareness of the benefits of early treatment – leading to an overall poor perceived cost–benefit ratio. Furthermore, poor awareness of early signs and symptoms will result in failure to recognise these as cues to action.

Rather than simply exhorting people to seek treatment if they experience any signs or symptoms, an HBM analysis indicates that the key issues to address are raising awareness of the risk of bowel cancer, the signs and symptoms which should prompt action and the benefits of early treatment. Similarly, efforts should be made to reduce the fear of diagnosis and the embarrassment associated with 'bowels'.

The HBM has been used extensively in planning programmes to encourage relatively simple preventive health actions. When the aim of the programme is more complex and it appears that a wider range of variables will influence the intended outcome, a more comprehensive theory or model will be needed. For example, the Health Action Model (HAM) (see Figure 10.1, page 286), probably the most comprehensive of the explanatory models of behaviour, considerably broadens the potential scope for health education.

If the HAM is applied hypothetically to the case of healthy eating, it suggests that in addition to specifically focusing on knowledge and beliefs about what constitutes a healthy diet and its benefits, the following should also be considered:

- beliefs about the cost of a healthy diet, including actual cost, preparation time and family reaction
- motivational factors, such as attitudes to healthy eating and junk food, snacking and dealing with hunger and the use of food as a reward
- normative beliefs about what constitutes a proper meal
- self-efficacy beliefs about the capacity to cook appetising, nutritious meals, stick to a healthy diet and avoid junk food
- self-esteem
- body image
- skill in cooking nutritious meals
- availability of affordable fruit and vegetables.

The skill, of course, is choosing the most appropriate theory or model. Knowing the community and the major determinants of behaviour helps ensure that the model selected incorporates these. The model can then be applied to unpicking the major determinants of behaviour in more detail and used as a framework for empirical research into their respective effects. Lay insights can also be incorporated and are particularly valuable in understanding what influences the choices people make and identifying key barriers to change.

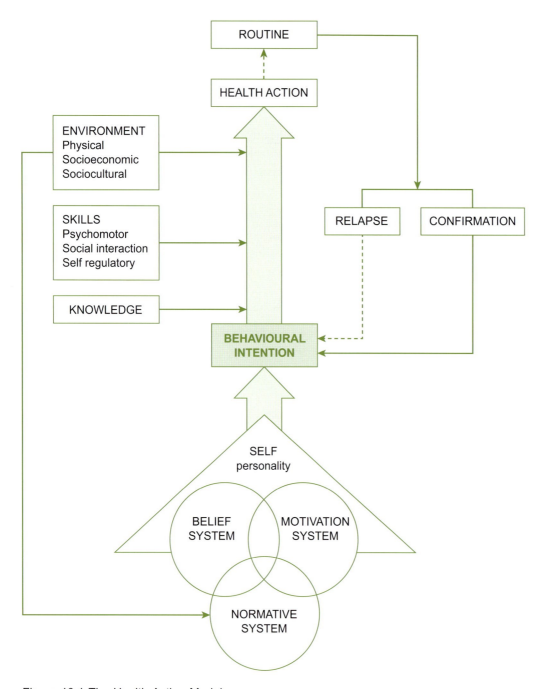

Figure 10.1 The Health Action Model

(Source: Green and Tones, 2010, p. 117)

A central tenet of health promotion has been that the healthy choice should be the easy choice. HAM recognises the fact that the environment – including the social environment – can determine whether or not behavioural intentions are put into practice. At the very least, any barriers to action should be removed and, ideally, the healthy choice be facilitated. Nudge theory takes this further by deliberately structuring the context in which people make decisions so that they are more likely to make the 'right' decision.

10.4 Nudge theory

Nudge theory (Thaler and Sunstein, 2009) is currently receiving considerable attention as a means for improving health choices. It is premised on the view that people cannot be trusted to do the 'right thing' and make decisions that are in their own best interest, but need to be manipulated or 'nudged' to do so. A central tenet of the theory is that decision making does not take place in a vacuum, but within a particular environment and that aspects of the environment will consciously or unconsciously influence choice. The 'choice architect has the responsibility for organising the context in which people make decisions' so that they are more likely to make the desired choice (Thaler and Sunstein, 2009, p. 3). A nudge is 'any aspect of the choice architecture that alters people's behaviour in a predictable way without forbidding any options or significantly changing their economic incentives' (Thaler and Sunstein, 2009, p. 6). For example, displaying fruit at eye level in a cafeteria is seen as a nudge, whereas banning junk food would not be. Marteau et al. (2011) note that nudging has certainly been effective in influencing purchasing behaviour. The placing of chocolates and sweets near supermarket checkouts is an obvious example and would support the argument for removing 'nudges' which have a negative effect on health. However, as yet, there is little evidence that nudging alone can improve public health in the longer term.

Ideologically, nudge theory has its origins in behavioural economics and is clearly linked to behaviourism (see Curtis, 2010). It is the antithesis of empowerment. The authors claim that nudge theory is located in the libertarian paternalist tradition. It is held to be libertarian because people have the freedom to choose, and paternalist because choices are steered to enhance lives. While the rhetoric may have some superficial appeal, there are clear ethical concerns. Deliberately engineering the environment to manipulate behaviour is entirely different from the notion of making the healthy choice easy for those who have selected it as their preferred option. Importantly, it fails to respect individual autonomy. This is particularly the case when the changes to the environment are so subtle that the population may be unaware of being the target of efforts to manipulate their behaviour. Respect for autonomy is a fundamental ethical principle as well as being central to empowerment and control. Nudge theory may therefore be focusing on achieving short-term behavioural goals at the expense of undermining empowerment and more sustainable longer-term change.

Nonetheless, the UK coalition government's approach to public health has been heavily influenced by behavioural economics and behavioural science, which have informed the development of the 'Mindspace' framework (see Table 10.1) for developing initiatives to change behaviour.

MINDSPACE	
Messenger	We are heavily influenced by who communicates information
Incentives	Our responses to incentives are shaped by predictable mental shortcuts such as strongly avoiding losses
Norms	We are strongly influenced by what others do
Defaults	We 'go with the flow' of pre-set options
Salience	Our attention is drawn to what is novel and seems relevant to us
Priming	Our acts are often influenced by sub-conscious cues
Affect	Our emotional associations can powerfully shape our actions
Commitment	We seek to be consistent with our public promises, and reciprocate acts
Ego	We act in ways that make us feel better about ourselves

Table 10.1 The 'Mindspace' framework

(Source: Behavioural Insight Team, 2010, p. 6)

10.5 Communication and education for health

Communication is an essential part of the educational process. Much of the literature on communication tends to be located within a top-down approach typical of traditional health education. Nonetheless, it still has relevance for an empowerment model. Communication is central to interaction and dialogue and is needed to develop awareness, knowledge and understanding. It may also develop values and attitudes and even skills which, as noted above, are elements of empowerment. Furthermore, convincing policy makers of the need for change may depend on the ability to communicate persuasively. This section begins by looking at the main features of effective communication before considering how the process of communication can contribute to both empowerment and learning.

Work on persuasive communication at Yale in the 1950s (Hovland et al., 1953) focused on three main elements, characterised as: Who says what? To whom? and How effective is it? The channel used for communication will also have an influence. The main elements or 'inputs' involved in communication are listed below and will provide the framework for a discussion of successful communication:

- sender or source
- message
- channel
- receiver or audience.

Drawing on McGuire (1989), the various stages of the communication process that must be successfully accomplished are:

- the message is presented and reaches the intended audience
- it attracts and maintains the attention of the audience
- the audience understands the message correctly
- the audience accepts the message
- the audience retains the message
- behaviour changes take place.

The first hurdle is ensuring that the message actually reaches the intended audience. For example, it may be easier to access men through initiatives in the workplace, football grounds, barbers or pubs than more conventional health service premises. Failure is possible at any stage and is best avoided by having sound knowledge of the characteristics of the target group – or, indeed, involving the target group in designing programmes.

Source factors

The credibility of the source is of fundamental importance. Moreover, it is not their actual credibility that really matters, but the audience's perceptions of their credibility.

Two key factors that appear to influence credibility are the perceived expertise and trustworthiness of the source.

 If Cancer Research UK and your local supermarket both produced leaflets on healthy lifestyle, which are you most likely to believe and why?

Expertise is generally associated with having relevant experience, expert knowledge or qualifications. However, some individuals who lack these qualities still seem able to exert a powerful influence by virtue of their personal charisma or celebrity. The attractiveness of the source is also a factor and will certainly help in gaining attention.

Celebrities can be used to deliver or endorse health-education messages. For example, Michelle Obama's anti-childhood-obesity campaign capitalised on her celebrity and on her experience as a mother. The inclusion of Regina Benjamin, the US Surgeon General, in the launch also added expert credibility. Celebrities will have greater credibility if they have relevant experience or some other legitimate association with the message.

Communication is generally likely to be easier between individuals who share similar backgrounds and culture. People are also more likely to be influenced by those with whom they identify, both in terms of accepting what they say as well as developing self-efficacy beliefs. 'Homophily' refers to 'the degree to which pairs of individuals who interact are similar in certain attributes, such as beliefs, values, education, social status and the like' (Rogers and Shoemaker, 1971, p. 14). This may, however, not always be possible. If there is little homophily, effective communication will be improved if the source has empathic understanding of the audience along with good communication skills. Furthermore, communication is more likely to be empowering if the source demonstrates respect for the audience.

The use of peers as educators is based on the view that peers are trusted and credible sources of information. 'Peer education' has been defined as 'the teaching or sharing of health information, values and behaviours by members of similar age or status groups' (Sciacca, 1987, cited in Milburn, 1995, p. 407). Peers can be more effective than outsiders in delivering health messages. Furthermore, being a peer educator can be an empowering experience in itself by enhancing the educator's knowledge, skills, self-confidence, self-esteem and social standing.

Message

Clearly, the message must address the communication objectives. However, the way it is constructed will influence whether it keeps the audience's attention, is understood and is persuasive. The *Pink Book – Making Health Communication Programs Work* (National Cancer Institute, undated) suggests that the following should be considered when designing messages:

- accuracy
- consistency
- clarity – messages should be simple and explicit
- relevance
- credibility
- appeal.

The appeal of the message can be either negative, to discourage people from particular behaviours such as smoking, or positive, to encourage them to take up new behaviours such as regular exercise. Whenever feasible, it is better to be positive.

A further consideration is the issue of 'sidedness' – should both sides of an argument be presented or just one side? One-sided arguments may work if the audience is never likely to be exposed to a counter argument. However a one-sided argument can still be questioned. If a one-sided argument is given, and people come across alternative arguments from different sources, this may undermine trust. If health education is about facilitating healthy choice, it follows that both sides of an argument should be presented and the audience be allowed to make up its own mind. Hubley (1993) notes that this is easier in face-to-face communication than when mass media is used. This does not mean that there necessarily has to be a balanced presentation of both sides. The message is more likely to be persuasive if the main argument is presented fully, then any counterarguments are briefly acknowledged and convincingly refuted, before reaching an explicit conclusion that endorses the original message. It also appears that, following exposure to both sides of an argument, people who already have positive attitudes to the proposed measure are more likely to maintain them when challenged. It acts as a form of 'social inoculation' (Pfau, 1995).

Many messages rely on their logical or factual appeal. While such messages may carry academic weight, they often have little appeal to the general public. Further, it is widely accepted that knowledge alone is unlikely to change beliefs, attitudes and behaviour. Generating some kind of emotional response may make messages more effective. The emotions may be either positive or negative. Lewis et al. (2007) found that road safety advertisements which aroused emotion were judged by drivers to be more persuasive. Although negative fear appeals are frequently used in this context, they found that positive emotional appeals including humour can also have a role in promoting safe behaviour. Some caution may need to be exercised when using humour, as what appears funny to one person may be offensive to another. Nonetheless, the use of positive appeal, which makes people feel good about engaging in the behaviour in question, raises few ethical objections in contrast to the use of negative affect or fear appeal.

There are widely divergent views about the use of fear appeal as a means of persuading people to change their attitudes or behaviour. Fear is the negative emotional response to a perceived threat. The threat itself is the product of perceived susceptibility or vulnerability and the perceived severity of the threat (Witte and Allen, 2000).

Conventional wisdom has for some time regarded the use of fear appeal as ineffective or even counterproductive. This stems from the influential work of researchers such as Janis and Feshbach (1953), who found that high levels of fear were least likely to result in behaviour change. However, there seems to be more recent evidence that fear can correlate positively with both attitude and behaviour change (Hale and Dillard, 1995). A meta-analysis by Witte and Allen (2000) shows that strong fear appeal is more persuasive than weak. However, the relationship is complex. Fear can motivate acceptance of the message and action to reduce the threat to the individual – so-called adaptive responses. It can, alternatively, lead to maladaptive responses in which the message itself is rejected as a means of denying the perceived threat. Witte and Allen conclude that 'fear can be a great motivator provided individuals believe that they are able to take action to protect themselves' (2000, p. 607).

It is clearly unethical to scare people unless due attention is also paid to developing efficacy beliefs about the solution. These include the effectiveness of action to reduce the threat and, importantly, self-efficacy beliefs about the individual's ability to take action. Those using fear appeal should also ensure that people are aware of any necessary services or goods and that these are readily accessible. For example, it would be entirely inappropriate to raise concerns about the danger of not attending for breast screening if there are long waiting lists or access to clinics is difficult.

10.6 Audience factors

Communication involves the encoding of a message by the source, transmission to the recipient and subsequent decoding by the recipient. The format of the message may be verbal, written, pictorial or any combination and, if the message is delivered face to face, non-verbal communication will also be a factor. If communication has been successful, the recipient will decode the message as the source intended. However, over and above whether the audience actually understands the message, a range of factors will influence its acceptability and interpretation. At a general level these include culture, social norms, social class, educational attainment, age, gender and ethnicity.

It is crucially important to pre-test messages with the intended audience to ensure that they are properly interpreted and understood, and are acceptable and relevant. This includes the use of images. When printed material is being used, the literacy of the audience is a key consideration. Clearly, it is the responsibility of those involved in producing written materials to ensure that they are consistent with the reading ability of the target group. Checking the readability of print materials is an essential part of pre-testing.

A closer match between the message and audience characteristics may be achieved through targeting and tailoring. 'Targeting' involves designing the message to suit the characteristics of particular defined subgroups (for example, by age, gender or ethnicity) whereas 'tailoring' focuses on the requirements of individuals. It is rather like comparing mass-produced clothes with bespoke tailoring. Tailoring is defined as:

> Any combination of information or change strategies intended to reach one specific person, based on characteristics that are unique to that person, related to the outcome of interest, and have been derived from an individual assessment.
>
> (Kreuter and Skinner, 2000, p. 1)

Tailoring offers the opportunity to deliver highly personalised messages. For example, anti-smoking messages could be adjusted in line with an individual's position in the stages of change model (Prochaska and DiClemente, 1984) discussed in Chapter 6 (see Figure 6.2). Those at the pre-contemplation stage could be urged to consider giving up smoking whereas those who are already trying to give up could be encouraged to maintain their efforts. The messages could be further refined in relation to psychosocial variables, such as self-efficacy, locus of control, perceived risk, and so on. Kreuter et al. (2000) note that, to date, comparatively few variables have been used. They predict that this is likely to develop further and also include personal characteristics such as:

- gender
- age or generation
- cultural-based identity, values and beliefs
- literacy level
- learning style.

The key challenge, of course, is identifying which variables to use for the purpose of tailoring and acquiring relevant data on individuals. Furthermore, a balance will need to be struck between the level of sophistication and number of variables used (and the attendant increase in cost) and what is actually needed to increase the effectiveness of the communication.

The growth in electronic communication increases the potential for delivering tailored messages. Users of some online stores will be familiar with the personalised 'Welcome back' greeting and an offer of items to consider based on previous purchasing patterns. Similarly, health education messages could be designed to match individual profiles, including both their behaviour and their psychosocial attributes.

10.7 Channel

A range of channels of communication is available. The National Cancer Institute (undated) identifies the following main groups:

- interpersonal
- organisational
- community
- mass media
- interactive digital media.

Some allow the source to have personal contact with the audience whereas others require the message to be mediated through, for example, posters or leaflets. The advantage of face-to-face communication is that it is a two-way process that provides some feedback to the source about the audience's understanding of the message and whether it is effective. There is an opportunity to respond to queries and modify the original message. Such approaches are more appropriate when the message is complex and are more likely to be effective in changing attitudes and behaviour or in developing skills. However, face-to-face communication is limited to relatively small audiences and dissemination can therefore be slow. In contrast, mass media can achieve a much more rapid spread of information. Mass media is discussed more fully below.

In what ways do you think interactive digital media such as the internet increase opportunities for health communication?

Interactive digital media open up a plethora of new opportunities for health communication. The internet, for example, can be a valuable source of health information. A study for the Health Education Board for Scotland by Susan Soloman Scott Porter Research and Marketing (2002) explored young people's views about health information and the internet (see Box 10.2, page 296).

While there are some similarities between mass media and interactive digital media, there are also important differences. These include the latter's capacity for tailoring messages, as noted above, the active involvement of the audience using the medium, and, in some instances, the opportunity to engage in online dialogue.

Box 10.2 Health information and the internet – young people's needs

The following needs of young people using the internet were identified by Susan Soloman Scott Porter Research and Marketing (2002, p. 31):

- both general information and the opportunity for more personalized data
- information presented in a relatively basic way, providing the option for increased complexity, if required
- interactive facilities, offering feedback with regards to health topics, e.g. online doctors, e-mail facilities, games, tailored programmes, chatrooms
- clearly signposted as information aimed at young people
- reliant more on (colourful) visuals than text
- small amounts of information
- clear, simple language
- ideally, aimed at different life stages within youth, e.g. pre-puberty, post-puberty
- reassuring and professional in tone
- provided by a known and trusted, ideally public sector, source
- for personal, rather than educational consumption
- communicated as an enjoyable, informative experience, rather than relating to health problems
- clearly communicated as entirely confidential and trustworthy.

The use of mass media

The mass media have the clear advantage of being able to reach large groups of people. They may also be able to reach groups that are not accessible through interpersonal methods, such as widely dispersed rural groups. A variety of media can potentially be used as channels for delivering health-education messages, including television, radio, print media (such as newspapers, magazines, billboards, leaflets and mass mail shots) and, as noted above, the full range of modern electronic communication. The message itself may be delivered directly, for example contained in leaflets, posters or advertisements, or be the subject of news items or television programmes. Alternatively, messages may be integrated into drama programmes such as soap operas – so-called 'edutainment', which capitalises on the audience identifying with the characters.

The key question is: how effective are the mass media in achieving health goals? Confidence in their capacity to achieve change is frequently misplaced and derives from the view that the message can act like a 'magic bullet'. The 'direct effects' or 'hypodermic' model of mass communication sees the audience as entirely passive and assumes that:

- mass media have a direct effect on the audience
- mass media act like a hypodermic syringe – the message is injected into the audience and uniformly triggers the desired effect among its members
- if the desired result is not achieved, a bigger syringe is needed (i.e. more exposure to the message) and/or a more powerfully persuasive message (Green and Tones, 2010).

Mendelsohn (1968) graphically challenged this view by describing the mass-media delivery of messages as more like an aerosol spray – most of it misses or drifts away, a small amount hits the target and only a small proportion of this actually penetrates. The key task for health educators using mass media is to maximise that proportion.

Over and above any direct effects mass-media campaigns may have, they may also operate through more indirect routes. These include:

- increasing discussion about the health issue within social networks
- influencing social norms and the acceptability (or otherwise) of the behaviour in question
- the effect on policy change (Yanovitzky and Stryker, 2001; Wakefield et al., 2010).

Wellings and MacDowall (2000) distinguish two basic models: the 'risk factor model' in which mass media focuses on changing individual behaviour and the 'social diffusion model' in which it activates the forces for social change (see Chapter 6, Figure 6.3).

The use of mass media to achieve public health goals clearly requires some form of learning among the audience and in many instances behaviour change. However, the evidence indicates that while the media can be very effective in conveying information and raising awareness, they are much less effective in achieving more complex learning or behaviour change. The WHO (2002, p. 42) notes that newspapers, magazines, radio and television are often 'the most influential sources for everyday information on risks to health' in industrialised countries and that this influence is also increasing in low- and middle-income countries due to the rapid growth of the media and general improvement in levels of literacy. However, in order to achieve behaviour change, mass media need to be accompanied – supplemented – by other interventions.

 Why and how do you think mass media health messages may need to be supplemented?

Wakefield et al. (2010) make the point that exposure to the health education message is generally incidental to people's use of the media. Furthermore, the health education message may fail to stand out from the background 'clutter' of other material. It follows, therefore, that in order to stand out and grab the attention of the intended audience, the content and style of the message should be sufficiently striking. Similarly, any campaign should be of sufficient intensity and duration to reach a significant proportion of the target audience.

A review by Wakefield et al. (2010) found that mass media were more likely to be successful in changing behaviour when:

- coupled with multiple other interventions
- the behaviour is one-off or episodic (e.g. screening, or vaccination) rather than habitual or ongoing (e.g. food choices, physical activity)
- any services or products needed to change behaviour are readily accessible
- policies support change (e.g. no-smoking policies).

Conversely, barriers to success include marketing campaigns delivering competing messages, unsupportive social norms and the drive of addiction.

Briefing on the effectiveness of public health campaigns, the Health Development Agency (2004, pp. 3–4) concluded that the use of mass media is appropriate when:

- wide exposure is desired
- the timeframe is urgent
- public discussion is likely to facilitate the educational process

- awareness is a main goal
- media authorities are 'on-side'
- accompanying back-up can be provided on the ground
- long-term follow-up is possible
- a generous budget exists
- the behavioural goal is simple
- the agenda includes public relations.

A characteristic of mass communication is that it is generally a one-way process with no opportunity for interpersonal contact and instant feedback. It is therefore not possible to adjust the message in response to the audience's reaction. Furthermore, communicating to large audiences means that the message cannot be tailored to suit individual needs. Considerable attention therefore needs to be given to ensuring that the message is appropriate. The design of the message should be based on a sound understanding of the audience characteristics and ideally involve them in the design process. As noted above, pre-testing is essential for all health communication, but it is particularly so for mass-media communication.

Social marketing offers a highly systematic approach to planning campaigns to promote health and this can usefully be applied to the stages in the development of mass-media campaigns. However, before moving on to consider the various elements of social marketing, this section concludes by briefly considering the two further ways in which mass media can influence public health: as a channel for advocacy and through its more incidental effects on health.

Media advocacy

Mass communication traditionally aims to achieve changes in individual attitudes and behaviour or the social norms that would support such change. However, it also has considerable potential for contributing to environmental, social and political change through media advocacy. 'Media advocacy' has been defined as 'the strategic use of media (usually the news media) to shape public opinion, mobilize community activists, and influence decision makers to create a change in policy' (The Health Communication Unit, 2000, p. 1). It moves the focus from 'the health behaviour of individuals to the behaviour of the policymakers whose decisions structure the environment in which people act' (Wallack and Dorfman, 1996, p. 293). It therefore involves changing the way a message is presented – so-called shifting the frame

– from personal to social responsibility. For example, encouraging pedestrians to cross roads safely frames road safety as an individual-behaviour issue whereas restricting the speed of traffic in residential areas re-frames it as a social responsibility.

Media advocacy has been variously interpreted. Stead et al. (2002) note that for some it is essentially a bottom-up approach that enables community groups to put pressure on those with the power to achieve policy or environmental change. For others – depending on the cause – it can additionally be a top-down approach used by public health authorities or professional associations to advocate for change. A guide produced by the International Council of Nurses (2008) identified three strategies for gaining access to the media: paying for it, asking for it or earning it. Media advocacy generally relies on the last and 'earns it' by using a whole range of strategies to attract media attention, particularly the news media (see Chapman and Lupton, 1994).

As well as getting the message directly across to powerful elites, the mass media has an important role in setting the public agenda. Media can also contribute to raising awareness and developing a groundswell of public opinion, which policy makers would be unwise to ignore. Media advocacy is essentially empowering because it gives communities a voice (Wallack, 1998).

Interactive digital media can also be hugely influential. The power of social networking sites and mobile phones to mobilise communities around a cause was witnessed, for example, in the 2011 uprising in Egypt.

Mass media as an environmental influence

Discussion has focused so far on the intended and planned use of mass media. Mass media can also have incidental positive and negative effects on health. Positive influences include exposure to positive role models and norms. Negative influences include the marketing of unhealthy products, such as 'junk food', and the portrayal of health-damaging behaviour that may have a direct effect on individuals and contribute to shaping social norms. For example, Hansen's (2003) analysis of British prime-time television found all the drama programmes and 92.6 per cent of soap operas included some reference to alcohol. Furthermore, because alcohol consumption generally formed the backdrop to the foreground story line, it became normalised as a frequent and common aspect of social interaction. Resistance to this type of influence will be improved by individuals having a good level of media literacy, including the skills to deconstruct these pervasive messages and identify any underlying motives. Codes of practice have been developed in relation to the advertising of products such as junk food and alcohol. However, controlling the more subtle background influences is challenging. Defoe and Breed (1989) have called for collaborative consultation between health promoters and programmers to achieve a responsible approach to programming.

Learning and empowerment: the importance of process

Communication can be about relatively trivial concerns, such as social pleasantries or day-to-day information. However, from the health-education perspective its purpose is to achieve some change in knowledge, beliefs, values, attitudes, skills or behaviour; that is, to achieve some learning. In line with the maxim 'I hear and I forget, I see and I remember, I do and I understand', approaches that require the active involvement of the audience are more likely to achieve learning – especially if the learning is complex and involves the acquisition of skills. The use of such participatory methods is favoured in situations that provide the opportunity for groups of people to work together over a period of time. Examples of methods that encourage participation include games, simulations, role play, group work, problem solving and community research projects.

Communication may also be either disempowering or empowering. What are the characteristics of empowering communication?

Communication that assumes that the learner has nothing to contribute or reinforces dependency of the learner on the teacher will undermine empowerment. Green and Tones (2010) identify the importance of process as well as content and particularly the contribution of participation to both achieving empowerment and maximising learning. Importantly, they note the need to recognise and respect the prior learning and experience of the learner rather than merely regarding them as empty vessels to be filled with knowledge. This shifts the role of the 'teacher' from expert to facilitator. Rather than informing, telling or advising, the facilitator will question, draw out, listen, reflect and clarify. The power relationship will also shift from top–down to one of mutual respect, which acknowledges the contribution of all and the potential of all to learn from the interaction. Clearly, such approaches are more likely to contribute to empowerment by building the general attributes of self-esteem, self-confidence and general health and life skills alongside addressing specific health issues.

Process is central to Freirian approaches to emancipatory education referred to earlier in this chapter (Freire, 1972). Freire is critical of traditional top-down education – referred to as 'banking' – which is seen to reinforce existing political structures and power relations. In contrast, Freirian pedagogy uses problem-posing techniques that encourage people to reflect critically on the world around them. Informal groups, known as culture circles, are presented with pictures, words or other triggers to stimulate dialogue that reflects on reality, searches for root problems and the implications of alternative courses of action. The cycle of reflection and action to achieve change is referred to as 'praxis'.

Fundamental to the approach is respect for the individual and their capacity to tackle oppressive structures and achieve change.

10.8 Social marketing for health

Social marketing is generally held to have its roots in Wiebe's (1952, p. 679) question, 'Why can't you sell brotherhood like you sell soap?' Or, to loosely paraphrase: why can't you use marketing principles to sell health-enhancing behaviour rather than products that damage health? Kotler et al. (2002, pp. 19–20) define social marketing as:

> the use of marketing principles and techniques to influence a target audience to voluntarily accept, reject, modify or abandon a behaviour for the benefit of individuals, groups, or society as a whole.

They identify the main strategies for changing behaviour as communication, education and economic measures and emphasise the voluntary aspect. However, they do not preclude the use of legislation as a last resort.

French and Blair-Stevens (2010, p. 36) note that the core characteristics of social marketing are a 'robust understanding and insight into the customer, and a clear focus on achieving and sustaining specific behaviours.' They review a number of definitions to pick out the key features:

- it is primarily concerned with achieving social good
- it focuses on behaviour
- it makes use of all forms of marketing
- understanding the target audience is of central importance.

French (2010, pp. 13–14) offers a technical definition of social marketing as:

> a highly systematic approach to social improvement that sets out unambiguous success criteria in terms of behavioural change alongside thorough and transparent planning about how to achieve it.

Stead et al. (2007) argue that social marketing is not a theory in itself, but a framework or structure. It does not rely simply on the application of marketing principles but draws from a number of bodies of knowledge including psychology, sociology, anthropology and communication theory. The main features of a social marketing approach to achieving behavioural goals are set out in Box 10.3.

Box 10.3 Main features of a social marketing approach

A consumer orientation that is concerned with understanding the consumer, what motivates them and what influences their behaviour within their own social context.

Exchange as the mechanism through which social marketing operates. In commercial marketing, goods are exchanged for money. In social marketing, the 'goods' are ideas or behaviour and the 'cost' to the consumer is assessed in terms of time, energy, loss of pleasure, and so on. Benefits may be either tangible or intangible. For example, walking rather than using a car will produce the tangible benefits of improved fitness and reduction in expenditure on fuel. It will also produce the intangible benefit of reduction in carbon emission. In order to be effective the cost-benefit ratio should be perceived as beneficial by the consumer.

Audience segmentation into groups that share key characteristics. This allows messages to be designed to appeal to specific groups and meet their needs.

Channel analysis to identify which channels are most likely to be successful in getting the message across to the intended target group.

Understanding the competition such as the marketing of 'unhealthy' products (e.g. alcohol, tobacco, junk food). It would also include external factors competing for time and attention and internal factors such as habit or addiction (National Social Marketing Centre, 2006).

Marketing mix which classically involves the four 'P's – product, price, place, promotion.

Understanding the marketing mix

In terms of 'product', there is the behaviour itself, which Kotler et al. (2002) refer to as the actual product. The core products are the associated benefits and the augmented products are the services or objects that are required to engage in the behaviour. Behaviour change is more likely to occur if the product appears attractive to the consumer, is accessible and the benefits are tangible. 'Price' may include some actual financial cost for the consumer, but is more likely to involve social and psychological cost. 'Place' in social marketing is generally held to be where the behaviour in question will be performed or services accessed. However, it is also sometimes used to refer to where the consumer can be reached. 'Promotion' is used to communicate what the benefits of the product are and information about availability.

Using a mix of intervention or marketing methods is more likely to be successful in changing behaviour than reliance on single methods. French and Blair-Stevens (2010) identify five primary intervention domains that should be considered to achieve an appropriate combination. These are:

- design – to alter the environment
- inform – to communicate facts and attitudes
- control – to regulate and enforce
- educate – to enable and empower
- service – to provide support services.

In order to establish some consistency about what constitutes social marketing and achieve better understanding of its basic principles, French and Blair-Stevens (2006) developed benchmark criteria based on Andreasen (2002). These include an emphasis on using behavioural theories, a customer focus, segmentation and research to identify 'actionable insights' that can shape interventions; understanding the competition, both for attention and influence on people's behavioural intentions; and considering the costs and benefits associated with adopting and maintaining the new behaviour. They also recognise the need for a mix of methods to bring about behaviour change.

In its early days, the focus of social marketing was principally on behavioural goals. The systematic application of social marketing processes provided the operational means for achieving them. This has therefore been referred to as 'operational social marketing' (French and Blair-Stevens, 2010). Because of its essentially downstream focus, social marketing, like the preventive model of health education, was open to criticisms of victim-blaming. Latterly, its strategic potential has begun to be recognised. Strategic social marketing can 'inform and enhance strategic discussions, and guide policy development and intervention option identification' (National Social Marketing Centre, 2006, p. 41). Up until now, the target has also principally been members of the public or communities, but it could equally be policy makers and professionals – in effect, reiterating the argument set out at the beginning of this chapter about the broader potential of health education.

What similarities and differences do you see between health education and social marketing?

Although they have separate origins, there has been considerable confluence between social marketing and health education and promotion. This raises a number of questions about social marketing for those working in public health and those commissioning services.

- Is it an alternative to health education/promotion?
- Is it a set of tools for use by health educators/promoters and those working in public health?
- Does it provide a complementary approach to health education/promotion?
- Is it just a re-badging of health education/promotion?

Scriven (2009) also questions whether it is a political diversion from tackling the socioeconomic determinants of health that would require an altogether more radical approach.

Clearly, there are technical lessons that can be derived from social marketing's highly systematised approach to achieving behavioural goals. These include:

- systematic planning
- understanding the determinants of behaviour
- understanding the audience and its motivations
- developing messages that tap into the audience's motivations
- pre-testing all materials.

Nonetheless, French and Blair-Stevens (2010, p. 30) claim that social marketing is more than simply a 'campaign development tool'; it brings a particular 'mindset' that informs the whole approach and way of working.

While there are undoubted similarities between health education and social marketing, there are also clear differences – especially if an empowerment model of health education is considered. A key issue is who decides which behavioural goals to tackle. Despite Lefebre and Flora's (1988) assertion that social marketing should address clients' needs, behavioural goals are frequently paternalistically defined. An empowerment model of health education, in contrast, enables individuals and communities to define their own health goals and achieve control over their own health.

The promise of social marketing to achieve behavioural targets and deliver 'measurable return on investment' (French, 2010, p. 14) has undoubtedly contributed to its popularity with government (DoH, 2008), those commissioning health services and managers responsible for achieving defined targets. It is also ideologically consistent with the thinking of liberal market economies. French (2009) attributed its rapid growth in England to an increasing understanding of what is involved in behaviour change and the close match between this and what social marketing can deliver. It also offered governments:

- an alternative to existing public health approaches, which were judged unlikely to achieve targets
- a solution to accusations of being a 'nanny state' through its focus on customers and contribution to developing joint responsibility.

However, public health practitioners have been more resistant to accepting the market philosophy on which it is based.

Buchanan et al. (1994, p. 53) are critical of the 'encroachment of technical and economic models of reasoning into social and political spheres of human experience.' They argue that social marketing's central tenet of exchange undermines the relationship between health professionals and the public. It results in the relationship being based on the pursuit of self interests by both parties with the risk of breakdown if poor cost-benefit ratios are perceived by either. It can also degenerate into a manipulative relationship in which the use of any means could potentially be justified on the basis of achieving desired ends. Ideologically, this would contrast starkly with an empowerment model, where the interaction is based on respect and mutual trust; the means are as important as the ends; and the end is empowerment rather than defined behavioural goals.

Griffiths et al. (2008) discussed the relationship between social marketing and health promotion and noted that while there are points of distinction, there is a core that is common to both (see Figure 10.2, page 308). They conclude that they offer complementary strengths:

> By coming together, specialised health promotion and social marketing for health can ensure that health improvement strategies and practice are as effective as they possibly can be.
>
> (Griffiths et al., 2008, p. 3)

The contribution of social marketing is held to be its focus on understanding people's lives and what motivates them; the systematic approach described above; and clearly defining and segmenting the audience. Specialised health promotion is characterised as bringing a rich theoretical tradition and a philosophy grounded in empowerment. It recognises the need to focus on inequality and address power differentials and also the importance of community engagement and building social capital.

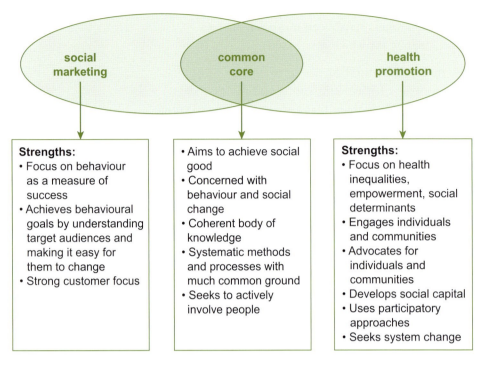

social marketing	common core	health promotion
Strengths: • Focus on behaviour as a measure of success • Achieves behavioural goals by understanding target audiences and making it easy for them to change • Strong customer focus	• Aims to achieve social good • Concerned with behaviour and social change • Coherent body of knowledge • Systematic methods and processes with much common ground • Seeks to actively involve people	**Strengths:** • Focus on health inequalities, empowerment, social determinants • Engages individuals and communities • Advocates for individuals and communities • Develops social capital • Uses participatory approaches • Seeks system change

Figure 10.2 Social marketing and health promotion compared

(Source: adapted from Griffiths et al., 2008)

The guide for commissioners on promoting health and wellbeing states:

> The commissioning of effective programmes to promote health and well-being will engage, empower and mobilise people to:
>
> ○ Implement structural solutions that help to make the healthier choices the easier choices, for example through making healthy food easily available, or developing social support networks;
>
> ○ Support them to change their behaviour if they wish.
>
> (Shircore, 2009, p. 9)

It goes on to say that social marketing and health-promotion programmes should be commissioned in an integrated way. Health education is not specifically mentioned. However, it is the health-education component of social marketing or health promotion that is the fundamental driver for achieving change – whether it be behaviour, empowerment or policy change.

Conclusion

Health education can play a part that goes well beyond its capacity to influence behaviour. It has a role in individual and community empowerment, professional development, policy development and, most radically, social change. In doing so, it must pay due regard to ethical principles – notably voluntarism and empowerment.

The design of health-education initiatives should draw on communication theory, be grounded in empirical research and make reference to psychosocial theory, which can identify key messages and target groups. Well-designed mass-media campaigns can raise public awareness and achieve simple behavioural goals, but more complex change requires supplementation by other interventions and personal interaction. Social marketing offers a highly systematic approach to achieving behaviour change. However, the broader scope of health education – particularly an empowerment model of health education – is needed to engage people and enable individuals and communities to achieve control over their health and health choices.

References

Andreasen, A. (2002) 'Marketing social marketing in the social change marketplace', *Journal of Public Policy and Marketing*, vol. 21, no. 1, pp. 3–13.

Bandura, A. (1986) *Social Foundations of Thought and Action: A Social Cognitive Theory*, Englewood Cliffs, New Jersey, Prentice-Hall.

Bandura, A. (1982) 'Self-efficacy mechanism in human agency', *American Psychologist*, vol. 37, no. 2, pp. 122–47.

Becker, M.H. (ed.) (1984) *The Health Belief Model and Personal Health Behavior*, Thorofare, New Jersey, Charles B. Slack.

Behavioural Insight Team (2010) *Applying Behavioural Insight to Health*, London, Cabinet Office. Available at: www.cabinetoffice.gov.uk/resource-library/applying-behavioural-insight-health (accessed 3 September 2011).

Buchanan, D.R., Reddy, S. and Hossain, Z. (1994) 'Social marketing: a critical appraisal', *Health Promotion International*, vol. 9, no. 1, pp. 49–57.

Chapman, S. and Lupton, D. (1994) *The Fight for Public Health: Principles and Practice of Media Advocacy*, London, BMJ Publishing Group.

Curtis, A. (2010) 'From pigeon to superman and back' in Adam Curtis – The Medium and the Message (blog on the BBC website). Available at: www.bbc.co.uk/blogs/adamcurtis/2010/11/ (accessed 3 September 2011).

Defoe, J.R. and Breed, W.R. (1989) 'Consulting to change media contents: two cases in alcohol education', *International Quarterly of Community Health Education*, vol. 9, pp. 257–72.

Department of Health (DoH) (2010) *Healthy Lives, Healthy People: Our Strategy for Public Health in England* (Cmnd 7985), London, The Stationery Office. Available at: www.dh.gov.uk/en/Publicationsandstatistics/Publications/PublicationsPolicyAndGuidance/DH_121941 (accessed 3 September 2011).

Department of Health (DoH) (2008) *Ambitions for Health*, London, Department of Health. Available at: www.dh.gov.uk/prod_consum_dh/groups/dh_digitalassets/documents/digitalasset/dh_086289.pdf (accessed 3 September 2011).

Freire, P. (1972) *Pedagogy of the Oppressed*, Harmondsworth, Penguin.

French, J. (2010) 'The case for social marketing' in French, J., Blair-Stevens, C., McVey, D. and Merritt, R. (eds) *Social Marketing and Public Health: Theory and Practice*, Oxford, Oxford University Press, pp. 1–18.

French, J. (2009) 'The nature, development and contribution of social marketing to public health practice since 2004 in England', *Perspectives in Public Health*, vol. 129, pp. 262–67.

French, L. and Blair-Stevens, C. (2010) 'Key concepts and principles of social marketing' in French, J., Blair-Stevens, C., McVey, D. and Merritt, R. (eds) *Social Marketing and Public Health: Theory and Practice*, Oxford, Oxford University Press, pp. 29–44.

French, J. and Blair-Stevens, C. (2006) *Social Marketing Benchmark Criteria*, London, The National Social Marketing Centre. Available at: http://thensmc. com/sites/default/files/benchmark-criteria-090910.pdf (accessed 3 September 2011).

Green, L.W. and Kreuter, M.W. (1999) *Health Promotion Planning: An Educational and Ecological Approach* (3rd edition), Mountain View, California, Mayfield.

Green, J. and Tones, K. (2010) *Health Promotion Planning and Strategies* (2nd edition), London, Sage.

Griffiths, J., Blair-Stevens, C. and Thorpe, A. (2008) *Social Marketing for Health and Specialised Health Promotion: Stronger Together – Weaker Apart. A Paper for Debate*, London, Royal Society for Public Health and The National Social Marketing Centre. Available at: http://thensmc.com/sites/default/files/ Social_marketing_for_public_health_and_specialised_health_promotion_sum-mary.pdf (accessed 3 September 2011).

Hale, J.L. and Dillard, J.P. (1995) 'Fear appeals in health promotion campaigns: too much, too little, or just right?' in Maibach, E. and Parrott, R.L. (eds) *Designing Health Messages*, Thousand Oaks, California, Sage, pp. 65–80.

Hansen, A. (2003) *The Portrayal of Alcohol and Alcohol Consumption in Television News and Drama Programmes*, London, Alcohol Concern.

Health Development Agency (2004) 'The effectiveness of public health campaigns', *HDA Briefing No. 7*, London, Health Development Agency. Available at: www.nice.org.uk/niceMedia/documents/CHB7-campaigns-14-7. pdf (accessed 3 September 2011).

Hovland, C.I., Janis, I.L. and Kelley, H.H. (1953) *Communication and Persuasion*, New Haven, Connecticut, Yale University Press.

Hubley, J. (1993) *Communicating Health: An Action Guide to Health Education and Health Promotion*, London, Macmillan.

International Council of Nurses (2008) *Promoting Health: Advocacy Guide for Health Professionals*, Geneva, International Council of Nurses. Available at: www. whpa.org/PPE_Advocacy_Guide.pdf (accessed 3 September 2011).

Janis, I.L. and Feshback, S. (1953) 'Effects of fear-arousing communications', *Journal of Abnormal and Social Psychology*, vol. 48, no. 1, pp. 78–92.

Kotler, P., Roberto, N. and Lee, N. (2002) *Social Marketing: Improving the Quality of Life*, Thousand Oaks, California, Sage.

Kreuter, M., Farrell, D., Olevitch, L. and Brennan, L. (2000) *Tailoring Health Messages: Customising Communication with Computer Technology*, Mahwah, New Jersey, Lawrence Erlbaum Associates.

Kreuter, M.W. and Skinner, C.S. (2000) 'Tailoring: what's in a name?' (editorial), *Health Education Research*, vol. 15, no. 1, pp. 1–4.

Lefebre, R.C. and Flora, J.A. (1988) 'Social marketing and public health intervention', *Health Education and Behavior*, vol. 15, no. 3, pp. 299–315.

Lewis, I.M., Watson, B., White, K.M. and Tay, R. (2007) 'Promoting public health messages: should we move beyond fear-evoking appeals in road safety?', *Qualitative Health Research*, vol. 17, no. 1, pp. 61–74.

Marmot, M. (2010) *Fair Society, Healthy Lives: A Strategic Review of Health Inequalities in England Post-2010 (The Marmot Review)*, London, University College. Available at: www.marmotreview.org/AssetLibrary/pdfs/Reports/FairSocietyHealthyLives.pdf (accessed 3 September 2011).

Marteau, T.M., Ogilvie, D., Roland, M., Suhrcke, M., Kelly, M.P. (2011) 'Judging nudging: can nudging improve population health?', *British Medical Journal*, vol. 342, no. 228, pp. 263–5.

McGuire, G. (1989) 'Theoretical foundations of campaigns' in Rice, R.E. and Atkin, C.K. (eds) *Public Communication Campaigns* (2nd edition), Newbury Park, California, Sage, pp. 42–65.

Mendelsohn, H. (1968) 'Which shall it be? Mass education or mass persuasion for health?', *American Journal of Public Health*, vol. 58, pp. 131–7.

Milburn, K. (1995) 'A critical review of peer education with young people with special reference to sexual health', *Health Education Research*, vol. 10, no. 4, pp. 407–20.

National Cancer Institute (undated) *Pink Book – Making Health Communication Programs Work*, Bethesda, National Cancer Institute. Available at: www.cancer.gov/pinkbook (accessed 3 September 2011).

National Health Service Scotland (undated) *West of Scotland Cancer Awareness Project Bowel Cancer Campaign*, London, Cancer Research UK. Available at: http://info.cancerresearchuk.org/prod_consump/groups/cr_common//@nre/@hea/documents/generalcontent/cr_044433.pdf (accessed 3 September 2011).

National Social Marketing Centre (2006) *It's Our Health (Summary Report)*, London, National Social Marketing Centre.

Nuffield Council on Bioethics (2007) *Public Health: Ethical Issues*, London, Nuffield Council on Bioethics. Available at: http://nuffieldbioethics.org/sites/default/files/Public%20health%20-%20ethical%20issues.pdf (accessed 3 September 2011).

Nutbeam, D. (2000) 'Health literacy as a public health goal: a challenge for contemporary health education and communication strategies into the 21st century', *Health Promotion International*, vol. 15, no. 3, pp. 259–67.

Nutbeam, D. (1998) 'Health promotion glossary', *Health Promotion International*, vol. 13, no. 4, pp. 349–64.

Pfau, M. (1995) 'Designing messages for behavioural inoculation' in Maibach, E. and Parrott, R.L. (eds) *Designing Health Messages*, Thousand Oaks, California, Sage.

Prochaska, J.O. and DiClimente, C.C. (1984) *The Trans-theoretical Approach: Crossing Traditional Boundaries of Therapy*, Homewood, Illinois, Dow Jones Irwin.

Rogers, E.M. and Shoemaker, F.F. (1971) *Communication of Innovations*, New York, The Free Press.

Rotter, J.B. (1966) 'Generalized expectancies for internal versus external control of reinforcement', *Psychological Monographs*, vol. 80, no. 1, pp. 1–28.

Ryan, W. (1976) *Blaming the Victim*, New York, Vintage Books.

Scriven, A. (2009) 'Social marketing: a toolkit, a profession or a political diversion?', *Perspectives in Public Health*, vol. 129, p. 242.

Shircore, R. (2009) *Guide for World Class Commissioners Promoting Health and Well-Being: Reducing Inequalities*, London, Royal Society for Public Health and The National Social Marketing Centre.

Stead, M., Gordon, R., Angus, K. and McDermott, L. (2007) 'A systematic review of social marketing effectiveness', *Health Education*, vol. 107, no. 2, pp. 126–91.

Stead, M., Hastings, G. and Eadie, D. (2002) 'The challenge of evaluating complex interventions: a framework for evaluating media advocacy', *Health Education Research*, vol. 17, no. 3, pp. 351–64.

Susan Soloman Scott Porter Research and Marketing (2002) *Young People, Health and the Internet: A Needs Assessment*, Edinburgh, Health Education Board for Scotland. Available at: www.healthscotland.com/uploads/documents/RE03520012002Final.pdf (accessed 3 September 2011).

Thaler, R.H. and Sunstein, C.R. (2009) *Nudge: Improving Decisions About Health, Wealth and Happiness*, London, Penguin Books.

The Health Communication Unit (2000) *Media Advocacy Workbook*, Toronto, Health Communication Unit. Available at: www.thcu.ca/resource_db/pubs/497736921.pdf (accessed 3 September 2011).

Tilford, S., Green, J. and Tones, K. (2003) *Values, Health Promotion and Public Health*, Leeds, Centre for Health Promotion Research, Leeds Metropolitan University.

Tones, K. (2002) 'Health literacy: new wine in old bottles?', *Health Education Research*, vol. 17, no. 3, pp. 287–90.

Tones, K. and Tilford, S. (2001) *Health Promotion: Effectiveness, Efficiency and Equity* (3rd edition), London, Nelson Thornes.

Wakefield, M.A., Loken, B. and Hornik, R.C. (2010) 'Use of mass media campaigns to change health behaviour', *The Lancet*, vol. 376, pp. 1261–71.

Wallack, L. (1998) 'Media advocacy: a strategy for empowering people and communities' in Minkler, M. (ed.) *Community Organizing and Community Building for Health*, New Brunswick, Rutgers University Press.

Wallack, L. and Dorfman, L. (1996) 'Media advocacy: a strategy for advancing policy and promoting health', *Health Education and Behavior*, vol. 23, no. 3, pp. 293–317.

Wellings, K. and Macdowall, W. (2000) 'Evaluating mass media approaches to health promotion', *Health Education*, vol. 100, no. 1, pp. 23–32.

Wiebe, G. (1952) 'Merchandising commodities and citizenship on television', *Public Opinion Quarterly*, vol. 15, pp. 679–91.

Witte, K. and Allen, M. (2000) 'A meta-analysis of fear appeals: implications for effective public health campaigns', *Health Education and Behavior*, vol. 27, no. 5, pp. 591–615.

World Health Organization (WHO) (1986) *Ottawa Charter for Health Promotion. First International Conference on Health Promotion, Ottawa 17–21 November*, Copenhagen, World Health Organization Regional Office for Europe. Available at: www.who.int/hpr/NPH/docs/ottawa_charter_hp.pdf (accessed 3 September 2011).

World Health Organization (WHO) (2002) 'Perceiving risks' in *World Health Report 2002 – Reducing Risks Promoting Healthy Life*, Geneva, World Health Organization, pp. 27–46. Available at: www.who.int/whr/2002/en/whr02_en.pdf (accessed 3 September 2011).

Yanovitzky, I. and Stryker, J. (2001) 'Mass media, social norms, and health promotion efforts: a longitudinal study of media effects on youth binge drinking', *Communication Research*, vol. 28, no. 2, pp. 208–39.

Chapter 11: Working at the local level

Jane Springett

Introduction

For the majority of public health practitioners, most public health work is done at the local level. Indeed, localism, seen as giving power to local authorities and local communities, was a key feature in 2010 of the English White Paper on public health (Department of Health [DoH], 2010). In other UK nations local involvement in decisions and initiatives related to their health is also seen as increasingly important. However, while public services are locally delivered and most agencies that contribute to the health of the population consider themselves to operate at local level, in practice agencies operate at many levels and against agendas that often do not lend themselves to the reality of communities and the way they live. This makes public health practice at the local level a complex process that involves not only working across sectors and engaging with activists and agencies beyond the healthcare sector, but also often simultaneously acting and networking at a number of levels. Most of all, it means working with local people directly.

This chapter focuses on how you work and who you work with, suggesting that this depends very much on context. There is no one formula for change. Indeed, the mistake of public health in the past has been to see action for health as a standardised administrative sequential process whereby issues are identified by statistical analysis, projects are developed based on 'evidence', outputs are specified and then local workers engage and organise local people towards the previously designated end and previously specified 'intervention'. This rather naïve approach ignores the complexity of engaging people in a process of personal and collective change. The greatest potential for change is through community-driven initiatives that create action from the bottom-up, while at the same time acting on those factors for which there are levers within the broader local context.

11.1 Going local: who should we be working with?

Defining 'local' and understanding 'community'

Different professions and agencies have their own definition of 'local', and the concept of 'community' is also highly contested and difficult to define (Jewkes and Murcott, 1996). Public agencies tend to rely on official data or ad hoc surveys to define and identify communities (see Table 11.1). Given the tendency for poor, excluded and marginalised people not to fill in questionnaires or respond to surveys, their voices are often not heard (Mander, 2010).

Moreover, people operate at different levels and in different social spaces depending on their access to resources, their background, the length of time they have lived in a place and their daily pattern of living. How they live will be constrained by the opportunities they have access to and their physical, social and economic environment, which is itself partly defined by history and geography (Popay et al., 2003). Social relationships become embedded over a period of time, but some areas will constitute a myriad of different and transitional communities due to the transitional nature of an immigrant population. Community identity emerges from the interplay of these different factors, many of which are related to the inherent inequalities in society. Where a population group shares a similar illness experience, they may form a community around their shared experience. But more often community, where it exists, will come from collective memories and the shared experiences of day-to-day living, whether it is a common experience of crime and drug violence or the local children's centre. So a community is not necessarily a geographical neighbourhood; it might be a collective identity around class, ethnicity, race, age, gender, etc.

Table 11.1 Definitions of community generated within health work

Definition of community	Examples
Geographical	A particular and clearly demarcated population
Shared characteristics	Young unemployed men; lone mothers
Communities of interest	People from minority ethnic groups
A numerically defined community	A census aggregate
An administrative area	The population within a health board/PCT
An at-risk group	Men who smoke and have high cholesterol
A GP's list	A practice population

(Source: adapted from Emmel and Conn, 2004)

What do you think the definitions in Table 11.1 fail to capture about the nature of 'community' as discussed above?

Table 11.1 offers some commonsense and useful definitions of 'community' but does not capture the social relationships and living patterns noted above. Communities are complex and take many forms and sensitivity to these issues must lie at the heart of public health practice. Communities are defined by a sense of identification and shared emotional connection, common symbol systems, shared values and norms, mutual influence, common interests and commitment to meeting shared needs (Diez-Roux, 2001; Bridger and Alter, 2006). Communities of identity may be geographically bound or be a geographically dispersed group with a common identity and fate. Furthermore, places contain many different and overlapping communities of identity. It is important either to identify and work with existing micro-communities of identity or work to strengthen a sense of community through collective engagement, while at the same time recognising that there may be benefits in drawing on the skills and resources that exist outside the immediate community of identity (Harris and Young, 2009).

This is not just about cultural competence but also about recognising the interwoven fabric of the multiple sites of deprivation and the social politics of marginalised people within society. Many so-called communities are inherently dysfunctional. Local leaders may hold power that they do not wish to give up or the patterns of social control have led to an inherent tribalism that makes intergenerational interaction or intercommunity engagement difficult (Ledwith, 2011). All these issues impact on a population's ability to engage in any public health activity or intervention.

Skills to support local public health work

An important element of working locally is to understand the complexities of who you are working with. This involves using a process of critical inquiry to explore together the complexities, assets and needs that the community possesses. Then, through listening and dialogue, what that group identifies as the key local issues can be drawn out. Some aspects of assessing need are discussed in Chapter 9, Section 9.4.

Public health action at the local level can involve acting as an advocate, a popular educator, a facilitator and a networker. It also means seeing the everyday world in a more critical light and helping others to do so as well. Box 11.1 sets out some of the skills used to build sustainable change at local level. Whether you are a health professional who wants to address obesity, a social activist who is concerned with the health of a particular marginalised group or a local authority employee who wants to increase the opportunities for physical activity, working locally is not just about your knowledge. It is as much about how you think and act in the world, the principles and values that underpin that thinking and acting, and the degree to which you incorporate critical reflection into your everyday practice.

Box 11.1 Skills and knowledge to support change at the local level

- Interpersonal skills: listening and dialogical skills, and facilitation
- Flexibility
- Critical analysis and reflexivity
- Knowledge of groups and group behaviour
- Understanding and working with power; managing conflict
- Popular education skills

Jones (1996) poses some useful questions that everyone working at a local level should ask of themselves.

- Whose reality counts?
- Whose knowledge counts?
- Whose criteria and values count?
- Whose appraisal counts?
- Whose analysis counts?
- Whose plans count?
- Whose monitoring and evaluation count?

The way in which you work is as important as what you work on. It is about putting local people at the heart of the health-development agenda and about being aware of the barriers and constraints you will have to work with and get round to achieve change. As a wise Chinese philosopher commented:

Go to the people. Live with them. Learn from them. Love them. Start with what they know. Build with what they have. But with the best leaders, when the work is done, the task accomplished, the people will say 'We have done this ourselves'.

(Lao Tzu, 600 BC)

Engaging local stakeholders

Most action for health requires operating at a number of levels at once and where you are located within the system can affect your ability to effect change and the level at which you need to advocate for change (Berkeley and Springett, 2006). For example, community health workers who support individuals to increase their physical activity will work alongside planners and others who make decisions about the physical environment that can impede or enhance a person's ability to make a daily healthy choice (Boyle et al., 2009). They need to influence not just the individuals but also their colleagues to prioritise health. Working to reduce obesity through healthy-eating programmes will only have an impact (or attract interest) if the levels of deprivation within an entire neighbourhood are addressed, for example through action on poverty or access to affordable shops.

Addressing the determinants of health locally requires the collective action of a range of different stakeholders. Bringing those stakeholders together and then getting them to accept their role in the generation of action to address health issues is an important challenge for the public health practitioner. One way forward is to explore the workings of a local health system (all the parts that deliver services) through a process of 'systems lens' analysis. This involves identifying key problems and generating a sense of urgency to find solutions. While there has been an increasing call for a systems approach to problem solving, there remain a number of institutional and professional barriers to operating in this way. Accountability issues within the public sector often limit the scope to operate in areas that are not recognised as the precise domain of a particular service or department. Competition for funding and the need to demonstrate outcomes in short-time horizons also impede progress. Top-down priorities change, either because of a change of minister or because of local political change. In addition, the effectiveness of partnership working between organisations in terms of health outcomes has yet to be established (Smith et al., 2009).

One way of engaging local stakeholders is to link health to wider cultural and social agendas. Health is increasingly becoming a useful banner under which to get people together to address some of the more intractable problems facing society. For example, in Liverpool a 2020 Decade of Health and Wellbeing has been adopted as an overarching local policy agenda. It brings together a wide range of stakeholders and organisations, including creative arts groups, to support people's health (see Box 11.2).

Box 11.2 Liverpool's 2020 Decade of Health and Wellbeing

In 2010 Liverpool celebrated a Year of Health and Wellbeing during which 2000 people took a pledge to 'lead a healthier life'. The Liverpool Primary Care Trust, Liverpool City Council and a range of other bodies work together to respond to evidence highlighting poor mental health. Forty-six grass roots organisations received a collective £200,000 to develop innovative approaches to improve mental health, including arts events, walking and language courses. Brazilian drumming sessions were among the activities on offer. Health and wellbeing was linked to transport, education, business and housing agendas.

In January 2011 Liverpool launched its 2020 Decade of Health and Wellbeing as an over-arching local policy agenda. The mantra associated with this initiative is, 'Connect, Be active, Take notice, Keep learning, Give.'

(Adapted from Liverpool Primary Care Trust and Liverpool City Council, 2010)

Initiatives such as Liverpool 2020 tap into people's instinctive understanding of health as something that encompasses all aspects of their lives. This can provide public health practitioners with imaginative ways of engaging reluctant stakeholders and connecting with communities. The creative arts, for example, have become an important component of local health action in many countries (see Sullivan and Lloyd, 2006). In England a National Strategy for the Arts, Health and Wellbeing, supported by the Arts Council and the DoH, announced itself as a legitimate arm of public health policy in 2007. The popularity of arts for health initiatives lies in the power of their engagement with the way people 'see' their world. Not only does the individual feel change and a sense of connection to the whole through the creative arts, but since the act of creation is also a social act, it encourages further social connections.

In what ways do you think community arts could contribute to enhancing health and wellbeing?

Community arts could be seen as a useful way of reaching out to people to solve a particular health or social problem, such as obesity, drug abuse or lack of physical activity. But it also links to much more holistic notions of health and wellbeing and this can create real conflicts. Many arts interventions find themselves with a foot in two camps. Public health imperatives may demand projects focusing on single issues, while an arts-based approach tends to focus on the personal and collective wellbeing of the whole. In negotiating these two realities, arts projects potentially provide a vehicle through which people renegotiate their notions of self, identity and how they feel, to a point where they are able to adopt the healthy lifestyle sought for them by health educators. Some examples of such projects are shown in Box 11.3 (page 322). But there are dangers: community arts may lose the creative fire that is their strength and, as this creativity is eroded, their capacity to support people's wellbeing and human flourishing may be weakened (Springett, 2009). Already, despite an enthusiasm for the arts for health, many such projects struggle with short-term funding and small budgets, as well as the need to demonstrate concrete outcomes in the form of narrow health-related targets.

Box 11.3 Community arts and health: urban and rural examples

The Vital Youth project worked with African and Afro-Caribbean youth in a part of inner London to develop a play about health and wellbeing issues at the centre of young people's concerns (Douglas et al., 2000). Young people were recruited through local radio and were involved in workshops run by core staff supported by specialists. The workshops covered script writing, dance and technical issues, like stage lighting. This health education initiative was relevant to the lives of young people and encouraged them to become interactive participants in the process, rather than passive recipients of health interventions.

Looking Well was a rural initiative that grew out of a community consultation in 1995, which revealed high levels of depression, loneliness and isolation among the farming community. Established as a charity by local artists living in North Yorkshire, the project was run on a shoestring from a rented shop in the local village of Higher Bentham. It was found that conversations about sensitive issues, such as depression, were able to take place more easily when the participants' eyes were focused on a creative activity. The resulting art was displayed and distributed in local locations, including a health centre. Within seven years, this arts-based activity regenerated the community, with over one-third of the population involved in its activities. One of the original mothers, who had been experiencing depression, is now employed along with five others and the local GP has been able to identify positive health outcomes in individual patients.

11.2 Bringing community views and agencies together

Change for health is not a short-term process. Box 11.4 highlights values and principles that, together with the skills and knowledge set out in Box 11.1, should be at the core of driving practice and working creatively at local level. In this section we explore these values, principles and skills in action using two case studies.

> **Box 11.4 Values and principles for practice at the local level**
>
> - Lived experience is the starting point of change and change is an emergent process. Start where people are at: transformative processes begin with the telling of stories.
>
> - Value all types of knowledge and ways of knowing. Bring the public health evidence to the table but recognise that visual and other data might have equal value as you construct a common understanding of the issues and solutions.
>
> - Treat people with dignity and respect, build and nurture trust and be prepared to address conflict.

Case study 1: Dovecot, Merseyside

In Dovecot, Merseyside problems are well entrenched and reinforced by top-down public sector action that has not addressed people's felt needs. As a deindustrialised social housing estate with high rates of unemployment, Dovecot has lost many of the connections it once had with external work and social networks. As a reaction to this, bonding networks to provide support increased in intensity, but these in themselves became ways in which some people controlled others. As opportunities for experience of the world outside decrease, the community closes down and opportunities for bridging networks to enable empowerment and social mobility gradually decrease.

Dovecot straddles the boundary of two wards, one of which is called Dovecot. However, Dovecot, as recognised by the people who live there, has an identity of its own but often loses out in local initiatives because of its location. Part of the area within one of the wards is the site of the previously famous television housing estate known as Brookside, which is mainly owner-occupied housing. The remainder of the area contains social housing and the population experiences a number of social problems around teenage pregnancy, drugs, youth crime and high unemployment. It often features in local surveys on substance use, hospital activity rates and alcohol abuse. Older people feel particularly threatened.

Over 15 years ago, local leaders and community workers within Dovecot undertook a local feasibility study for a proposed community centre. The centre was eventually designed and built by the city council, but with little involvement of the local population. It was also managed by the council and housed services and private businesses that bore no relationship to local needs but served other groups elsewhere in the city. Young people were banned from using the centre and there was no sense of local ownership. The local health centre also did not engage with the population or the city council.

In 2009, a local youth and community worker contacted the local university asking for help to engage young people. A participatory research process was started (see Chapter 9, Section 9.4) that saw community development workers working alongside university researchers to engage the population in a local survey, driven by and executed by trained local people, to identify key issues. Critical consciousness-raising sessions (Freire, 1972; see Chapter 10, Section 10.2) were held with young and older people and the two groups were brought together in a major discussion session. Over time, the intergenerational conflict started to be understood locally, and tension eased. At the same time, the community workers also started to engage local organisations delivering services in the local area, including police, social services, housing and transport. Eventually, a locally driven community forum was developed. During this period, the local primary care trust (PCT) was developing its policy for local neighbourhood service delivery around local problems of teenage pregnancy and binge drinking, and efforts were made to integrate the new recognised community within the process (Woods, personal communication, 2010).

 In what ways are the values and principles set out in Box 11.4 being applied in the Dovecot case study?

Initially, it seems local people had things 'done to them' and felt no ownership of the amenities provided. Later on, their direct involvement in the local survey and participation in discussion sessions enabled them to share their lived experience, bring issues into the open and begin to change their situation. The process used suggests that people were respected and listened to, their knowledge was valued, a common understanding of issues was reached and trust began to be built.

Subsequent events demonstrated how local people had gained confidence to determine their own priorities. When local university researchers applied for funding to work with the new initiatives, they were restrained by the new local forum, who said they were not ready to address the primary-care agenda before their own concerns had been addressed. The forum decided to focus on youth crime, intergenerational conflict and the need for a locally driven community centre. They were, however, willing to engage in local research around the issues of binge drinking among the local young people, but from their own and not the PCT's perspective (Woods, personal communication, 2010).

Case study 2: Partington, Manchester

Using Sure Start resources, a local health visitor worked with a group of mothers in a local centre to explore how they fed their children. Adopting a Freirean approach (Freire, 1972) using story dialogue techniques, the group explored their priorities and decisions around feeding their children. The health visitor's original agenda was obesity among young children and the development of an appropriate health-education programme. However, the process started to build the mothers' self-esteem, and they decided to produce a cookery book for their peers to encourage them to provide healthy but cheap meals based on their experience and that of their own mothers.

What also emerged in the exploration was that the mothers were making sensible decisions within their own lives while trying to address the media messages received around health and safety and feeding their children their breakfast. On health and safety grounds, having been told that it was dangerous to cook while having your children around, the mothers insisted that their children watched television. This increased the propensity for children becoming 'couch potatoes' and also undermined the link between nurturing and learning about cooking. Meanwhile, the mothers'

> battle to make children eat their breakfast had led to an association of food with conflict rather than love for both mothers and children.
>
> This project is ongoing but suffered a setback due to reductions in funding for Sure Start under recent English government cuts, resulting in the early retirement of the health visitor and the disappearance of a local source of employment for two of the mothers involved.

In Case study 2, the values of respect for local people and trust-building are evident. The telling of stories was deliberately used to elicit their lived experience and the public health agenda was then adapted to respond to the mothers' expressed needs. Operating intensively with small groups of people is often the only way of working locally.

Community-based or community development?

Taken together, the skills, values and principles set out in Boxes 11.1 and 11.4 underpin much of what has been termed a 'community development' approach to health (Amos, 2002), reflected in part in the case studies above. Indeed, in the Dovecot case study the community workers themselves played a significant role in involving the local population and engaging local services. Community development has a focus on participatory processes, bottom-up planning and capacity-building. It has a strong commitment to communitarian values (see Chapter 6, Figure 6.2), to remedying inequalities and distributing resources more fairly. While it has also been criticised for excluding or marginalising groups, it highlights ways of working that go beyond the community-based models often used in health. Table 11.2 summarises some key distinctions between community-based and community development models.

Table 11.2 Key distinctions in approaches to 'community'

Community-based models	Community development models
Problem, targets and action defined by sponsoring body	Problem, targets and action defined by community
Community seen as medium, venue or setting for intervention	Community itself the target of intervention in respect of capacity building and empowerment
Notion of 'community' relatively unproblematic	Community recognised as complex, changing, subject to power imbalances and conflict
Largely target individuals within either geographical area or specific subgroup in geographical area defined by sponsor	Target may be community structures or services and policies that impact on the health of the community
Activities largely health oriented	Activities may be quite broad-based, targeting wider factors with an impact on health, but with indirect health outcomes

(Source: adapted from Hills, 2004)

11.3 Participatory action research as emancipatory public health practice?

So far, we have focused on community action. But some of the examples discussed earlier also reveal a participatory action-research approach being used as part of health development. We now consider what this involves.

Traditionally, research, learning and practice have been separated out as different activities. Research is undertaken by experts in universities, and the knowledge is disseminated or translated through courses and papers. It is then assumed that the evidence base is taken on board by practitioners to plan actions. However, Chapter 8 highlights how qualitative methods can steer practitioners towards more participatory, respectful and reflexive ways of engaging in research with people. Participatory action-research (or what is termed 'community-based participatory research' in North America) takes us a step further. Research learning and action are not separate but are part of an integrated whole. This integrated reflection and action process encourages the ownership of the findings of any research by all participants and a commitment to action, as well as encouraging transformative learning by integrating the evaluation of action into the process of change. Thus, the research underpinning any action is not undertaken by a researcher operating in isolation but by the community-based or public health practitioner in collaboration with the people who have a stake in the outcome of any intervention or action. This does not negate formal basic intervention research but embeds it in the locality. Using such an approach to health action makes sense when a systems approach to understanding health is adopted. Given that any social system is under a constant state of flux and any change in a part is connected to the whole, envisaging research as something separate from any intervention into that system, and taking a linear approach to evidence and practice, immediately becomes an anachronism. In this way, practice becomes inquiry-based and embedded within the system (see Box 11.5).

Box 11.5 Participatory approaches to local change

A participatory approach seeks to integrate formal knowledge with local contextual knowledge and people's lived experience, and such real-time research is crucial for generating appropriate and sustainable change for health. It should:

- incorporate a local understanding of the issue (research)
- come up with a contextually sensitive solution (intervention/project)
- reflect on how that solution is working (evaluation)
- modify it appropriately (continual responsive change).

So, how does the process in Box 11.5 work in practice? Let us assume that a local public health team has identified high rates of diabetes in a particular ethnic group within an area's population. There is a whole range of evidence of the biomedical causes of type 1 diabetes and the preventive measures that can be adopted to prevent its onset – many to do with lifestyle issues. There are also measures that can be taken by individuals to control their dependence on insulin and provide social support and help to those suffering from this type of diabetes. The current response is to provide diabetes clinics within GP practices. While this deals with those individuals who have acquired the disease, it does little to prevent it.

So what would the participatory action-research approach lead you to do in this situation? The first step would be to engage with community members in the ethnic group to explore the nature of the problem and their own understanding of it within that community. This would mean bringing together a review of the formal research undertaken in the area and exploring with the community through workshops their perceptions and experience of the issue. This exploration would include local agencies delivering services that are relevant to the issue. It is likely that some of the cultural barriers to change will surface, but also the community may have ideas for overcoming those barriers or alternative solutions to addressing the issue. Together, you will formulate a plan of action, maybe setting out through the use of a logic model the expected short-, medium- and long-term outcomes. As part of the evaluation process, you would revisit the model as the action is evaluated. That evaluation would be done by the stakeholders themselves. In this example, the driving force is the health sector's concern about diabetes, and the challenge will be to identify those who are willing to explore this issue and take action on it locally as well as the resources to take that action. By adopting this way of working, a culturally appropriate intervention will be developed and local people who are involved will have broadened their understanding of the issue and own the change.

Does a public health practitioner have to have a specific medical issue to address to initiate this type of approach? The answer, of course, is no. Indeed, in any community development approach to change, it is important to address the issues a local community thinks are important rather than those prioritised by the health sector. Often there will be a burning issue to address or the process can be kick-started by a rapid-appraisal exercise involving representatives from the community identifying local needs or a local survey that they themselves have developed. A lot of groundwork is needed to engage people in the process and to make sure marginalised voices are heard. The inquiry process does not have to be a traditional survey but an inquiry process using the wide range of participation tools that have been developed, such as an open space event, a world café or a future search exercise (see Box 11.6, page 330).

> **Box 11.6 Useful techniques for participation and action planning**
>
> These approaches aim to avoid vested interests or more powerful groups managing agendas and priorities by creating situations in which everyone is enabled to speak and contribute.
>
> **Open space event** – gathers individuals together; agenda is not pre-defined but developed within event through careful process of discussion and adjusted as event progresses.
>
> **World café** – series of short discussions in small groups at café tables. Focus on value-creating conversations; harvesting of all ideas in order to build shared ways forward.
>
> **Future search** – focus on mutual learning sessions over two or three days; people tell stories about past, present and future hopes to discover common ground and only then build concrete plans.

The key is to involve as many people as possible from different interests in the process. Health, disease and other formally collected data can be included alongside people's stories. From this, an action group can be formed that can commit to taking action on behalf of the larger group on some of the issues identified. Here the role for the public health practitioners as advocate is called on to engage and make links with key players in service, both public and private provision. So, for example, if the issue that comes to the fore is about lack of affordable and accessible food, then the role of the public health practitioner is to engage with local companies or support a cooperative to achieve the change. Or it may be that the issue that comes up is intergenerational conflict. This may well in the first instance not immediately be perceived as a health issue. However, it is an issue of mental wellbeing, which in the longer term may cause physical problems. So community action to enhance intergenerational understanding has wider benefits beyond that immediate problem. What is required is a mix between responding to emergent issues and having a structured and systematic approach to change. It should be a constant process of search and re-search (Freire, 1972).

A key part of the process is community capacity building and enabling empowerment. Thus, there is a balance to be achieved between enabling the community to articulate its own needs and network, advocate and engage in decision making for itself, and building community capacity and engaging decision makers to act on key issues. This does not mean acting alone: there are people who have community development training who can support such work. However, a central role for the public health practitioner is to act as bridge builder between the organisations, between the community and the organisations, and between different groups within the community. In this process, the key element is that the focus is not on deficit but on what assets the community has that can be enhanced and capitalised on to bring about change (Minkler, 2000). Table 11.3 highlights community assets as well as needs.

Table 11.3 Needs and assets-based community development

	Needs	**Assets**
Community	Crime reduction; alcohol and drugs strategy; employment; sexual health/ pregnancy services; etc.	Networks; activists; employers; associations/clubs; public spaces; schools and other institutions; etc.
Personal	Lose weight; get a job; give up smoking; develop skills; engage in local community and democracy; etc.	Aspirations; abilities; interests; relationships; resources; commitment; knowledge; etc.

(Source: Chitty, 2011)

What difficulties do you think there might be in trying to focus on community assets (see Box 11.3)?

This is sometimes difficult because of the mindset of the health and social sectors in particular. They are concerned not so much with development as with fixing problems. Equally, local people may hold entrenched positions about what is possible. Marginalised communities and members are often angry, apathetic and overwhelmed with the challenges of everyday living. This might require conflict management or the introduction of alternative approaches and ideas from outside the group. Often the latter can be achieved by linking particular types of community with other groups who share their problems but have come up with solutions. No matter how much evidence base there is for a particular intervention, people learn most from seeing their peers address similar issues successfully. This encourages community learning and 'provides a powerful way of turning alienation into engagement' (Community Development Exchange, 2006, p. 1).

The LEAP approach

In Scotland, the Community Development Foundation and National Health Service (NHS) Health Scotland have collaborated to produce a resource for developing such community learning partnerships. Called the LEAP framework (learning, evaluation and planning), it is designed to support a partnership approach to achieving change and improvement in the quality of community life (see Box 11.7). It is specifically directed at those who work in community settings to plan and evaluate their work in partnership with one another and the members of the community they seek to help. The framework emphasises evaluation as an integral part of the process because evaluation can be more than proving something works: it can act as a process of systematic reflection for change. It also encourages critical thinking about what works and what does not work, as well as whether what is being proposed will actually solve the issues in the first place (see Figure 11.1).

Box 11.7 The LEAP approach

The LEAP approach is based on five simple but important principles.

1 We should plan and act according to **need**.

2 We should be clear about what we hope to achieve and whether we have achieved it – planning and evaluation should be **outcome focused**.

3 We should recognise that achieving change depends on building on and using people's strengths and abilities – planning and evaluation should seek to **build on capacity and develop assets**.

4 We should plan, act and evaluate in partnership, and involve communities as key stakeholders.

5 We should be committed to learning from what we do and from each other, and applying this learning to improve our effectiveness and efficiency.

The LEAP planning and evaluation cycle is based on seven simple but important questions.

---

1   What is the need we are trying to address?

2   What specifically needs to change?

3   How will we know if change has taken place?

4   What will we actually do?

5   How will we make sure we are doing it as planned?

6   How successful have we been and what have we learned?

7   What now needs to change?

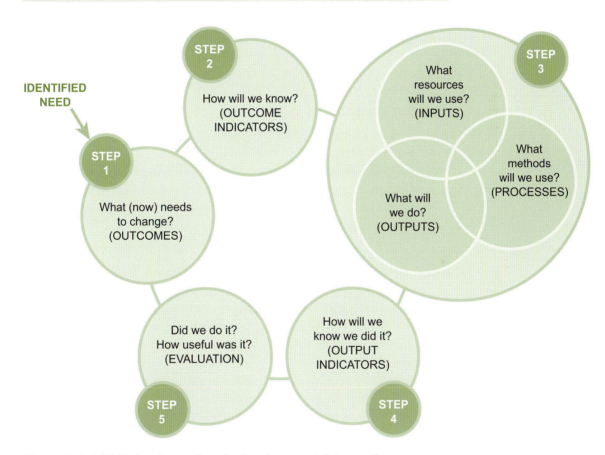

Figure 11.1 LEAP planning and evaluation framework into practice

(Source: NHS Health Scotland, 2003, p. 2)

This type of community-led approach to health improvement is now a significant feature of health improvement and health-equity policy and practice, both in the UK and internationally. It is an approach that is concerned to support communities experiencing disadvantage and poor health outcomes to identify what is important to them about their health and wellbeing and the factors that impact on their wellbeing, and help them take the lead in identifying and implementing solutions. It situates community capacity building as a core approach to health improvement/promotion.

However, working with local people in this way is much more than following through a structured process. As Ledwith and Springett (2010) argue, a set of principles and values about the way you work with people has to be at the centre of any practice. The approach outlined above will only encourage transformative change if certain key elements are present. These key elements include the use of story, engaging in real dialogue and encouraging critical reflection alongside the fundamental values of treating everyone with dignity and respect.

Building transformative change

Story is the first strand of an integrated process of story, dialogue, reflection and action. Stories can be personal, interpersonal and collective/organisational (Torbert, 2001). It is through story that the community is engaged in self-inquiry and self-knowledge. The process takes people towards being co-creators of their own community and can be used as rituals for healing and moving forward. As you have seen, such a process can also be achieved through popular theatre or art.

Once the story strand is complete, dialogue becomes possible. Trust is at the centre of dialogue – where there is no dialogue, mistrust develops. Dialogue is about with-ness rather than one-ness. Historically, there has been a lack of dialogue between those in poverty and suffering from poor health, and the agencies that serve them (Lasker and Weiss, 2003). Authentic dialogue is central to equality – it creates an interruption in everyday experience by opening up the space for change through engaging people in a respectful experience. At its best, authentic dialogue encourages people to relate to each other in ways that are mutual, reciprocal, trusting and cooperative. It requires listening from the heart with true compassion rather than the act of hearing. Dialogue can never work as a top-down process. Successful dialogue requires the participation of all stakeholders in a process of full reciprocity. Arenas for dialogue are opened up through common participatory techniques (see Box 11.6). Different perspectives are allowed to be heard and reflected on. That reflection can be superficial, but it can also be critical. That is, as dialogue continues, things taken-for-granted start to be questioned.

Reflection and critical questioning form the basis of change and action. This critical pedagogy is the underpinning of perspective change. This is not an easy process (Lee Sohng, 1996). It is often an uncomfortable and challenging process that will be consciously and unconsciously resisted. It is not just a matter for the community; professionals also have to engage completely in the process and can find it particularly threatening because it can unsettle, identify and expose insecurities. But it can also be productive. Jacobs (2008), drawing on the work of Barnett (1997), has shown how a group of health-promotion practitioners moved through levels of reflection towards deeper insights during a development project and criticality changed the way they worked. They started asking, 'Whose voices are heard?' and 'What is not seen, not said or acknowledged as relevant?' This extended their practice and the way they worked with communities, leading them to adopt approaches that allowed more voices and experiences to be heard and acted on through dance, art and other media.

Action is linked with the reflective process. Reflection without action results in actionless thought, while action without reflection results in thoughtless action. Through the combined elements of story reflection, dialogue and action, a spiral of learning develops, through which meaning is made (see Figure 11.2).

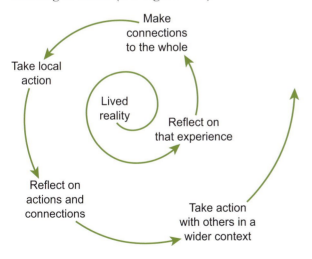

Figure 11.2 New spiral of learning and action: connection to the whole

(Source: adapted from Peat, 2008, pp. 168–9)

Through this process, groups of people, for example, can start to construct their own indicators of change – indicators that really mean something to people. This has been the approach of the New Economics Foundation (NEF). NEF has adopted a holistic approach supporting new ways of looking at practice, providing indicators of wellbeing and environmental sustainability developed from the bottom up.

An example of this practice is Sustainable Seattle, which convened a panel of over 150 civic leaders – environmental groups, city and county government representatives, unions, the religious community, business leaders, educators, students and social activists – to create indicators of change. Currently, they are engaged in a process at neighbourhood level:

> We believe that the sustainable community will be promoted where many players in different roles and with differing interests and values are all provided with a flow of meaningful information, and where they have the opportunity for joint learning and innovative responses to this feedback from the environment and from other changes.
>
> (Innes cited in Van Gelder, no date)

In the Sustainable Seattle model, citizen values and needs drive the process, but scientific data and methods provide the foundation for indicators so that the selected metrics are understandable and valid. The process is iterative, with information moving among and being discussed by the general public, a group of civic leaders and a group of technical advisers. The process of developing and selecting indicators is as important as publishing them. For example, Innes and Booher (2005, p. 230) believe that 'the process of debating the design of indicators shapes the players' thinking about the policies.' Innes also believes that if 'an indicator is to be useful, it must be clearly associated with a policy or set of possible actions ... policy can be advanced by discussion of how to design suitable indicators.' In this way the local and the strategic can be integrated. Normally, indicators are developed centrally and then handed down to the local level, where priorities and context may be very different. If indicators are developed from the bottom-up, then issues of relevant and appropriate policy can be debated as part of the dialogical process. Diverse and appropriate indicators can be developed to help all parties, strategic and local, see how things that they view as important are changing. A participatory process has the added advantage of creating shared values and understanding among people who are working together through the process.

> Indicators a society chooses to report to itself about itself are surprisingly powerful. They reflect collective values and inform collective decisions. A nation that keeps a watchful eye on its salmon runs or the safety of its streets makes different choices than does a nation that is only paying attention to its GNP. The idea of citizens choosing their own indicators is something new under the sun – something intensely democratic.
>
> (Meadows, 1991, p. 5)

11.4 Transforming ourselves: the final piece in the equation

It is often assumed that development work only needs to occur in the community, but often the development work needs to take place in organisations themselves (Pickin et al., 2002). For public health action to lead to sustainable change, attitudes of the powerful as well as the marginalised need to be brought into a process of thinking differently and acting differently. Foucault (1980) drew attention to the localised techniques and tactics for domination of those officials and functionaries who carry out the exercise of power and the specific manifestations of that power: the forms of subjection, the infection of localised systems and the strategic apparatus.

Those of us who are currently immersed in these structures as people who provide or receive services have to begin this task. It requires a high level of reflexivity about how we act and encourage such reflexivity in others. Local solutions to problems are often dependent on the nature of local sense-making by local practitioners and agents. There is evidence that shows that no matter how much a public service is reorganised, local sense-making encourages a repeat of ways of working and action that remain despite organisational change (Stensaker et al., 2008). Local groups may be incorporated into areas of control and spaces for dissent might be reduced by reinforcing the status quo (Barnes, 2007).

Public health practitioners need to be politically astute. This requires an understanding of how the micropolitics of engagement can subvert even the best institutional designs (Gaventa, 2007). Paying attention to and changing the rules and processes by which decisions are made can help encourage and support good local practice. For example, there are many things taken for granted in the way meetings are conducted in existing bureaucracies. How a room is set out, how the agenda is set, who records the discussion, whose voices are heard, what is talked about and how decisions are reached contain the very essence of liberation/domination. In such contexts, even the simplest changes, like renaming chairs as facilitators, change the dynamics. Incrementally changing such practices within the existing world can start a cultural change. It is such 'spaces for change' (Cornwall and Coelho, 2007) that are the small steps to the creation of new democratic arenas. It is in the area of local government that new experiments have started, such as participatory budgeting. These experiments are instructive in how the rules of engagement enable more participatory practices. Therefore, the use of an emergent approach to community approaches to health through emancipatory action research does not imply structureless practice, but involves structures that enable participation and the development of critical connections with others in ever-widening networks. Box 11.8 provides an international example from Kyrgyzstan, a poor ex-Soviet state.

Box 11.8 Integrating participation, health promotion and primary care: learning from an international example from Kyrgyzstan

In the poor region of Naryn Oblast in Kyrgyzstan, where the health system had all but collapsed, the Swiss Red Cross (funded by the Swiss and Swedish governments) has been implementing a project to improve primary healthcare using participatory action research. The process starts with an analysis of the health situation in each village, with the people using a tool specifically designed for this purpose based on principles of participatory reflection and action (PRA). The PRA project staff train local primary care staff as facilitators and they work with small groups in sessions of one to two hours on the question, 'What do you need to stay healthy and live a healthy life?'

Groups list their views and compare them with World Health Organization (WHO) statements on primary healthcare. People have invariably named all or most of the same determinants of health in their own list. The facilitator then asks the group to list the most common and important diseases in the area. The group ranks them and identifies the five diseases that are the most burdensome for people in this village. Graphs are created charting these determinants and diseases alongside villagers' views about their prevalence in the village. The result is a profile of the village's own concerns and priorities, which also incorporates the WHO dimension. The elected village health committees (VHCs) are then supported to act on those diseases that emerge as priorities. Their intimate knowledge of the neighbourhoods means they can help people with specific problems that have gone undetected by the primary care team and can act as a vehicle for spreading health promotion messages about good practices, for example, hygiene. Through such capacity building, the VHCs can become sustainable organisations and partners in the health system.

What do you see as the strengths and risks of the type of approach discussed in Box 11.8?

The initiative engages people in a rural health and healthcare development process at grassroots level, and then integrates it into a developing health system, suggesting that when the health system was stripped of its resources, it was also stripped of its institutional constraints on participation. External evaluation indicates that the approach has had a substantial impact in the development of skills within rural communities. However, as the process has developed, agencies, government departments and the medical profession (with their own agendas) have tried to coerce communities into addressing needs that reflect their interests or perceptions. The project leaders have had to work to ensure that community-identified needs are not subsumed under these external agendas, and support local people to strike a balance between their own priorities and the opportunities for resources from such agencies.

The challenges of democratising health development

There is considerable rhetoric about engaging communities, but much of public-sector practice pays lip service to this notion, preferring to consult rather than engage and to drive through their own agendas rather than adapting and facilitating actions to fit local needs and resources (Mitchell and Shortell, 2000). Adopting a more democratic approach to health development through adopting participatory practices is also not a cure-all. It presents some major challenges in a world where capitalist and market values dominate the political sphere and everyday life. The participatory approach has been criticised as naive, over-idealistic and potentially a tyranny in itself, actually recolonising and reinforcing the very inequalities it is trying to address (Kothari, 2001; Pain and Francis, 2003). It is also not easy to achieve in a climate that seeks constant accountability for outcomes from its public sector servants and where there is a medical model that fails to acknowledge the role of human relationships and sees health action as an intervention rather than a change process (Jackson and Kassam, 1998).

Public health practitioners need to be aware of institutional practices within the public sector, which often create the conditions for non-participation and work towards their improvement, for example:

- dependence on grants and short-term funding – the health sector and urban regeneration are replete with 'project-ism' and competitive tendering not only takes a great deal of energy, but also sets up poor communities against each other in a bidding war
- the tendency of governmental institutions to focus on target groups and indicators determined by top-down processes
- the silo nature of governmental institutions divides life into separate entities: environment is separated from economy, and economic development from social and spiritual wellbeing
- the reverence in some domains for certain forms of knowledge at the expense of other forms, with scientific knowledge perceived as superior
- the entanglement of much of so-called community engagement with service delivery, with consequent devaluing by consumer speak and notions of customer satisfaction
- the power sharing, high levels of trust and giving up the need to control that is required in a participative approach.

Working at the local level requires sustainable action over many years, while at the same time trying to improve the impact of the structural causes of ill health and increase the agency of local populations. Much of the work often involves a small group of people rather than large-scale work with mass impact. However, when you connect such local intense interventions with a systemic approach to change, then sustainability becomes possible. Burns (2007) provides a number of examples of what happens if you work in this way and connect action-research approaches to decision making and local and national policy. The key is to follow the interconnecting threads in a particular problem area and be committed to open boundary thinking, effectively scaling-up the processes outlined in this chapter and adopting multiple inquiry processes at multiple levels in the system and then inquiries across these levels. Mapping these connections is often the first stage of the process. Burns gives an example of a project in Melbourne, Australia, which started as a small project about the poor experience of mental health service users in acute psychiatric care and which eventually impacted on state and federal mental-health policy. He also illustrates how policy initiatives that do not attend to local social norms will be unsustainable because what is important is not the facts but what people believe is possible. This may mean replacing the commonly held notion of 'consistency' in public service with the idea of 'appropriate action'. Moreover, it means moving from traditional models of stakeholder involvement, where the representatives come from key agencies, to models that start with representatives from stakeholders who are experiencing the problem themselves.

Conclusion

Working at the local level for health in the way outlined in this chapter means addressing the social determinants of health for, as Popay et al. (2010) argue, social injustice kills. It moves us beyond a focus on individual behaviour change alone, but an individual focus can still be relevant at the collective level. If participatory development approaches are well integrated into topic-based work, changes in community wellbeing can support positive change in individual health. An empowered community can start to influence and network for the wider changes required and begin to assert control over their everyday lives in such a way as to enhance health (Wallerstein, 2006).

Working locally in public health means engaging in the act of co-creating other possibilities through cultures of organisational learning, dialogue, integrative thinking and systematic problem solving, thereby expanding the spaces for change in existing practice, however small (Ledwith and Springett, 2010). It is about social processes as much as health outcomes, and it is about changing the behaviour of those in positions of power as much as about behaviour change in local people themselves. In the end, it is about how all of us learn to think and act differently.

References

Amos, M. (2002) 'Community development' in Adams, L., Amos, M. and Munroe, J. (eds) *Promoting Health: Politics and Practice*, London, Sage, pp. 63–71.

Barnes, M. (2007) 'Whose spaces? Contestations and negotiations in health and community regeneration forums in England' in Cornwall, A. and Coelho, V.S.P. (eds) *Spaces for Change? The Politics of Citizen Participation in New Democratic Arenas*, London, Zed Books, pp. 240–59.

Barnett, R. (1997) *Towards a Higher Education for a New Century*, London, Institute of Education, University of London.

Berkeley, D. and Springett, J. (2006) 'From rhetoric to reality: barriers faced by Health for All initiatives', *Social Science and Medicine*, vol. 63, no. 1, pp. 179–88.

Boyle, M., Lawrence, S., Schwarte, L., Samuels, S. and McCarthy, W.J. (2009) 'Healthcare providers' perceived role in changing environments to promote healthy eating and physical activity: baseline findings from healthcare providers participating in the healthy eating, active communities program', *Pediatrics*, vol. 123, no. 5, pp. S293–300.

Bridger, J.C. and Alter, T.R. (2006) 'The engaged university, community development, and public scholarship', *Journal of Higher Education Outreach and Engagement*, vol. 11, no. 5, pp. 163–78.

Burns, D. (2007) *Systemic Action Research: A Strategy for Whole System Change*, Bristol, The Policy Press.

Chitty, M. (2011) 'Asset based community development (26 January)' in *Community Development* [blog]. Available at: http://leedscd.wordpress.com (accessed 4 September 2011).

Community Development Exchange (2006) *The Community Development Challenge*, Wetherby, Communities and Local Government Publications. Available at: www.communities.gov.uk (accessed 4 September 2011).

Cornwall, A. and Coelho, V.S.P. (eds) (2007) *Spaces for Change? The Politics of Citizen Participation in New Democratic Arenas*, London, Zed Books.

Department of Health (DoH) (2010) *Healthy Lives: Healthy People*, London, Department of Health. Available at: www.dh.gov.uk/en/ Publicationsandstatistics/Publications/PublicationsPolicyAndGuidance/ DH_121941 (accessed 4 September 2011).

Diez-Roux, A.V. (2001) 'Investigating neighborhood and area effects on health', *American Journal of Public Health*, vol. 91, no. 11, pp. 1783–89.

Douglas, N., Warwick, I., Whitty, G. and Aggleton, P. (2000) 'Vital Youth: evaluating a theatre in health education project', *Health Education*, vol. 100, no. 5, pp. 207–15.

Emmel, N. and Conn, C. (2004) *Towards Community Involvement: Strategies for Health and Social Care Providers*, Leeds, University of Leeds/Nuffield Institute for Health.

Foucault, M. (1980) *Power/Knowledge: Selected Interviews and Other Writings*, Brighton, Harvester Wheatsheaf.

Freire, P. (1972) *Pedagogy of the Oppressed*, Harmondsworth, Penguin.

Gaventa, J. (2007) 'Foreword' in Cornwall, A. and Coelho, V.S.P. (eds) *Spaces for Change? The Politics of Citizen Participation in New Democratic Arenas*, London, Zed Books, pp. x–xviii.

Harris, M. and Young, P. (2009) 'Developing community and social cohesion through grassroots bridge-building: an exploration', *Policy and Politics*, vol. 37, no. 4, pp. 517–34.

Hills, D. (2004) *Evaluation of Community-level Interventions for Health Improvement: A Review of Experience in the UK*, London, Health Development Agency.

Innes, J.E. and Booher, D.E. (2005) 'Reframing public participation: strategies for the 21st century', *Planning Theory and Practice*, vol. 5, no. 4, pp. 419–36.

Jackson, E.T. and Kassam, Y. (1998) *Knowledge Shared: Participatory Evaluation in Development Cooperation*, West Hartford, Connecticut, Kumarian Press.

Jacobs, G.C. (2008) 'The development of critical being? Reflection and reflexivity in an action learning programme for health promotion practitioners in the Netherlands', *Action Learning: Research and Practice*, vol. 5, no. 3, pp. 221–35.

Jewkes, R. and Murcott, A. (1996) 'Meanings of community', *Social Science and Medicine*, vol. 43, no. 4, pp. 555–63.

Jones, C. (1996) *PRA in Central Asia: Coping with Change*, Brighton, IDS Sussex University.

Kothari, U. (2001) 'Power, knowledge and social control in participatory development' in Cooke, B. and Kothari, U. (eds) *Participation: The New Tyranny?*, London, Zed Books, pp. 139–52.

Lasker, R. and Weiss, E.S. (2003) 'Broadening participation in community problem solving: a multidisciplinary model to support collaborative practice and research', *Journal of Urban Health*, vol. 80, no. 1, pp. 14–60.

Ledwith, M. (2011) *Community Development: A Critical Approach*, Bristol, The Policy Press.

Ledwith, M. and Springett, J. (2010) *Participatory Practice: Community-based Action for Transformative Change*, Bristol, The Policy Press.

Lee Sohng, S.S. (1996) 'Participatory research and community organizing', *Journal of Sociological and Social Welfare*, vol. 23, no. 4, pp. 77–97.

Liverpool Primary Care Trust and Liverpool City Council (2010) *2020 Decade of Health and Wellbeing* website. Available at: www.2010healthandwellbeing.org.uk/index.php (accessed 4 September 2011).

Mander, H. (2010) '"Words from the heart": researching people's stories', *Journal of Human Rights Practice*, vol. 2, no. 2, pp. 252–70.

Meadows, D. (1991) *The Global Citizen*, Boston, Island Press.

Minkler, M. (2000) 'Using participatory action research to build healthy communities', *Public Health Reports*, vol. 115, nos 2–3, pp. 191–7.

Mitchell, S. and Shortell, S. (2000) 'Evaluating partnerships for community health improvement', *Journal of Health Politics, Policy and Law*, vol. 27, no. 1, pp. 49–92.

NHS Health Scotland (2003) *LEAP for Health: Learning, Evaluating and Planning*, Glasgow, M&M Press. Available at: www.healthscotland.com/documents/308.aspx (accessed 4 September 2011).

Pain, R. and Francis, P. (2003) 'Reflections on participatory research', *Area*, vol. 35, no. 1, pp. 46–54.

Peat, F.D. (2008) *Gentle Action: Bringing Creative Change to a Turbulent World* (new edition), Pari, Italy, Pari Publishing, pp. 168–9.

Pickin, C., Popay, J., Staley, K., Bruce, N., Jones, C. and Gowman, N. (2002) 'Developing a model to enhance the capacity of statutory organisations to engage with lay communities', *Journal of Health Services Research and Policy*, vol. 7, no. 1, pp. 32–42.

Popay, J., Thomas, C., Williams, G., Bennett, S., Gatrell, A. and Bostock, L. (2003) 'A proper place to live: health inequalities, agency and the normative dimensions of space', *Social Science and Medicine*, vol. 57, no. 1, pp. 55–69.

Popay, J., Whitehead, M. and Hunter, D.J. (2010) 'Injustice is killing people on a larger scale – but what is to be done about it?', *Journal of Public Health*, vol. 32, no. 2, pp. 148–9.

Smith, K.E., Bambra, C., Joyce, K.E., Perkins, N., Hunter, D.J. and Blenkinsopp, E.A. (2009) 'Partners in health? A systematic review of the impact of organizational partnerships on public health outcomes in England between 1997 and 2008', *Journal of Public Health*, vol. 31, no. 2, pp. 210–21.

Springett, J. (2009) 'Kultur: att införliva den holistika och mänskliga' ['The arts: putting the human back into public health'] in Ejlertsson, G. and Andersson, I. (eds) *Folkhäls som tvärvetenskap* [*Interdisciplinary Public Health*], Lund, Studentlitteratur, page numbers unavailable.

Stensaker, I., Falkenberg, J. and Grønhaug, K. (2008) 'Implementation activities and organizational sensemaking', *Journal of Applied Behavioral Science*, vol. 44, no. 2, pp. 162–85.

Sullivan, J. and Lloyd, R.S. (2006) 'The forum theatre of Augusto Boal: a dramatic model for dialogue and community-based environmental science', *Local Environment*, vol. 11, no. 6, pp. 627–46.

Torbert, W. (2001) 'The practice of action inquiry' in Reason, P. and Bradbury, H. (eds) *Handbook of Action Research: Participative Inquiry and Practice*, London, Sage Publications, pp. 250–60.

Van Gelder, S. (no date) 'Fourth set of indicators' on Sustainable Seattle website. Available at www.sustainableseattle.org/programs/124-fourth-set-of-indicators (accessed 4 September 2011).

Wallerstein, N. (2006) *What is the Evidence on Effectiveness of Empowerment to Improve Health?*, Copenhagen, WHO Regional Office for Europe. Available at: www.euro.who.int/__data/assets/pdf_file/0010/74656/E88086.pdf (accessed 4 September 2011).

Chapter 12: Settings for promoting health

Mark Dooris

Introduction

The settings approach moves beyond just delivering interventions in a setting and recognises that the places and contexts in which people live their lives are themselves crucially important in determining health and wellbeing (Dooris et al., 2007). It has its roots within the World Health Organization (WHO) Health for All strategy and, more specifically, the Ottawa Charter for Health Promotion, which stated that: 'health is created and lived by people within the settings of their everyday life; where they learn, work, play and love' (WHO, 1986, p. 3). Subsequent international health promotion conferences lent further support and legitimacy to the settings approach. Within the UK, it received varying degrees of endorsement and validation through government policy initiatives.

This chapter presents an overview of the settings movement by reviewing international and national programme development and reflecting critically on its progress and achievements. It focuses on four areas in which the settings approach has operated over time and for which there is significant evidence of outcomes: local environments, focusing on healthy cities; education, focusing on healthy schools; workplaces; and health-promoting hospitals. In doing so, cross-cutting challenges are explored and conclusions are drawn about the relevance of the settings approach to twenty-first-century public health.

12.1 The settings approach: conceptual underpinnings

The WHO has defined 'settings for health' as:

> The place or social context in which people engage in daily activities in which environmental, organisational and personal factors interact to affect health and wellbeing ... where people actively use and shape the environment and thus create or solve problems relating to health. Settings can normally be identified as having physical boundaries, a range of people with defined roles, and an organisational structure.
>
> (WHO, 1998, p. 19)

However, this rather instrumental view of settings as sites for health interventions has been criticised on the grounds that:

> most settings are usually oriented to goals other than health and are arenas of sustained interaction, with pre-existing structures, policies, characteristics, institutional values, and both formal and informal sanctions on behaviours.
>
> (Green et al., 2000, p. 23)

A broader view would see the settings approach as an investment in social systems and settings as contexts that influence wellbeing directly and indirectly (Poland et al., 2009). The complexity of settings work has been recognised to some extent in health strategies. The 2002 Northern Ireland strategy, for example, acknowledged that since many risk factors are inter-related they 'can be best tackled through comprehensive, integrated programmes in appropriate settings where people live, work and interact' (Department of Health, Social Services and Public Safety [DHSSPS], 2002, p. 124).

Theorising the settings approach

The settings approach, emerging from the health-promotion movement, has been underpinned by values such as equity, participation, empowerment, partnership and sustainability (Dooris, 2005). It embraces the following.

- An ecological model of health promotion: focusing on what creates health in populations and on a holistic vision of health and wellbeing determined by a complex interaction of environmental, organisational and personal factors within the contexts and places in which people live their lives.

- A systems perspective: viewing settings as open complex systems, mapping relationships and synergy between different components, and recognising that although organisation development and change can to an extent be planned, they must also allow for unpredictability.

- Whole system development and change: applying 'whole system thinking' to create living and working environments that promote health and productivity, integrate health within a setting's culture and core business, and connect with and improve wider community wellbeing.

However, in practical terms, settings work varies considerably, not least because approaches might differ (or even conflict with each other) in their models of intervention, analysis of the 'problem' and 'solution', organisational contexts and degrees of opportunity and constraint encountered. In a critical review of the literature, Whitelaw et al. (2001) identified five types of practice ranging from a 'passive' model of settings work, in which the problem and solution both target individual behaviour, through to what they termed a 'comprehensive' model, in which both the problem and the solution are seen to lie within the setting (see Table 12.1, page 349). In some cases they suggest a settings model turned out to be little more than repackaging individualistic health education in a particular setting.

Table 12.1 Typology of settings-based health promotion

Type/model	Core perspective/ analysis of problem solution	Relationship between the health promotion and the setting	Practical focus of activity
Passive	The problem and solution rest within the behaviour and action of individuals	Setting is passive: only provides access to participants and medium for intervention; health promotion occurs in setting independent of settings features	Mass media and communication, individual education
Active	The problem lies within the behaviour of individuals; some of the solution lies in the setting	Setting provides 'active' and comprehensive resources to fulfil health promotion goals; health promotion utilises setting resources	Mass media and communication, individual education plus complementary work on policy development and structure change around the specific topic area
Vehicle	The problem lies within the setting; the solution is learning from individually-based projects	Health promotion initiatives provide an appropriate means for highlighting the need for broader setting development; health promotion seen as a vehicle for setting change	Principal focus on developing policies and bringing about structural change using feeder activity from mass media and communication, individual education
Organic	The problem lies within the setting; the solution in the actions of individuals	Organic setting processes involving communication and participation are inherently linked to health and are thus 'health promoting'	Facilitating and strengthening collective/ community action
Comprehensive/ Structural	The problem and the solution lie in the setting	Broad setting structures and cultures inherently linked to health and are thus 'health promoting'; health promotion as central component of comprehensive setting development	Focus on developing policies and bringing about structural change

(Source: adapted from Whitelaw et al., 2001, p. 346)

What conclusions can you draw from Table 12.1 about the tensions inherent in implementing the settings approach?

Table 12.1 indicates that tensions may exist at various stages. They might exist in the initial conceptualisation of the 'problem', in assumptions about the setting itself and what it might deliver or about what should be the main focus of activity. This suggests that conflicts might arise in spite of what we have noted is an underlying commitment to values such as empowerment and partnership. Practitioners and local residents might have rather different ideas about what these values mean in practice.

In addition, on the ground, settings work will involve a series of balancing acts in which trade-offs are likely to be required (Dooris, 2004). There is a balance to be struck between engaging in high-profile projects and ensuring long-term commitment; between getting high-level support and ensuring bottom–up involvement; and between being driven by current public health agendas and being responsive to the setting's core business needs. Figure 12.1 (page 351) sets out these three balancing acts as part of a whole system approach. It also draws attention to the diversity of methods that might be used and to the core underpinning values.

There is as yet no overarching theory for healthy settings but the frameworks that have emerged highlight some key tensions and potential conflicts in settings practice. The case studies investigated below explore some of the complexities and challenges faced in a settings approach, but also identify tangible benefits.

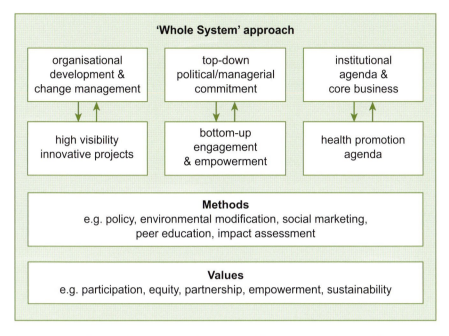

Figure 12.1 A model for conceptualising and operationalising the healthy settings approach

(Source: adapted from Dooris, 2004)

12.2 A whole environment focus: healthy cities

The Healthy Cities movement emerged in the mid 1980s, articulating a vision of a healthy city as one:

> that is continually creating and improving those physical and social environments and expanding those community resources which enable people to mutually support each other in performing all the functions of life and in developing to their maximum potential
>
> (Hancock and Duhl, 1988, cited in Tsouros, 1991, p. 20)

It was initiated by WHO as a small-scale European project that aimed 'to put health on the agenda of decision-makers in the cities of Europe' (Tsouros, 1995, p. 133) and translate the rhetoric of Health for All and the Ottawa Charter into tangible action. It was seen as a testing ground for developing new public health approaches at local level and focused on the process of development, recognising that success required experimentation, learning, adaptation and change (Tsouros, 1991). The healthy city would emerge through a combination of political commitment, visibility for health, institutional change and innovative action, supported by partnership working, networking, evaluation and dissemination.

Expansion and further development

The approach quickly fired the imagination of professionals, politicians and citizens worldwide. By the early 1990s, Healthy Cities was fast becoming a major global movement for the new public health, having not only expanded within Europe but also taken root within other parts of the developed world such as Australia, Canada, Japan, New Zealand and the United States of America (Tsouros, 1991; Baum, 2002; WHO, 2003). There followed expansion into Latin America, south-east Asia and Africa.

Why do you think the Healthy Cities programme proved so popular?

Looking back, three interrelated factors help explain the popularity of the approach. First, rapid urbanisation particularly affected developing countries. By 2000, the world's population had exceeded six billion, with much of this growth occurring in developing countries and being absorbed by urban areas (United Nations Human Settlement Programme, 2011). Second, the focus on health and equity, combining top-down political commitment, bottom-up community participation and intersectoral collaboration to bring about change. Third, it brought together the health and sustainable development agendas, which proved both influential and challenging for Healthy Cities (Price and Dubé, 1997; WHO, 1997a; Dooris, 1999).

Within Europe, Healthy Cities is now in its fifth five-year phase (see Box 12.1, 356) and 14 UK cities have been designated. At the start of each new phase, a set of criteria are issued, and European cities and towns have the opportunity to apply to become a designated city. The application involves cities demonstrating competence and commitment against a range of requirements and showing that they are committed to partnership working, capacity building, networking and evaluation. They must have multi-sectoral support for Phase V principles and goals, identify a coordinator and high-level steering group, provide a city health profile and have integrated strategic planning mechanisms in place.

Box 12.1 WHO European Healthy Cities Network Phase V (2009–2013)

Strategic goals of the WHO European Healthy Cities Network

1 To promote policies and action for health and sustainable development at the local level and across the WHO European Region, with an emphasis on the determinants of health, people living in poverty and the needs of vulnerable groups.

2 To strengthen the national standing of Healthy Cities in the context of policies for health development, public health and urban regeneration with emphasis on national–local cooperation.

3 To generate policy and practice expertise, good evidence, knowledge and methods that can be used to promote health in all cities in the region.

4 To promote solidarity, cooperation and working links between European cities and networks and with cities and networks participating in the Healthy Cities movement.

5 To play an active role in advocating for health at the European and global levels through partnerships with other agencies concerned with urban issues and networks of local authorities.

6 To increase the accessibility of the WHO European Network to all member states in the European Region.

Overarching aim of Phase V

To strengthen political commitment and solidarity to achieve health and health equity in all local policies.

Core themes of Phase V

1 Caring and supportive environments: a healthy city should be a city for all its citizens; inclusive, supportive, sensitive and responsive to their diverse needs and expectations.

2 Healthy living: a healthy city provides conditions and opportunities that support healthy lifestyles.

3 Healthy urban environment and design: a healthy city offers a physical and built environment that supports health, recreation and wellbeing, safety, social interaction, easy mobility, a sense of

> pride and cultural identity and is accessible to the needs of all its citizens.

Drawing on the experience of Healthy Cities, a range of other geographical or area-based programmes have emerged, including Healthy Villages initiatives in Africa and the eastern Mediterranean (Howard, 2002), Healthy Districts and Healthy Islands projects in the western Pacific and other regions (Galea et al., 2000), as explored in Box 12.2.

Box 12.2 Healthy Islands

A vision for Healthy Islands was first proposed in the Yanuca Declaration (WHO, 1995). Focused on national-level developments and reflecting a holistic and ecological model of health promotion and a respect for cultural and environmental diversity, Healthy Islands were conceptualised as places where:

- children are nurtured in body and mind
- environments invite learning and leisure
- people work and age in dignity
- ecological balance is a source of pride.

This initial concept of Healthy Islands – based on a commitment to community empowerment, capacity building and cultural sensitivity – proved to be a powerful catalyst for change. Ministers reaffirmed their commitment to the pursuit of Healthy Islands in the Rarotonga Agreement (WHO, 1997b), which presented a framework for co-ordinating health promotion strategies, health protection strategies and issue-based programmes across the island setting (Galea et al., 2000).

(WHO, 1995)

Assessing progress

Within Europe, evaluation has formed an integral part of Healthy Cities since its inception. Building on case studies and evaluations exploring key features of the approach (e.g. Goumans and Springett, 1997; de Leeuw, 1999), the WHO-led evaluation of Phase III was more formalised and comprehensive, and drew on data collected through self-reporting questionnaires, interviews and documentary analysis. It addressed themes such as partnership, equity, participation, healthy urban planning and municipal strategic development – concluding that cities have gained much from their membership of the European Healthy Cities Network and that the network has contributed more widely to innovative urban health practice through the production and dissemination of tools and other resources (Tsouros, 2009).

Other evaluations have concluded that the healthy cities approach can bring benefits. For example, a multi-method multiple case study and cross-case analysis of 20 participating communities in the California Healthy Cities and Communities programme concluded that the healthy cities and communities model had the potential to: increase community participation; strengthen the leadership and organisational infrastructure of communities to promote health; catalyse policy changes reflecting increased commitment to intersectoral collaboration and community engagement; and enhance skills development among coordinators and coalition members (Kegler et al., 2003, 2007, 2008a, 2008b, 2009). Evidence from Australia has indicated that strong social health vision, inspirational leadership, meaningful community involvement and adaptability all contribute to sustainable progress (Baum et al., 2006).

In developing countries, however, the evidence is much weaker. Although stakeholders appreciated the links between environment and health and the importance of community involvement and intersectoral collaboration, there was less success in mobilising resources and political commitment and minimal influence on municipal policy development (Harpham et al., 2001). Awofeso (2003) contends that Healthy Cities has failed to be truly effective outside the developed world due to the entrenched nature of urban problems in developing countries, limited understanding of health promotion, and social class polarisation caused by capitalist globalisation and the growth of neoliberal ideology.

The importance of the Healthy Cities approach lies partly in its appreciation of the influence of the physical, built, social and work environment on people's health. This understanding of the social determinants of health is essential in any health improvement. The goals and themes for Phase V in Europe (see Box 12.1) emphasise tackling inequalities and creating supportive environments: both are key objectives for public health across the UK today. In addition, the requirement to have multisectoral planning mechanisms, a city health profile and designated leadership is key to enabling effective analysis and action. All public health systems in the UK identify such features as important.

Although progress has been patchy and evaluation has been fragmented and challenging, there is a growing body of literature that points to the overall success of the Healthy Cities approach. In future, it is argued, it will be important to prioritise evaluation studies that are appropriate, rigorous and capture the added value of the whole system approach, elucidating what works, in which contexts, and why. This may require drawing on realist and other theory-based approaches to evaluation (Baum et al., 2006; de Leeuw and Skovgaard, 2005; Green and Tsouros, 2007).

12.3 An education focus: healthy schools

The second case study relates to places where people learn. Schools have provided the main focus for international and national programme development but there has also been interest in applying the settings approach across the educational spectrum, most recently to higher education (Dooris, 2010).

The European Health Promoting Schools Network was established in 1992 by WHO, the European Commission and the Council of Europe (Barnekow Rasmussen, 2005). It was influenced by ideas from health promotion and went beyond a focus on the formal curriculum to highlight the importance of school ethos and environment, health-related services and interrelationships between staff, pupils and the wider community in building the Health Promoting School. This later became known as the 'whole school approach'. As with Healthy Cities, the concept quickly expanded and the network – now known as Schools for Health in Europe – currently involves more than 45 countries. European developments were paralleled worldwide: the Australian Health Promoting Schools Association was launched in 1994; the WHO Global School Health Initiative was established in 1995; and further Health Promoting Schools and Healthy Schools programmes took shape across other regions. More widely, the International School Health Network has been established to support the health, learning and social development of young people through effective school-based and school-linked programmes, policies and practices.

National developments

The UK signed up to Healthy Schools in the mid 1990s and a strong but diverse set of initiatives then developed in each of the UK nations. England, for example, launched the National Healthy Schools Standard, later reconfigured and rebranded as National Healthy School Status in 2005. The programme aims to support children and young people to develop healthy behaviour, help raise achievement, reduce health inequalities and promote social inclusion (National Healthy Schools Programme, 2009). It promotes a whole school approach to health (see Box 12.3).

Box 12.3 A 'whole school' approach to health

A healthy school requires a focus on:

- leadership, management and managing change
- policy development
- curriculum planning and resources, including working with outside agencies
- learning and teaching
- school culture and environment
- giving children and young people a voice
- support services for children and young people
- staff professional development needs, health and welfare
- partnerships with parents/carers and local communities
- assessing, recording and reporting children and young people's achievement.

(Adapted from National Healthy Schools Programme, 2009)

Schools have been supported at a local level by health and education partnerships and can engage with the Healthy Schools process by completing an audit tool and then developing an action plan. All schools achieving National Healthy School status have had to demonstrate that they are using a whole school approach across the four themes of: personal, social, health and economic education; healthy eating; physical activity; and emotional health and wellbeing (see Figure. 12.2, page 358). Once a school felt that its activity (and evidence of that activity) met national criteria, it could complete an online assessment and submit an application.

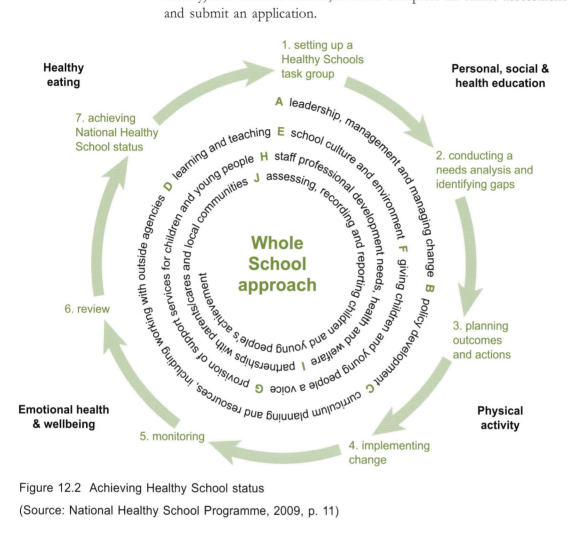

Figure 12.2 Achieving Healthy School status

(Source: National Healthy School Programme, 2009, p. 11)

 Review the components of a Healthy School in Box 12.3. What advantages do you think might exist for children in such a school?

Assessing progress

In a major review of the evidence on Health Promoting Schools, St Leger et al. (2010) conclude that:

- both education and health outcomes are improved if the school uses the Health Promoting Schools approach to address health-related issues

- multi-faceted approaches are more effective in achieving health and educational outcomes than classroom only or single intervention approaches

- the factors affecting learning are mostly influenced by social–emotional factors, which are pivotal to the Health Promoting Schools approach

- a whole school approach, where there is coherence between the school's policies and practices that promote social inclusion and commitment to education, facilitates learning outcomes, increases emotional wellbeing and reduces health-risk behaviours.

This suggests that children would be advantaged by being in a healthy school. However, the evidence is mixed. An evaluation of the impact of the National Healthy Schools Standard in England (Warwick et al., 2004) concluded that quantitative outcomes revealed few significant differences between schools at level 3 (the most intensive level of Healthy Schools) and other schools. On the other hand, its analysis of Ofsted inspection ratings showed that level 3 schools were rated higher on relevant scales after controlling for other background factors. Barnard et al. (2009) reported in an interim evaluation that schools within the programme accepted that promoting physical and emotional health was part of their core role in adopting a 'whole child' approach and preparing pupils for life. There was, however, variation in the extent to which the 'whole school' approach was adopted, which has implications for achieving whole system cultural change.

In some ways, healthy schools can be seen as easier to deliver than healthy cities. They are, after all, relatively coherent, small-scale and malleable compared with sprawling urban environments. This may be why evaluation has delivered more precise output and governments have provided more support for healthy schools. Our third investigation focuses on workplace health, which is an area where the boundaries and priorities are shifting in favour of a greater focus on health issues.

12.4 Workplace health

Workplace health interventions, traditionally focused on individual behaviour, had by the late 1990s incorporated a broader understanding of the complex determinants of workers' health (Chu et al., 2000). A European Network for Workplace Health Promotion (ENWHP) was created in 1996 and members signed up to the Luxembourg Declaration, which defined workplace health promotion as requiring the combined efforts of employers, employees and society. Healthy workplaces would be achieved through improving the work organisation and the working environment, promoting active participation and encouraging personal development (ENWHP, 1997).

WHO's Global Healthy Work Approach (WHO, 1997c) also called for the development of a comprehensive approach towards the promotion of the health of all working populations. Emerging networks for health-promoting workplaces were supported by the publication of guidelines for healthy workplaces (WHO, 1999), which encouraged the exchange of information and experiences, joint studies of common problems and mutual support.

The economic imperative: national developments

In the early twenty-first century, economic arguments for health interventions in the workplace became more powerful. In the UK, the Wanless Report (2004) stated that employers have much to gain from considering the revenue implications of preventative health for their businesses. The Institute of Directors (2006) emphasised the importance of prioritising workplace health and the UK government-commissioned report, *Working for a Healthier Tomorrow*, has made a strong economic and social case to act decisively to improve the health of the working-age population (Black, 2008). Black estimates that between 150 and 175 million working days were being lost each year due to illness, with around 7 per cent of the working-age population on incapacity benefits and an additional 3 per cent off work sick at any one time. The annual cost of sickness, absence and worklessness associated with working-age ill health is over £100 billion – greater than the annual budget for the National Health Service (NHS) at that time. In a supporting report, PriceWaterhouseCoopers LLP (2008) concluded that sickness absence costs approximately £495 per employee per year and that 'presenteeism' – people being in the workplace but performing at a suboptimal level due to ill health or lack of motivation – could cost the economy many times more. Black (2008) concluded that:

- for individuals and their families, health impacts on the quality and length of life people lead and affects their capacity to work and provide for their family
- for employers, a healthier workforce is a more productive workforce

- for society as a whole, the consequences of ill health lead to social exclusion, lower output and reduced tax revenues and higher costs in terms of healthcare and social security benefits.

The report proposed shifting the focus from reactive services to proactive preventive interventions but it largely overlooked the broader potential of the workplace as a setting and context. Little attention was paid to the role of management styles, employer-employee relationships, involvement in decision making, level of job security and the social organisation of work in determining health and wellbeing. This is reflected in the government's response to the report, although commitments were made to introduce and extend services and programmes (see Box 12.4).

Box 12.4 The government's response to *Working for a Healthier Tomorrow* – key initiatives

Creating new perspectives on health and work
- An electronic 'fit note', replacing the medical certificate and helping GPs switch the focus of their advice to what people can do rather than what they cannot.
- An education programme aimed at improving GPs' knowledge, skills and confidence when dealing with health and work issues and enabling them to adapt the advice they give to help people stay in or return to work.

Improving work and workplaces
- A business HealthCheck tool that will enable businesses to estimate the costs of sickness absence, turnover, worker ill health and injury in their organisation; enable employers to identify the savings that could be generated by investing in health and wellbeing programmes; and help them measure the return on investment.
- The National Strategy for Mental Health and Employment aims to bring employment and health services closer together, support employers and healthcare professionals and tackle issues such as stigma and discrimination.
- A review of the NHS workforce to consider the evidence for where the priorities for whole system improvement should be and recommend action that will enable local delivery.

Supporting people to work

- A range of early intervention services that aim to help individuals by making access to work-related health support more widely available (including: Fit for Work service pilots; the embedding of employment advisers within the Improving Access to Psychological Therapies programme; and the extension of the Pathways Advisory Service, which places employment advisers in GP surgeries).

- Extending the Access to Work service makes it as flexible and timely as possible and ensures that it is reaching more of the people who need it, particularly those who have fluctuating conditions.

(Adapted from Health, Work and Wellbeing Programme, 2009)

Assessing progress

The alignment of public health and core business agendas has begun to convince employers of the business benefits of prioritising workplace health, showing that improved work conditions lead to a healthier workforce, which in turn lead to improved organisational performance and productivity. In relation to evaluation, although it is widely recognised that interdisciplinary, comprehensive approaches are essential for effective workplace health promotion (Breuker and Schröer, 2000), it is also evident that few studies have examined integrated, comprehensive strategies as a whole, focusing instead on the effectiveness of individual components (Dugdill and Springett, 2001). Bauer (2007) suggests that future research needs to focus on comprehensive workplace health programmes covering a range of health issues and intervention levels, moving beyond the mere question of effectiveness to examine adoption, implementation, reach and sustainability, thereby increasing the utility of the evidence for informing future practice.

12.5 Health-promoting hospitals

Hospitals were an obvious and early candidate for the settings approach, not least because the Ottawa Charter called specifically for the reorientation of health services, arguing that:

> The role of the health sector must move increasingly in a health promotion direction, beyond its responsibility for providing clinical and curative services. Health services … should support the needs of individuals and communities for a healthier life, and open channels between the health sector and broader social, political, economic and physical environmental components.
>
> (WHO, 1986, p. x)

WHO initially focused on trying to integrate health promotion and education, disease prevention and rehabilitation services within curative care. The rationale for this was an appreciation that hospitals represent the main investment of health service resources and that there was enormous potential to reorient their focus on 'sickness', thereby promoting the health of patients, staff and the wider community. More broadly, it was recognised that:

- as major institutions, hospitals can reach large numbers of service users, staff and visitors
- as centres of modern medicine, research and education, they can influence professional practice
- as producers of large amounts of waste, they can contribute to the reduction of environmental pollution
- as large-scale consumers, they can develop socially and environmentally responsible procurement and institutional management practices.

Getting started: the European picture

The WHO Health Promoting Hospitals Network was launched in 1990 and 17 criteria were developed to judge a healthy hospital. The criteria covered clinical tasks, the physical environment, living and working conditions, educational programmes and collaboration with the community (WHO, 1991). By the end of the 1990s, largely through the work of the European Pilot Project of Health Promoting Hospitals, these had been refined into an insightful set of principles and implementation strategies that have influenced thinking and driven the initiative forward (see Box 12.5, page 364). A key requirement was for integration of the initiative into the organisation's management system and core processes, and coordination with primary and secondary goals and structures, like quality, sustainability or corporate social responsibility (Pelikan, 2007).

Box 12.5 Vienna recommendations for health-promoting hospitals

Fundamental principles

- Promote human dignity, equity and solidarity, and professional ethics, acknowledging differences in the needs, values and cultures of different population groups.
- Be oriented towards quality improvement, the wellbeing of patients, relatives and staff, protection of the environment and realisation of the potential to become learning organisations.
- Focus on health with a holistic approach and not only on curative services.
- Be centred on people providing health services in the best way possible to patients and their relatives, to facilitate the healing process and contribute to the empowerment of patients.
- Use resources efficiently and cost-effectively, and allocate resources on the basis of contribution to health improvement.
- Form the closest links possible with other levels of the healthcare system and the community.

Strategies for implementation

- Fostering participation and creating commitment.
- Improving communication, information and education by using methods and techniques from organisational development and project management.
- Learning from experience.

(WHO, 1997c)

As with Healthy Cities, embedding the work into mainstream business was seen as being crucial to its success. Although more limited in scope and vision, WHO's Standards for Health Promotion in Hospitals (WHO, 2004) provide a useful self-review tool for hospitals to assess progress in certain fields, such as management policy, patient assessment, patient information and intervention, staff health, and multi-service and multi-sectoral cooperation.

Branching out

Alongside European developments, Health Promoting Hospitals took root in other regions of the world such as south-east Asia. An ambitious project in Adelaide, Australia attempted to combine infrastructure development to support health promotion and organisational change with health-promotion activity related to patients and families, staff, organisation, physical environment and community (Johnson and Paton, 2007). Research into this project led to the development of a typology of health-promoting hospitals, based on degree of organisational commitment and types of health-promotion activities undertaken. Johnson and Baum (2001) identified four distinct approaches:

- doing a health-promotion project
- delegating health promotion to the role of a specific division, department or staff
- being a health-promotion setting
- being a health-promotion setting and improving the health of the community.

What similarities can you find between this typology and the findings of Whitelaw et al. in Table 12.1?

Whitelaw et al. (2001) drew a similar distinction between a 'passive' approach – doing a project in a setting – and more 'organic' and 'comprehensive' approaches in which the setting itself was centre-stage and action was linked to community and policy development. You might also have noted that work by WHO on healthy workplaces focused on a comprehensive approach as opposed to the rather more constrained initiatives launched in the UK in 2009 (see Box 12.4).

Health Promoting Hospitals has had some success in extending the concept and practice across the wider healthcare system. The WHO European Network of Health Promoting Hospitals has evolved into the International Network of Health Promoting Hospitals and Health Services. This currently has more than 800 member institutions from over 40 countries, and works in partnership with WHO through two collaborating centres. Scotland's Health Promoting Health Service is perhaps the best-known example of a programme that has shifted its focus from the specific hospital setting to this wider system. It aims to ensure that health promotion is an integral and sustainable part of healthcare, service delivery and organisation development – and advocates a whole system approach to health improvement, with all NHS sectors and all staff groups having a role to play. Underpinned by principles of equity, participation, empowerment and sustainability, the framework provides a tool to guide the development of consistent standards in health promotion practice across health service sectors (NHS Health Scotland, 2009).

Assessing progress

In relation to Health Promoting Hospitals, a review carried out for the European Commission by the International Union for Health Promotion and Education found 'little empirical evidence of a measurable health impact of such policies' although 'the message that they transmit is likely to reinforce the ethos of health promotion and to make it easier to introduce specific interventions' (McKee, 2000, p. 127). More recent research has found 'better and stronger evidence for many health promotion interventions directed at patients, staff and the community' but notes that 'the process of extending and incorporating these activities at a broader level has been slow' (Groene and Garcoa-Barbero, 2005, pp. 11, 17). It may be that the healthy hospitals philosophy adds value in giving health a higher profile in hospital settings but a 'whole hospital' approach in the NHS (as in the Healthy Schools initiative) seems quite a distant prospect.

 What do you think might increase the likelihood of a 'whole hospital' approach in the NHS?

As in any settings work, embedding health philosophy and action into the infrastructure of NHS organisations – into their DNA as it were – is crucial to success. If managers and practitioners are not involved and do not incorporate it into their work, little progress can be made. For example, evaluation of Scotland's Health Promoting Health Services framework suggests that its effective use depends on managerial commitment, leadership, coordination and training. Progress depends on developing the necessary infrastructures to facilitate appropriate organisational change and support programme delivery, not just on planning and implementing health promotion activities (Johnson and Paton, 2007).

12.6 Challenges for the settings approach

Settings were a marked feature of WHO's approach in the 1990s and this helped to foster a wide range of settings-related work. As initiatives developed, the complexity and challenges of settings work has become clearer. In particular, health issues (and people) spilled across boundaries and between settings, structures and power relations were notably difficult to influence, and new agendas emerged and needed to be incorporated. These are each briefly assessed below.

Settings and boundaries

Health issues do not necessarily 'respect' organisational or geographical boundaries, and a particular problem manifest in one setting may have its roots in a different setting (for example, bullying in schools may have its roots in neighbourhood relationships). People's lives may be divided between home, work and leisure pursuits, and they will also interact with and be influenced indirectly by other settings. Someone might spend time in prison before resettlement into the community, or in hospital before moving back to home and work.

Our understanding of settings needs to expand to embrace broader systems. We need to reject the tendency to operate along tramlines and begin to network horizontally as well as vertically. This involves making links across settings, seeking to understand more fully the synergies or contradictions between them, and maximising their potential contribution to public health beyond their own boundaries by exploring joined-up delivery (Dooris, 2004, 2009).

Settings also operate at different levels and one may nest within another, like Russian dolls; for example, a healthy hospital or school will sit within a healthy city. This challenges the overly simplistic conceptualisation of settings as homogeneous and discrete:

> The range of settings has grown to the extent that the concept itself … requires further clarification. It is clear that cities are not to be compared to marketplaces, or schools to islands. There is no common frame of reference between many of the settings that are being used as the basis of health promotion.
>
> (Galea et al., 2000, p. 170)

In south-east Asia, a technical report on healthy settings (WHO, 2002) conceptualised healthy settings as an approach or process informed by community development. The report proposed the development of healthy districts as the key contextual setting and suggested the districts have a key role in coordinating the development of a range of other healthy settings, such as schools, hospitals, markets, workplaces and villages. This recasting of settings as 'community development' recognises the need for clearer conceptualisation of the settings approach, as signalled in Section 12.1, and its close alignment with community-based work.

Settings and power relations

The settings approach, it is claimed, has too often ignored issues relating to power. By aligning itself with management, it has marginalised less powerful groups such as students or patients and 'inadvertently played into existing power relations and alliances' (Green et al., 2000, p. 24). While it is important to build senior management commitment, it is also vital to develop broad-based ownership: 'the politics of this dual process can be extremely challenging' (Dooris, 2001, p. 59). In area-based settings, initiatives such as healthy cities, which involve working across organisations with stakeholders from public, private, voluntary and community sectors, power relations are even more complex to manage (Costongs and Springett, 1997).

A second issue relates to participation: who spends time in which settings and who is left out; who benefits and who loses out (Green et al., 2000). For example, with a few exceptions such as prisons, 'the settings in which one is to find the unemployed, the homeless, the disenfranchised youth, the illegal immigrants, and so forth are not as well defined' (Green et al., 2000, p. 25). There may be an inverse care law operating for settings so that those with the greatest needs get the least access.

A third issue concerns the relationship of settings initiatives to other approaches and macro-policy. A criticism of the settings approach has been that is has tended to fragment action to promote public health and divert attention from the underlying determinants of health. It is therefore important that healthy settings initiatives look upwards and outwards, focusing on the organisational structures, policies and practices that will create supportive environments and make a difference (St Leger, 1997), while at the same time explicitly addressing broader social, economic and political contextual factors (Baum, 2002).

Settings and sustainable development

Sustainable development is of major concern to public health bodies (Griffiths and Stewart, 2008). Integrated action on issues such as food and transport has the potential to deliver long-term public health benefits through carbon reduction and climate change mitigation. Could the settings approach help to deliver such change?

Poland and Dooris (2010) suggest that settings and sustainability agendas are closely interrelated. Both seek to create health-enhancing environments; both acknowledge that health is determined by a diversity of environmental, social and economic influences and that the health of people, places and the planet are interdependent. Moreover, the causes and manifestations of unsustainable development and poor health are interrelated and frequently pose further interconnected challenges.

However, there is little evidence as yet that settings programmes are alert to these opportunities. Poland and Dooris (2010) note that:

> There have, however, been relatively few signs of such connectedness becoming central ... whilst health-oriented programmes may include an environmental component and sustainability-oriented programmes may include a healthy living component, the kind of hoped-for synergistic collaboration between the initiatives of healthy and sustainable settings has in reality not yet materialized.
>
> (Poland and Dooris, 2010, p. 288)

While there has been increased rhetoric about integrating health and sustainable development since the 1990s, Bentley (2007) concludes that initiatives at the city level have less clearly embraced eco-social sustainability as a central aim or made explicit their connectedness to the climate-change agenda. Davis and Cooke (2007, p. 352) critique the lack of connectedness between Health Promoting Schools and Sustainable Schools in Australia. In the health sector, health and sustainable development initiatives and networks – specifically those for health and climate change mitigation and adaptation – operate separately, although Hancock (2007) noted encouraging signs of increased liaison and joint working.

Conclusion

Having been developed and applied in diverse contexts over the past 25 years, the settings approach still has much to offer, including the potential to address the challenges outlined in Section 12.6. However, the approach has arguably struggled to generate a robust evidence base to demonstrate and articulate its effectiveness. Although a number of evaluation and evidence reviews have included a focus on settings (International Union for Health Promotion and Education, 2000; Rootman et al., 2001), there is still truth in the claim that 'the settings approach has been legitimated more through an act of faith than through rigorous research and evaluation studies ... much more attention needs to be given to building the evidence and learning from it' (St Leger, 1997, p. 100).

Conversely, we might argue for a more realistic assessment of the inherent problems in conducting complex, multi-dimensional interventions that do not lend themselves easily to evaluation through randomised controlled trials. Funding for evaluation is often a problem and a continuing focus on specific diseases and single risk-factor interventions militates against the settings approach. Evaluation of settings is not linear and reductionist, but has to wrestle with the interrelationships, interactions and synergies within and between settings, different groups of the population, different components of the system and different 'health' issues. However, the lack of conceptual clarity and variety of real-life practice brought together under the banner of the settings approach present obvious difficulties in generating a substantive body of research that allows comparability and transferability.

Settings will remain an important feature of public health work, but it needs to demonstrate its ability to improve and enhance health and wellbeing in more robust ways.

References

Awofeso, N. (2003) 'The Healthy Cities approach – reflections on a framework for improving global health', *World Health Bulletin*, vol. 81, no. 3, pp. 222–3.

Barnard, M., Becker, E., Creegan, C., Day, N., Devitt, K., Fuller, E., Lee, L., Neil, H., Purdon, S. and Ranns, H. (2009) *Evaluation of the National Healthy Schools Programme: Executive Summary of the Interim Report*, Nottingham, National Centre for Social Research.

Barnekow Rasmussen, V. (2005) 'The European Network of Health Promoting Schools – from Iceland to Kyrgyzstan', *Promotion and Education*, vol. XII, no. 3–4, pp. 169–72.

Bauer, G. (2007) 'Worksite health promotion research: challenges, current state and future directions', *Italian Journal of Public Health*, vol. 4, no. 4, pp. 238–47.

Baum, F. (2002) *The New Public Health* (2nd edition) Oxford, Oxford University Press.

Baum, F., Jolley, G., Hicks, R., Saint, K. and Parker, S. (2006) 'What makes for sustainable Healthy Cities initiatives? A review of the evidence from Noarlunga, Australia after 18 years', *Health Promotion International*, vol. 21, no. 4, pp. 259–65.

Bentley, M. (2007) 'Healthy Cities, local environmental action and climate change', *Health Promotion International*, vol. 22, no. 3, pp. 246–53.

Black, C. (2008) *Working for a Healthier Tomorrow*, London, The Stationery Office. Available at: www.dwp.gov.uk/docs/hwwb-working-for-a-healthier-tomorrow.pdf (accessed 7 September 2011).

Breuker, G. and Schröer, A. (2000) 'Settings 1 – health promotion in the workplace' in International Union for Health Promotion and Education, *The Evidence of Health Promotion Effectiveness. Shaping Public Health in a New Europe. Part Two: Evidence Book*, Brussels, International Union for Health Promotion and Education, pp. 98–109.

Chu, C., Breucker, G., Harris, N., Stitzel, A., Gan, X., Gu, X. and Dwyer, S. (2000) 'Health promoting workplaces – international settings development', *Health Promotion International*, vol. 15, no. 2, pp. 155–67.

Costongs, C. and Springett, J. (1997) 'Joint working and the development of a city health plan: the Liverpool experience', *Health Promotion International*, vol. 12, no. 1, pp. 9–15.

Davis, J. and Cooke, S. (2007) 'Educating for a healthy, sustainable world: an argument for integrating Health Promoting Schools and Sustainable Schools', *Health Promotion International*, vol. 22, no. 4, pp. 346–53.

Department of Health, Social Services and Public Safety (DHSSPS) (2002) *Investing for Health*, Belfast, DHSSPS.

Dooris, M. (1999) 'Healthy cities and local agenda 21: the UK experience – challenges for the new millennium', *Health Promotion International*, vol. 14, no. 4, pp. 365–75.

Dooris, M. (2001). 'The "health promoting university": a critical exploration of theory and practice', *Health Education*, vol. 101, pp. 51–60.

Dooris, M. (2004) 'Joining up settings for health: a valuable investment for strategic partnerships?', *Critical Public Health*, vol. 14, pp. 49–61.

Dooris, M. (2005) 'Healthy settings: challenges to generating evidence of effectiveness', *Health Promotion International*, vol. 21, pp. 55–65.

Dooris, M. (2009) 'Holistic and sustainable health improvement: the contribution of the settings-based approach to health promotion', *Perspectives in Public Health*, vol. 129, no. 1, pp. 29–36.

Dooris, M. (2010) *Healthy Universities: An Introduction*, Preston, UCLan. Available at: www.healthyuniversities.ac.uk (accessed 7 September 2011).

Dooris, M., Poland, B., Kolbe, L., de Leeuw, E., McCall, D. and Wharf-Higgins, J. (2007) 'Healthy settings: building evidence for the effectiveness of whole system health promotion – challenges and future directions' in McQueen, D. and Jones, C. (eds) *Global Perspectives on Health Promotion Effectiveness*, New York, Springer Science and Business Media, pp. 327–52.

Dugdill, L. and Springett, J. (2001) 'Evaluating health promotion programmes in the workplace' in Rootman, I., Goodstadt, M., Hyndman, B., McQueen, D., Potvin, L., Springett, J. and Ziglio, E. (eds) *Evaluation in Health Promotion: Principles and Perspectives*, Copenhagen, WHO Regional Office for Europe, pp. 285–308.

European Network for Workplace Health Promotion (1997) *Luxembourg Declaration of Workplace Health Promotion in the European Union*, Brussels, European Network for Workplace Health Promotion.

Galea, G., Powis, B. and Tamplin, S. (2000) 'Healthy islands in the western Pacific – international settings development', *Health Promotion International*, vol. 15, no. 2, pp. 169–78.

Goumans, M. and Springett, J. (1997) 'From projects to policy: "Healthy Cities" as a mechanism for policy change for health?', *Health Promotion International*, vol. 12, no. 2, pp. 311–22.

Green, G. and Tsouros, A. (2007) 'Evaluating the impact of healthy cities in Europe', *Italian Journal of Public Health*, vol. 4, no. 4, pp. 255–60.

Green, L.W., Poland, B.D. and Rootman, I. (2000) 'The settings approach to health promotion' in Poland, B.D., Green, L.W. and Rootman, I. (eds) *Settings for Health Promotion: Linking Theory and Practice*, London, Sage, pp. 1–43.

Griffiths, J. and Stewart, L. (2008) *Sustaining a Healthy Future: Taking Action on Climate Change*, London, Faculty of Public Health.

Groene, O. and Garcia-Barbero, M. (eds) (2005) *Health Promotion in Hospitals: Evidence and Quality Management*, Copenhagen, WHO Regional Office for Europe.

Hancock, T. (2007) 'Greening healthcare: looking back, looking forward', *Healthcare Quarterly*, vol. 8, no. 1, pp. 40–41.

Harpham, T., Burton, S. and Blue, I. (2001) 'Healthy city projects in developing countries: the first evaluation', *Health Promotion International*, vol. 16, no. 2, pp. 111–25.

Health, Work and Wellbeing Programme (2009) *Improving Health and Work: Changing Lives. The Government's Response to Dame Carol Black's Review of the Health of Britain's Working Age Population*, London, The Stationery Office. Available at: www.mentalhealthpromotion.net/?i=portal.en.policydocuments.938 (accessed 7 September 2011).

Howard, G. (2002) *Healthy Villages: A Guide for Communities and Community Health Workers*, Geneva, World Health Organization.

Institute of Directors (2006) *Wellbeing at Work*, London, Director Publications Ltd. Available at: www.director.co.uk/content/pdfs/wellbeing_guide.pdf (accessed 7 September 2011).

International Network of Health Promoting Hospitals and Health Services website. Available at: http://hphnet.org (accessed 7 September 2011).

International School Health Network website. Available at: www.internationalschoolhealth.org (accessed 6 September 2011).

International Union for Health Promotion and Education (2000) *The Evidence of Health Promotion Effectiveness. Shaping Public Health in a New Europe. Part Two: Evidence Book* (2nd edition), Brussels, International Union for Health Promotion and Education.

Johnson, A. and Baum, F. (2001) 'Health promoting hospitals: a typology of different organizational approaches to health promotion', *Health Promotion International*, vol. 16, no. 3, pp. 281–87.

Johnson, A. and Paton, K. (2007) *Health Promotion and Health Services: Management for Change*, Oxford, Oxford University Press.

Kegler, M.C., Ellenberg Painter, J., Twiss, J.M., Aronson, R., and Norton, B.L. (2009) Evaluation findings on community participation in the California Healthy Cities and Communities Program', *Health Promotion International*, vol. 24, no. 4, pp. 300–10.

Kegler, M.C., Norton, B.L. and Aronson, R. (2008a) 'Achieving organizational change: findings from case studies of 20 California Healthy Cities and Communities coalitions', *Health Promotion International*, vol. 23, no. 2, pp. 109–118.

Kegler, M.C., Norton, B.L. and Aronson, R. (2008b) 'Strengthening community leadership: evaluation findings from the California Healthy Cities and Communities Program', *Health Promotion Practice*, vol. 9, no. 2, pp. 170–79.

Kegler, M.C., Norton, B.L. and Aronson, R. (2007) 'Skill improvement among coalition members in the California Healthy Cities and Communities Program', *Health Education Research*, vol. 22, no. 3, pp. 450–57.

Kegler, M.C., Norton, B.L. and Aronson, R. (2003) *Evaluation of the Five-Year Expansion Program of California Healthy Cities and Communities (1998–2003), Final Report*, Atlanta, Georgia, Emory University Rollins School of Public Health.

de Leeuw, E. (1999) 'Healthy cities: urban social entrepreneurship for health', *Health Promotion International*, vol. 14, pp. 261–69.

de Leeuw, E. and Skovgaard, T. (2005) 'Utility-driven evidence for healthy cities: problems with evidence generation and application', *Social Science and Medicine*, vol. 61, pp. 1331–41.

McKee, M. (2000) 'Settings 3 – health promotion in the healthcare sector' in International Union for Health Promotion and Education, *The Evidence of Health Promotion Effectiveness. Shaping Public Health in a New Europe. Part Two: Evidence Book*, Brussels, International Union for Health Promotion and Education, pp. 123–33.

National Healthy Schools Programme (2009) *Whole School Approach to the National Healthy Schools Programme*, London, Department of Health and Department for Children, Schools and Families.

NHS Health Scotland (2009) *Overview of Health Promoting Health Service*, Edinburgh, NHS Health Scotland.

Pelikan, J. (2007) 'Health Promoting Hospitals – assessing developments in the network', *Italian Journal of Public Health*, vol. 4, no. 4, pp. 261–70.

Poland, B. and Dooris, M. (2010) 'A green and healthy future: a settings approach to building health, equity and sustainability', *Critical Public Health*, vol. 20, no. 3, pp. 281–98.

Poland, B., Grupa, G. and McCall, D. (2009) 'Settings for health promotion: an analytic framework to guide intervention design and implementation', *Health Promotion Practice*, vol. 10, no. 4, pp. 505–16.

Price, C. and Dubé, P. (1997) *Sustainable Development and Health: Concepts, Principles and Framework for Action for European Cities and Towns*, Copenhagen, World Health Organization Regional Office for Europe.

PriceWaterhouseCoopers LLP (2008) *Building the Case for Wellness. Report Prepared for the Department for Work and Pensions*, London, PriceWaterhouseCoopers LLP. Available at: www.dwp.gov.uk/docs/hwwb-dwp-wellness-report-public.pdf (accessed 26 May 2011).

Rootman, I., Goodstadt, M., Hyndman, B., McQueen, D., Potvin, L., Springett, J. and Ziglio, E. (eds) (2001) *Evaluation in Health Promotion: Principles and Perspectives*, Copenhagen, World Health Organization Regional Office for Europe.

Schools for Health in Europe website. Available at: www.schoolsforhealth.eu (accessed 6 September 2011).

St Leger, L. (1997) 'Health promoting settings: from Ottawa to Jakarta', *Health Promotion International*, vol. 12, no. 2, pp. 99–101.

St Leger, L., Young, I., Banchard, C. and Perry, M. (2010) *Promoting Health in Schools: From Evidence to Action*, Paris, International Union for Health Promotion and Education.

Tsouros, A. (ed.) (1991) *World Health Organization Healthy Cities Project: A Project Becomes a Movement. Review of Progress 1987–1990*, Copenhagen/Milan, FADL Publishers/SOGESS.

Tsouros, A. (1995) 'The WHO Healthy Cities project: state of the art and future plans', *Health Promotion International*, vol. 10, no. 2, pp. 133–41.

Tsouros, A. (2009) 'City leadership for health and sustainable development: the World Health Organization European Healthy Cities Network', *Health Promotion International*, vol. 24, no. S1, pp. i4–i10.

United Nations Human Settlement Programme (2011) 'Global trends' in the *UN-habitat website*. Available at: ww2.unhabitat.org/habrdd/global.html (accessed 6 September 2011).

Wanless, D. (2004) *Securing Good Health for the Whole Population*, London, HM Treasury. Available at: www.dh.gov.uk/en/Publicationsandstatistics/Publications/PublicationsPolicyAndGuidance/DH_4074426 (accessed 7 September 2011).

Warwick, I., Aggleton, P., Chase, E., Zuurmond, M., Blenkinsop, S., Eggers, M., Schagen, I., Schagen, S. and Scott, E. (2004) *Evaluation of the Impact of the National Healthy School Standard. Final Report*, London, Thomas Corum Research Unit, University of London.

Whitelaw, S., Baxendale, A., Bryce, C., Machardy, L., Young, I. and Witney, E. (2001) 'Settings based health promotion: a review', *Health Promotion International*, vol. 16, no. 4, pp. 339–53.

World Health Organization (WHO) (1986) *The Ottawa Charter for Health Promotion*, Geneva, WHO.

World Health Organization (WHO) (1991) *Budapest Declaration for Health Promoting Hospitals*, Copenhagen, WHO Regional Office for Europe.

World Health Organization (WHO) (1995) *Yanuca Island Declaration for Health Promoting Hospitals*, Copenhagen, WHO Regional Office for Europe.

World Health Organization (WHO) (1997a) *City Planning for Health and Sustainable Development (European Sustainable Development and Health Series: 2)*, Copenhagen, WHO Regional Office for Europe.

World Health Organization (WHO) (1997b) *WHO's Global Healthy Work Approach*, Geneva, WHO.

World Health Organization (WHO) (1997c) *Vienna Recommendations for Health Promoting Hospitals*, Copenhagen, WHO Regional Office for Europe.

World Health Organization (WHO) (1998) *Health Promotion Glossary*, Geneva, WHO.

World Health Organization (WHO) (1999) *Regional Guidelines for the Development of Healthy Workplaces*, Manila, WHO Regional Office for the Western Pacific.

World Health Organization (WHO) (2002) *Integrated Management of Healthy Settings at the District Level. Report of an Intercountry Consultation* (Gurgaon, India, 7–11 May 2001), New Delhi, WHO Regional Office for South-East Asia.

World Health Organization (WHO) (2003) *Healthy Cities Around the World: An Overview of the Healthy Cities Movement in the Six WHO Regions*, Copenhagen, WHO Regional Office for Europe.

World Health Organization (WHO) (2004) *Standards for Health Promotion in Hospitals*, Copenhagen, WHO Regional Office for Europe.

World Health Organization (WHO) (2009) *Phase V (2009–2013) of the WHO European Healthy Cities Network: Goals and Requirements*, Copenhagen, WHO.

Chapter 13: Building partnerships and alliances

Angela Scriven

Introduction

At the public health policy level, partnership working can appear attractively simple, economically expedient and is often presented as an unqualified good. This chapter focuses on unpacking the rhetoric of partnership working and investigates what drives it, how far and in what circumstances it can succeed, what it is best used for and what its limitations are. Examples of UK and international partnerships will be used to inform this analysis and the future prospects for partnerships will be evaluated in the light of recent public health policies.

13.1 The imperative of partnership working

There are a range of imperatives for building partnerships and alliances for health (Scriven, 2007; 2010; 2011). A plethora of national and international policy directives have highlighted over time the importance and the need for agencies to work in partnership to improve public health and a wide range of policy initiatives have been implemented with partnership approaches at their core (Baggott, 2010). The UK government has driven partnership working, with Jupp (2000) documenting an expansion in the use of the term 'partnership' in parliament, from a total of 38 times in 1989 to 6197 times in 1999. Interest in partnership working intensified and became a central feature of New Labour's approach to the delivery of health and social policy (Perkins et al., 2010; see also Baggott, 2010, for a detailed evaluation of New Labour public health policy).

Knight et al. (2001) point out that partnership engagement is no longer simply an option for some health and social services, but a requirement. The evidence to support this argument is clearly set out in the policies of the last decade, which have consistently advocated a move to partnership working. The Northern Ireland public health strategy, for example, *Investing for Health* (Department of Health, Social Services and Public Safety Northern Ireland [DHSSPSNI], 2002) created four Investing for Health locality-based public service partnerships, focused around a set of health and welfare-related targets. In England, *Our*

Health, Our Care, Our Say (Department of Health [DoH], 2006) strengthened the momentum for partnership and *Health Challenge England* (DoH, 2007a) prioritised new national alliances for good health and wellbeing with government, industry, voluntary organisations and local alliances between public services, business and third sector partners. In *Partnerships for Better Health* (DoH, 2007b), the underlying message was that future healthcare will be underpinned by partnerships between individuals, communities, business, voluntary organisations, public services and government. Subsequent plans to devolve public health prevention services to local government in England (DoH, 2010) were predicated on increased collaboration across the public sector, with local partnerships seen as critical to the reconfiguring of services (Local Government Improvement and Development, 2011a). The value of such multi-layered partnership working has also been a strong theme in policy making in Wales and Scotland over the past decade.

Partnership working, therefore, has remained a constant feature of national policy and the focus of a significant range of activities at a local level. All the indications are that this will remain the case for the foreseeable future.

Why do you think that partnership working is so popular with government and policy sectors?

The reason for this policy emphasis is because of the assumed benefits of partnership working, which are displayed in their most simplistic form in Figure 13.1). The primary purpose of partnership working is ultimately to improve the experience and health outcomes of people who use services, and the general health, wellbeing and quality of life of communities. There is an expectation that interagency collaboration will provide more seamless services, achieve joined-up effective solutions and prevent silo working of agencies that share the same public health goals. The principles of community participation and empowerment are core to this way of working, as previous chapters have indicated.

Defining partnerships

Developing a shared understanding of what constitutes a partnership and partnership working is a key starting point for all organisations and groups wanting to work together for health gain. One problem is that there is no consensus on what the 'partnership' concept means and the term is often misunderstood and used interchangeably and synonymously with other terminology, such as 'joint working' and

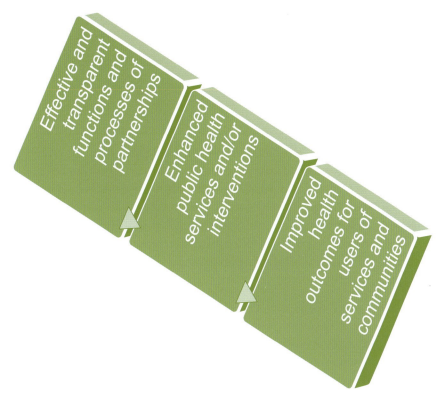

Figure 13.1 Assumed benefits of public health partnership working

(Source: based on an idea by Glasby et al., 2006b)

'collaboration', which have different connotations (for a full discussion of the meaning of the range of terms used in partnership discourses see Scriven, 2011). Reflecting on what the word and the work denote is a useful starting point for those establishing a partnership. Many public-sector organisations define what partnership working implies for them on their web pages. This often reflects what is also present on government websites. So, for example, a partnership is deemed to be a joint working arrangement where the partners:

- are otherwise independent bodies
- agree to cooperate to achieve common goals or outcomes
- create a new organisational structure or process to achieve this goal
- plan and implement a jointly agreed programme, often with joint staff or resources

- share relevant information, and pool risks and rewards.

(Thanet District Council, 2011)

This is an unambiguous and coherent explanation of what partnership working involves, although it omits community engagement. Other definitions emphasise similar characteristics. Eilbert and Lafronza (2005), for example, stress the sharing of benefits and risks, as well as resources and power. Brinkerhoff (2002) introduces the notion of comparative advantage and views partnerships as dynamic relationships, based on mutually agreed objectives, pursued through a shared division of labour based on the respective comparative advantages of each partner. Partnerships involve a careful balance between synergy and respective autonomy, which incorporates mutuality in terms of respect, equal participation in decision making, accountability and transparency.

Partnerships therefore incorporate notions of balanced power, absolute interdependence (El Ansari and Phillips, 2001) and pooled resources, including skills. The collaboration across different organisations and with different stakeholders that is inherent in a partnership is more than a mere exchange; it is the creation of something new and a long-term approach requiring flexibility and openness (World Health Organization [WHO], 2009).

The principle of participation

A fundamental principle that is embedded in partnership discourse is participation. While Lowndes (2001) makes a rather controversial point by arguing that there is no real reason why partnerships and participation should go together, partnership and the principle of public participation have co-evolved. There are different levels of participation, and in some partnerships there is a requirement for community representation. For this to work, the community and community stakeholders must be prepared and capable of taking on active decision-making roles and there must be a readiness on the part of public health professionals to share power and decision-making processes with lay community members. Table 13.1 is an adjusted ladder of participation from Scriven (2007) related to partnership engagement.

Table 13.1 Degree of community participation in public health partnership

Community participation	Public health partnership	Examples of involvement
High	Full membership	Community identifies the public health need and takes a leading part in establishing and managing the partnership
	Delegated authority	Professional members present a problem to the community and ask the community to make a series of decisions which can be embodied in a plan which it will accept
	Community is consulted, receives information	Professional members promote a service or an intervention. Seek to develop support to facilitate acceptance or give sufficient sanction so that compliance can be expected
Low	No membership	Community not part of the partnership

(Source: adapted from Scriven, 2007)

Do you think high levels of community participation are always preferable to low engagement?

The ladder metaphor helps clarify the different levels of participation, with the top rung of the ladder denoting an empowered community fully engaged in public health partnerships and the bottom rungs reflecting little or no participation. While one could make the case for striving for full community participation in all public health partnerships, Burton (2003) suggests that in some there may be reduced, but still appropriate, levels to which communities can be involved. Butterfloss (2006) takes this further and suggests that not all health problems or social issues require a community-participative approach, especially if there is an easier way to get the work done and achieve community health goals. The various levels of community engagement outlined in Figure 13.2 (page 382) supplement the ladder metaphor and illustrate how public health professionals can engage communities from a very minimal level to full partnership or to the point where decision making is handed over to them.

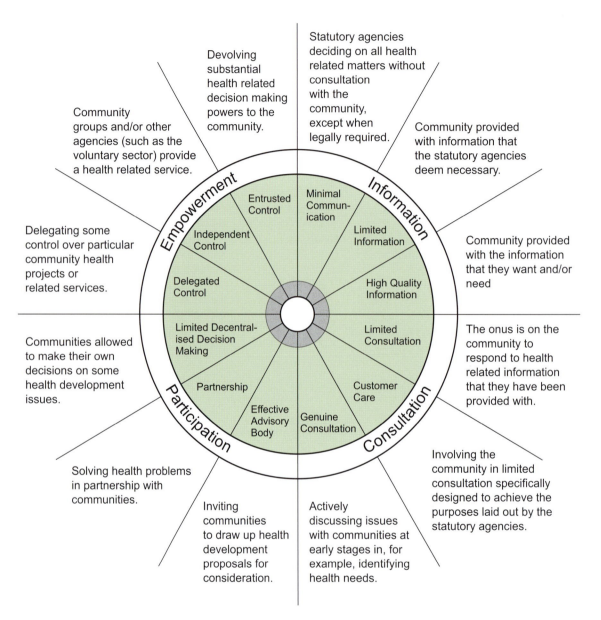

Figure 13.2 The wheel of participation

(Source: adapted from WHO, 2002; Davidson, 1998, first published in Scriven, 2007)

The extent to which the community engages in public health partnerships and alliances will generally be governed by a number of factors, including the character and overall purpose of the partnership, but also by a number of potential barriers or inhibitors. One study found a range of barriers to full participation, and from this there emerged a number of suggestions about how community participation could be developed (Skidmore et al., 2006). Recommendations included:

- Changing partnership structures so they fit a community's preferred participation mode. This is likely to be more productive than attempting to change people's participation so it fits existing structures.

- Giving more attention to the incentives for participation, and fundamentally about the devolution of power. Community participants will find it much easier to mobilise their networks if the formal structures they inhabit are places where real power lies.

- Building new approaches that develop trust in the community participation process. Trust is a vitally important prerequisite to enhancing the culture of participation. The building of social capital will be intrinsically linked to the development of trust.

- Long-term capacity building and empowerment, which promotes community participation among larger numbers of people and more diverse population groups. Capacity building will increase the pool of people from the community who are skilled in participatory approaches and who can work with existing stakeholders to create succession plans for the various partnerships where community participation is required.

Enhancing the overall culture of participation in the long term is likely to be more effective than inventing more structures of participation. To influence change in attitudes to participation, it must become a national priority in policy and something that is expected of all communities.

This latter point is interesting, because Evans et al. (2010) argue that while there has been a philosophical commitment to participation in public health since the 1970s, and UK government policy rhetoric on community participation in public health has been particularly marked since 1997 (see Baggott, 2011), it is less clear that participatory approaches have been pursued in practice. Evans et al. go on to demonstrate that there is very little evidence of participatory approaches by UK public health units and also little evidence of such approaches having any noteworthy impact on health and social outcome. One possible reason for this is that mobilising community members to the full participation level in the ladder and wheel metaphors is both difficult and complex. Butterfloss (2006) maintains that a better understanding of the benefits and the pitfalls is needed to ensure that community participation is valued and used effectively. How communities are defined and who represents the community are critical factors in participation. Key questions are:

- Who is left out of community partnerships?
- How are participants relating back to their organisations and/or communities?
- How well do community participants in partnership working represent the actual community and get held accountable to the actual community?

Another interesting question is whether participation is seen by public health professionals as utilitarian and a means to an end (public health outcomes gained more effectively and efficiently) or as an end in itself (empowered communities), or both (Morgan, 2001; Scriven, 2007). Some argue that participatory approaches are being used to simply legitimate the decisions made for communities (Baggott, 2005). Participation that did not automatically impact on partnership decision making would ultimately be regarded as pointless (Milewa, 2004).

Despite some of the issues outlined above, participation (and the extent to which communities are recognised and included in health partnerships) is still seen as one of the critical factors determining the course of public health (WHO, 2001). For those wishing to enable participatory approaches, Involve offer a number of case studies and provide a database of ideas for a large number of participatory methods, outlining their strengths and weaknesses (Involve, 2005; 2011).

13.2 Different types of partnerships for health

In public health and health promotion, there are many different types of partnerships with different goals. Some partnerships are based on a voluntary agreement between two or more partners to work cooperatively on a shared health agenda. Such partnerships may be limited by the pursuit of one or more clearly defined goals, such as the successful development and introduction of a health service, or may be ongoing, covering a broad range of issues and initiatives. Some partnerships are statutory and seek to affect the structural determinants of health, such as Health Action Zones (DoH, 2003; Barnes, et al., 2005), and some partnerships are strategic and local, and are employed to deliver a complex range of services that change as community needs change.

Local strategic partnerships

Local strategic partnerships (LSPs) bring together organisations from public, private, community and voluntary sectors and exist in nearly all of the local authority areas in England and in an analogous form in Northern Ireland. In Scotland, the equivalent to LSPs are called community planning partnerships (Improvement Service, 2011; Scottish Government, 2011) and in Wales, local service boards (Welsh Assembly Government, 2011). The key objective of an LSP is to develop strategies and initiatives at a local level to meet local need and improve the quality of life within communities, and as such they are linked with the neighbourhood renewal agenda (Department of Environment, Transport and the Regions [DETR], 2001). LSPs aim to encourage joint working and community involvement and because they are locally based, the community is well placed to influence its decision making. The structure of an LSP is flexible and is decided at the local level. This has resulted in a diverse collection of partnerships, in terms of both who is represented and how they work (see Box 13.1 on page 386 for an example of an LSP). For those establishing an LSP there are a set of tools produced as part of the Audit Commission's national study *Working Better Together? Managing Local Strategic Partnerships* (Improvement Network, 2011a). The tools are designed to help LSPs develop using a whole-systems approach to performance improvement and provide case studies and guidance materials.

In England, the function of LSPs in coordinating and bringing together local public health services has been acknowledged and supported (DoH, 2010), although policy may change. Meanwhile many LSPs have found themselves in a rapidly changing environment. In this new context, some are reviewing how they work, including streamlining and refocusing on subgroups and thematic partnerships (Local Government Improvement and Development, 2011b). New issues have appeared on the agenda, such as the need to form relationships with the proposed clinical commissioning groups and health and wellbeing boards. The latter suggests a greater need for strategic partnerships in the new policy environment (Clews, 2011). In Scotland, community planning partnerships are well entrenched, with formal targets, specific strategies for community engagement and national-level guidance on their development (Improvement Service, 2011).

> **Box 13.1 The East Riding of Yorkshire Local Strategic Partnership**
>
> Founded in 2001, the East Riding LSP is comprised of partner organisations from the public, private, voluntary and community sectors. Its key function is to develop and deliver a plan for the ongoing sustainable development of the area. Through this jointly developed sustainable community plan, partners work together for the benefit of all residents and visitors, both now and in the future. The LSP is comprised of an LSP board and four LSP action groups; all these groups are comprised of wide-ranging networks that aim to achieve the objectives set out in the sustainable community plan. The delivery mechanism for the plan is the East Riding Local Area Agreement 2008–2011. The East Riding LSP Board is responsible for overall partnership policy and decision making.
>
> The four action groups are as follows:
>
> - sustainable communities and transport action group
> - children and young people action group
> - healthier communities and older people action group
> - safer and stronger communities action group.
>
> (East Riding Local Strategic Partnership, 2007)

Health alliances

The term 'healthy alliances' first emerged in the England White Paper *The Health of the Nation* (DoH, 1994), and it was to dominate partnership terminology for a number of years. The WHO subsequently defined a health alliance as 'a partnership between two or more parties that pursue a set of agreed upon goals in health promotion' (WHO, 1998, p. 5). The term still prevails in some of the UK-policy arenas, particularly in Wales, where the concept of local health alliances has been developed as a means for bringing together all those who have a part to play in influencing the health of communities (Scriven, 2011). Local health alliances exist in most local authority areas across Wales and the term is also used within other health-related non-statutory partnerships, such as the Welsh Tobacco Control Alliance (WTCA) (ASH Wales, 2011). See Box 13.2 for an example of a health alliance.

> ### Box 13.2 The Food and Health Alliance
>
> The Food and Health Alliance is managed by the National Health Service (NHS) Health Scotland and supported by the Scottish Government and Food Standards Agency Scotland. The alliance is a partnership of key stakeholders involved in implementing a multi-sector food and health strategy. Membership includes a broad range of sectors, such as national and local government, NHS health boards and community healthcare partnerships, community planning, voluntary and community organisations, national governance organisations, research and academia, media, local enterprise companies and all food chain organisations.
>
> (NHS Health Scotland, 2011)

Public–private partnerships for public health

Public–private partnerships (PPPs) for health have increased over recent years, in part due to resource constraints in the public sector, resulting in the blending of public and private sector resources and skills for economic advantage (Ridolfi, 2004; Goel et al., 2007). This type of partnership seeks to complement rather than substitute for public health services and many such partnerships are said to be positively contributing to health outcomes, particularly in low-income countries, linked to such issues as reproductive health and communicable and tropical diseases, including HIV/AIDS (see, for example, US Government, 2011) and malaria (Kaminiski, 2011).

The growth of public health PPPs has arisen against a backdrop of perceived failure on the part of the public sector to provide public good in an efficient and effective manner. This has led to the evolution of a range of interface arrangements that bring together organisations with the mandate to offer public good on the one hand, and those that could facilitate this goal through the provision of resources, technical expertise or outreach, on the other. Although such partnerships create a powerful mechanism for addressing difficult problems by leveraging on the strengths of different partners, they also present multifaceted ethical and process-related challenges. The complex transnational nature of some of these partnership arrangements necessitates that they be guided by a set of global principles and norms (see, for examples and further discussion, the Global Forum for Health Research, 2011).

Njau et al. (2009) and Nishtar (2004) offer a useful definition of what constitutes the public and private sector when it comes to public–private partnership working. 'Public sector' refers to national and local government and sectors which are paid by national and local government to deliver public goods, such as health and education services. The private sector can be divided into two categories: for-profit commercial enterprises or businesses, ranging from small businesses and microenterprises to cooperatives and large national and multinational companies; and it also means business associations, coalitions and corporate charitable foundations directly funded and/or governed by business and not-for-profit enterprises, including non-governmental organisations (NGOs) and charities (WHO, 2006). Many NGOs operate as not-for-profit providers of healthcare, public health and health-promotion services within the UK and globally. PPP architectures across these public and private organisations can be complex. Several components have been found to be fundamental in their development and success (Njau et al., 2009). These include trust, the presence of champions, clear operating principles, action-orientated ethos, operational efficiency and effective time management. Njau et al. (2009) argue that if these components are in place then PPPs can become powerful advocates for meeting prescribed health agendas. The same arguments and drivers can be used when establishing PPPs locally and nationally in the UK. The following list (adjusted from Nishtar, 2004) outlines the potential operational and process-related challenges in PPPs.

1   Governance structures and operational strategies must be established: arrangements must not develop on an *ad hoc* and opportunistic basis with resultant questionable credibility. Workable partnerships require a well-defined governance structure to be established to allow for the distribution of responsibilities to all the stakeholders. Public–private partnerships may run into problems because of ill-defined governance mechanisms.

2   Participatory approach to decision making – the term 'partnership' gives the impression of equality. However, adopting a fully participatory approach to the partnership's decision-making process can be difficult to accomplish (see Table 13.1). Decision making may be biased, and in the case of relationships with the for-profit private sector, there is the danger of the financially stronger partner

influencing the public or not-for-profit sector's decision-making process.

3   Power relationships: skewed power relationships are a major impediment to the development of successful partnerships. In some cases there are more serious issues relating to power relationships, such as who assumes the leadership role.

4   Risks to reputation by choosing the wrong partner: it is particularly problematic to collaborate with partners whose activities are infringing or violating environmental, social or other standards (Martens, 2007). The criteria for selection and screening of partners are important issues, from both an ethical and a process-related perspective, as they raise the questions of competence and appropriateness.

5   Accountability: partnerships must ensure that all stakeholders are held accountable for the delivery of efficient, effective and equitable services in a PPP arrangement. To hold partners accountable for their actions, it is imperative to have clear governance mechanisms and clarify partners' rights and obligations.

6   Impartiality in health: if public–private partnerships are not carefully designed, there is a danger that they may reorient the mission of the public sector, interfere with organisational priorities, and weaken their capacity to uphold norms and regulations.

These types of operational and process-related challenges can equally occur in partnerships between the public sector and the voluntary sector and the private for-profit and the voluntary sector. Shelter's partnership approach to homelessness is outlined in Box 13.3 (page 390). As a charity, Shelter is a not-for-profit private sector organisation that engages with both private and public sector partners and may therefore be confronted by the challenges outlined above.

Box 13.3 Shelter – a partnership approach to homelessness

Shelter is a national housing and homelessness charity that helps people find and keep a home, and campaigns for decent housing for all. The organisation has set a specific aim to work in partnership with other local and national agencies, and public and private bodies, therefore partnership working is the mainstay of its operations (Shelter, 2010). Shelter has developed a number of national partnerships to improve their range of services to clients, including those which combine the functions of advice services to deliver combined debt, welfare benefits, housing and community care advice services. In addition, the organisation has worked at a local authority level to establish a series of partnerships across England that focus on the key issues of health, social services, criminal justice and personal safety. These partnerships aim to understand the needs and experiences of homeless people, so that statutory agencies and other organisations can plan services to meet the needs of homeless people in their local area. The partners differ in each area. In most cases, these partnerships involve key agencies, including local housing providers, social work services, the probation service, advice agencies, support providers, day centres, youth projects, hostels, resettlement projects and lodging schemes. These multi-agency partnerships have been successful in identifying trends and experiences amongst the homeless population. This means that partners can develop a better understanding of the underlying reasons for homelessness across the county, and at a regional and local level.

The list of partners includes commercial and other charitable organisations. For example, Shelter, Bob the Builder and HIT Entertainment have been working in partnership since the beginning of 2010 to raise awareness of the problems faced by homeless and badly housed children and families throughout the UK, and to generate support for positive change. Shelter and HIT Entertainment harnesses the power of Bob the Builder's creative, can-do spirit to show how Shelter's expert advice and support can make life better for families in housing need.

(Shelter, 2011)

13.3 Implementing partnerships

Public health and other health and social care professionals are often asked to work together across traditional agency boundaries and with third-sector and private organisations. Such partnerships are not easy to implement but can be helped by applying some key principles.

What do you think would need to be in place to make Shelter's partnerships (Box 13.3) successful?

Shelter's own view is that the success of their partnerships has been driven by trust, understanding, commitment and focus.

- Trust – time has to be dedicated to establishing relationships. For example, when establishing a health and homelessness partnership in Richmond, the partners spent two years networking and sharing good practice before the partnership was formally established.

- Understanding – agencies involved in the partnerships also went to lengths to ensure they understood the priorities, working practices, organisational structure and legal obligations of partner agencies. This meant that any false perceptions could be eliminated before misunderstandings led to resentment and confusion.

- Commitment – the importance of regular attendance at meetings of designated staff from each agency has been critical in the establishment of trust between partners and demonstrating the priority each organisation attaches to being a partner.

- Focus – the most effective homelessness partnerships appear to be those that focus on key issues, and ensure activities link with and complement the strategies of partner organisations.

Nonetheless, doing such work can be difficult and complex. In many cases, practitioners and managers in health and social care are often tasked with making partnerships work without the necessary support (Glasby and Dickenson, 2008). Smith et al. (2008) also identified that for implementation to be successful local champions are crucial to drive the public health policy agenda forward. There are, therefore, a number of processes that have to be undertaken to ensure that partnerships are shaped effectively.

Before establishing or entering into any partnership, the potential benefits need to be assessed. This can be done by comparing the objectives and intended outcomes of the proposed arrangement with your organisation's own priorities and any other policy or agency agendas. Useful questions are:

- Why do we need to work in this partnership?
- What will the partnership deliver that we could not deliver on our own?
- Are the aims and objectives of the partnership clear and what are the links between the partnership's aims and objectives and the organisation's aims and objectives?

If the responses to the questions above suggest that a partnership approach is beneficial then the following elements are important for establishing a public health partnership:

- identify key stakeholders and local champions
- set up a steering group
- canvass all sectors for support (public, voluntary, private, community and academic)
- enlist top-level management support
- bring existing partnerships in, where relevant
- build capacity and capability among members
- develop a shared vision of what the partnership could achieve
- undertake a review or an audit of health indicators and existing provision
- define roles and responsibilities
- draw up a partnership agreement template and terms of reference.

For partnerships to be effective they must be transparent and accountable and be based on agreed ethical principles, mutual understanding and respect (see Standards for England, 2011), for an ethical behaviour protocol designed to enhance partnerships with adherence to professional partnership guidelines (see Markwell et al., 2003 and International Union of Health Promotion and Education [IUHPE], 2011). Partnership agreements with procedural terms of reference may be needed, as the guidance in Box 13.4 indicates, to ensure that partners deliver on their commitments.

Box 13.4 Key dimensions of partnership agreement

Partnership agreement templates might include sections on:

- aims, objectives and purpose of the partnership
- roles, responsibilities and accountability
- members (include selection criteria) and terms of office
- governance, including ethics
- declarations of interest
- anticipated life of partnership and exit strategy.

Terms of reference might include components of the agreement template plus:

- frequency of meetings
- process for changes to the terms of reference.

Managing and sustaining partnerships

The management of public health partnerships is likely to involve consideration of most of the elements set out in Box 13.4. Partnerships may also require formal procedures to deal with issues such as risk management, insurance, fraud and corruption, legal issues and accountability (see Thanet District Council, 2011 for further details).

In terms of sustainability, some public health partnerships may only require formation for a limited period, whereas others may require ongoing commitment, so it is important at the outset to establish a timeframe and an exit strategy, and to keep reviewing the relevance and effectiveness of the partnership processes and outcomes. There are many reasons for sustaining partnerships, which usually reflect the overall purpose of setting it up in the first instance. Baldwin et al. (2005) argue that the perceived personal and public health benefits the representatives receive for their efforts are crucial to sustainability. Drawing on a range of literature, Baldwin et al. identify a number of important issues relating to managing and sustaining partnerships, including the need for flexibility to allow for change and the requirement of good communication, including the use of information technology, to maintain commitment and involvement of partners. Having a coordinator in place and ensuring there are regular reviews of the ongoing work are also key factors linked to sustainability. Despite the availability of guidelines, many partnerships at a local level will prove difficult to sustain. Evaluating the work of the partnership is fundamentally important to understanding maintenance and sustainability issues.

Evaluating partnerships

There is a dearth of evaluation of partnership working, despite the Verona Benchmarking initiative (Watson et al., 2000; Scriven, 2011). This might be in part because of the complexity of partnerships as an approach to achieving public health gain and in terms of their structural diversity. The majority of the partnership evaluation literature focuses on structures and processes and not outcomes, argue Dowling et al. (2004), with evidence focusing on the process of partnership working (how well are partnerships working together?), not on the outcomes of partnerships (do they make a difference to services or to health outcomes?). Smith et al. (2008) contend that too little emphasis has been placed on evaluating the partnerships themselves with regard to their purpose in achieving better outcomes in improved health and support for recipients of interventions and/or services. The dominance of process evaluation has led Glasby and Dickinson (2008) to argue that existing partnership working remains essentially faith-based. Corbin and Mittelmark (2008) share the view that when partnerships are promoted as an approach to public health, with little research undertaken to identify factors and processes that promote as well as inhibit the production of synergistic outcomes, what is demonstrated is a leap or act of faith. The systematic review undertaken by Perkins et al. (2010) of public health partnerships poses the question: 'How long is it necessary or acceptable to wait in order to be able to establish whether partnerships are having any tangible effects?' In the spirit of evidence-based policy, they suggest the time may have come for a bolder assessment of not merely the alleged benefits of partnership working, but also their limits.

Another issue relating to evaluation of partnerships is introduced by Glasby et al. (2006a; 2006b). They suggest that when it comes to assessing the effectiveness of partnership functioning, there is too great a tendency to focus on the perspectives of policy makers and managers without adequately exploring the views and experiences of service users and frontline staff. There is also very little evaluation that examines partnerships in the context of the existing theory around organisational behaviour or that analyses the dynamics of the relationships that develop over time. Finally, Glasby et al. (2006b) also claim there is a tendency to view health and social care partnerships in isolation without locating them in wider partnerships, such as local strategic partnerships. More needs to be done, therefore, to measure the effectiveness of public health partnerships in terms of outcomes, organisational effectiveness and their synergy, within and across other partnerships.

13.4 Challenges in partnership working

It is important for those who wish to create a partnership or who are working members of a partnership to be aware from the outset of potential challenges.

From your reading so far, what do you think are the most challenging aspects of partnership work?

Competition between organisations can result in a barrier to cooperation. Part of the issue of competition is a battle for authority or power – a real concern discussed under private public partnerships earlier in the chapter. Another pitfall is losing sight of the purpose of the partnership. The broad-ranging and competing responsibilities and agendas of partner organisations can mean that the specific purpose of the partnership can be forgotten. Partnerships might aim for short-term high-profile goals, and not tackle fundamental problems or address critical need. It can be difficult to get the balance of communication right. Too many meetings can put partners off attending, while too little communication can result in duplication of effort, lack of understanding and mistrust among partners. There might also be a lack of outcome orientation, with some health partnerships existing in form but not contributing to improvements in quality and efficiency (Nishtar, 2004).

Hidden agendas can also cause problems if organisations get involved in partnerships for other motives, such as to access funding. Coulson (2005) highlights culture clash, citing incompatibility in the aims of the different partners, or cultures and histories that are too diverse to be brought into harmony. A general lack of understanding of their different organisational structures can also cause problems, particularly when local informal groups are engaging with larger statutory organisations. Finally, there may be an issue of time. It takes time to develop trust between partners, which can slow up the process of making decisions and using resources. Community representation may result in unequal power relations and there may be an imbalance in what each partner brings to and takes from the partnership. Entwistle

(2006) claims that partnership working generates frustration and disappointment; too many partnerships are created to address all manner of problems which overstretch capacity and may result in collaborative fatigue or even cynicism.

Box 13.5 highlights these issues and offers some solutions, which reinforce some of the comments from Shelter about PPPs that were noted earlier. Of fundamental importance is building trusting relationships and, through these, a shared purpose, vision and set of priorities.

Box 13.5 The top ten partnership killers

1 For ever and ever …

The problem: The partnership lives on beyond its purpose.

The solution: For project-based partnerships and those based on limited funding, agree an exit strategy, know when the job is done and what you might leave in place. End the partnership with a party and thank everyone for their input.

2 One-upmanship

The problem: Competition between organisations leads to blame, self-righteousness and a trench mentality.

The solution: Ensure you spend time early on team building and developing a sense of shared purpose – build relationships between organisations to blur the boundaries.

3 Right place, wrong people

The problem: Representatives from constituent bodies constantly have to go back to their parent organisations for decisions.

The solution: Make sure the people put on your partnership have delegated authority to decide much of the business at the meetings.

4 Pulling rank

The problem: Higher-paid or higher-graded officers pulling rank around the table will silence others who have just as much to give.

The solution: The principle of 'equality around the table' should be agreed and written into your terms of reference.

5 Mission creep

The problem: People come up with hundreds of other ideas that can be tackled beyond the partnership's original brief.

The solution: Agree a clear vision and underpin this with a clear focus on five or six priorities. Allow some flexibility for one or two priorities to change over time.

6 Only here for the cash

The problem: Organisations attracted to a partnership for the money may be unwilling to do much work, volunteer for shared activities, etc.

The solution: Set out clear shared common ground from the start and focus on your shared priorities and outcomes.

7 Target? What target?

The problem: Failure to set real targets around the shared vision. Starting vague will mean you will never know what you have achieved.

The solution: Set clear targets to support your shared priorities and agree a simple but shared performance management system that everyone signs up to.

8 Death by drudgery

The problem: Endless business meetings that no-one wants to attend.

The solution: Keep business meetings short and focused on what you need to do. Would a workshop or brainstorm be a better use of time? Build in time to celebrate success.

9 We know what's best for you

The problem: Many partnerships are based in consultation but fail to continually engage. Building your work plan on historical information is not enough.

The solution: Establish your partnership based on a solid foundation of genuine consultation and ensure that you have built in activities that continually engage your client group.

10 Strictly on a need-to-know basis ...

The problem: Lack of communication between partners and beneficiaries will breed suspicion and resentment and will fuel personal agendas.

The solution: Set up good processes to network and share information. Evidence shows that the more you inform, the more satisfied people will be.

(Adapted from Improvement Network, 2011b)

Partnership working as an approach often takes longer to produce results than most organisations or policy makers anticipate. Partnerships deemed to have failed to deliver may simply not have been allowed enough time to succeed. A study that evaluated partnership working (Smith et al., 2008) found that constantly changing policy priorities and organisational restructuring could have a detrimental impact on partnerships. This results from having to renegotiate the partnership with new or reconfigured agencies, or partnerships suddenly finding themselves faced with a new policy framework. In the same study, several other areas were seen as detrimental to partnership working, including not having the key personnel with authority to act on behalf of their respective organisations or not having the capacity to fulfil their policy priorities due to the lack of appropriate, or adequate, financial and human resources. It is important, therefore, to address the problems that partnership working might result in and to fully understand how to establish and maintain partnerships for health (Perkins et al., 2010). Figure 13.3 summarises the key process (in the interacting circle) and outcome inhibitors (in the boxes) that partnerships have to overcome.

Conclusion

The clear deduction from various reviews of public health partnerships is that partnership working is not an entirely successful approach to achieving public health outcomes. However, partnership working appears still to have political support across the UK, so health providers, local authorities and social services departments with remits for public health will need to continue to collaborate across agency boundaries. Public health practitioners at all levels are therefore likely to

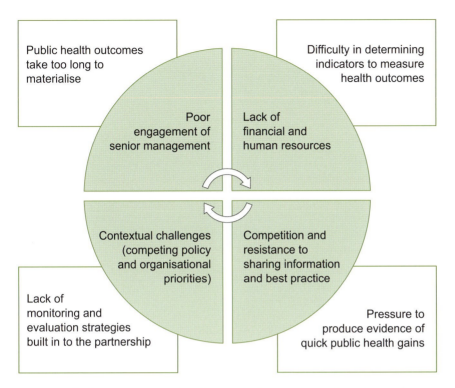

Figure 13.3 Key process and outcome challenges for partnership working (Source: based on the findings of Perkins et al., 2010)

be involved in partnership work. They will need to continue to engage other public and private organisations and the local communities which they serve.

Public health does not have the luxury of organisational stability, so partnerships need to be established and sustained in the shifting sands that reflect political will. Against this background, those with a responsibility to support partnership development should be more active (Markwell et al., 2003). To improve the quality of partnership working, sponsors need to invest in an assessment process to demonstrate partnership achievements, build on good practice, identify areas for improvement and capacity building, and track progress in delivering shared objectives and improving services. Only then will partnerships and the policies that drive them be able to claim effect.

References

ASH Wales (2011) www.ashwales.org.uk/ (accessed 22 September 2011).

Baggott, R. (2011) *Public Health: Policy and Politics* (2nd edition), Basingstoke, Palgrave Macmillan.

Baggott, R. (2010) *Public Health: Policy and Politics*, Basingstoke, Palgrave.

Baggott, R. (2005) 'A funny thing happened on the way to the forum? Reforming patient and public involvement in the NHS in England', *Public Administration*, vol. 83, no. 3, pp. 533–51.

Baldwin, L., Abernethy, P. and Roberts, L. (2005) 'Forming, managing and sustaining alliances for health promotion', *Health Promotion Journal of Australia*, August, vol. 16, no. 2, pp. 138–42.

Barnes, M., Bauld, L., Benzeval, M., Judge, K., MacKenzie, M. and Sullivan, H. (eds) (2005) *Health Action Zones: Partnerships for Health Equity*, London, Routledge.

Brinkerhoff, J.M. (2002) 'Government–non profit partnership: a defining framework', *Public Administration and Development*, vol. 22, pp. 19–30.

Burton, P. (2003) 'Community involvement in neighbourhood regeneration: stairway to heaven or road to nowhere?' London, Economic and Social Research Council Centre for Neighbourhood Research.

Butterfloss, F.D. (2006) 'Process evaluation for community participation', *Public Health*, vol. 27, pp. 323–40.

Clews, G. (2011) 'Health boards need greater powers, says King's Fund', *Health Service Journal*, 31 March.

Corbin, J.H. and Mittelmark, M.B. (2008) 'Partnership lessons from the Global Programme for Health Promotion Effectiveness', a case study, *Health Promotion International*, vol. 23, no. 4, pp. 365–71.

'Coulson, A.C. (2005) A plague on all your partnerships: theory and practice in regeneration', *International Journal of Public Sector Management*, vol. 18, no. 2, pp. 151–63.

Davidson, S. (1998) 'Spinning the wheel', *Planning*, vol. 1262, pp. 14–15.

Department of Environment, Transport and the Regions (2001) *Local Strategic Partnerships: Government Guidance*, London, The Stationery Office.

Department of Health (DoH) (2010) *Equity and Excellence: Liberating the NHS* (Cmnd 7881), London, The Stationery Office. Available at: www.dh.gov.uk/en/Healthcare/LiberatingtheNHS/index.htm (accessed 9 September 2011).

Department of Health (DoH) (2007a) *Health Challenge England*, London, The Stationery Office. Available at: www.dh.gov.uk/en/Publicationsandstatistics/Publications/PublicationsPolicyAndGuidance/DH_4139514 (accessed 9 September 2011).

Department of Health (DoH) (2007b) *Partnerships for Better Health: Small Change, Big Difference: Healthier Choices for Life*, London, The Stationery Office. Available at: www.dh.gov.uk/en/Publicationsandstatistics/Publications/ PublicationsPolicyAndGuidance/DH_075758 (accessed 9 September 2011).

Department of Health (DoH) (2006) *Our Health, Our Care, Our Say*, London, The Stationery Office. Available at: www.dh.gov.uk/en/ Publicationsandstatistics/Publications/PublicationsPolicyAndGuidance/ DH_4127602 (accessed 9 September 2011).

Department of Health (DoH) (2003) *Working in Partnership to Reduce Inequalities: A Programme for Action*, London, The Stationery Office.

Department of Health (DoH) (1994) *The Health of the Nation*, London, The Stationery Office.

Department of Health, Social Services and Public Safety Northern Ireland (DHSSPSNI) (2002) *Investing for Health – Report 2002*, Belfast, DHSSPSNI. Available at: www.dhsspsni.gov.uk/show_publications?txtid=10415 (accessed 9 September 2011).

Dowling, B., Powell, M. and Glendinning, C. (2004) 'Conceptualising successful partnerships', *Health and Social Care in the Community*, vol. 12, no. 4, pp. 309–17.

East Riding Local Strategic Partnership (2007) www.lsp.eastriding.gov.uk/ccm/ navigation/home/ (accessed 9 September 2011).

Eilbert, K. and Lafronza, V. (2005) 'Working together for community health – a model and case studies', *Evaluation and Program Planning*, vol. 28, pp. 185–99.

El Ansari, W. and Phillips, C. (2001) 'Empowering healthcare workers in Africa: partnerships in health – beyond the rhetoric towards a model', *Critical Public Health*, vol. 11, no. 3, pp. 231–52.

Entwistle, T. (2006) 'The distinctiveness of the Welsh partnership agenda', *International Journal of Public Sector Management*, vol. 19, no. 3, pp. 228–37.

Evans, D., Pilkington, P. and McEachran, M. (2010) 'Rhetoric or reality? A systematic review of the impact of participatory approaches by UK public health units on health and social outcomes', *Journal of Public Health*, vol. 32, no. 3, pp. 418–26.

Glasby, J. and Dickinson, H. (2008) *Partnership Working in Health and Social Care*, Bristol, Policy Press.

Glasby, J., Dickinson, H. and Peck, E. (eds) (2006a) 'Partnership working in health and social care', *Health and Social Care in the Community*, vol. 14, no. 5, pp. 373–444.

Glasby, J., Dickinson, H. and Peck, E. (2006b) *Effective Partnership Working: An International Symposium*, Birmingham, Birmingham University Health Services Management Centre.

Global Forum for Health Research (2011) 'Initiative on public-private partnerships for Health (IPPPH)' in Global Forum for Health Research website. Available at: www.globalforumhealth.org/research-issues/research-initiatives/initiative-on-public-private-partnerships-for-health-ippph/ (accessed 6 April 2011).

Goel, N.K., Galhotra, A. and Swami, H.M. (2007) 'Public private partnerships in the health sector', *The Internet Journal of Health*, vol. 6, no 2.

Improvement Network (2011a) *Working Better Together? Managing Local Strategic* Partnerships, London, Improvement Network. Available at: www.improvementnetwork.gov.uk/imp/aio/1098422 (accessed 9 September 2011).

Improvement Network (2011b) *The Top Ten Partnership Killers*, London, Improvement Network. Available at: www.improvementnetwork.gov.uk/imp/aio/11465 (accessed 9 September 2011)

Improvement Service (2011) 'Community planning' in Improvement Service website. Available at www.improvementservice.org.uk/community-planning/ (accessed 9 September 2011).

International Union of Health Promotion and Education (2011) 'Tools for partnership activities in health promotion and evaluating interventions that aim to reduce social inequalities in health' in International Union of Health Promotion and Education website. Available at: www.iuhpe.org/?page=508&lang=en (accessed 9 September 2011).

Involve (2011) www.peopleandparticipation.net/display/Involve/Home (accessed 9 September 2011).

Involve (2005) *People and Participation: How to Put Citizens at the Heart of Decision-making*, London, The Stationery Office.

Jupp, B. (2000) *Working Together. Creating a Better Environment for Cross-sector Partnerships*, London, Demos.

Kaminiski, M. (2011) 'Case study of medicines for malaria venture', *International Affairs Review.* Available at: www.iar-gwu.org/node/296 (accessed 9 September 2011).

Knight, T., Smith, J. and Cropper, S. (2001) 'Developing sustainable collaboration: learning from theory and practice', *Primary Health Care Research and Development*, vol. 2, pp. 139–48.

Local Government Improvement and Development (2011a) 'Coalition government plans – implications for local partnership working' in Local Government Improvement and Development website. Available at: www.idea.gov.uk/idk/core/page.do?pageId=20784973#contents-19 (accessed 9 September 2011).

Local Government Improvement and Development (2011b) 'How do you know partnership working is effective?' in Local Government Improvement and Development website. Available at: www.idea.gov.uk/idk/core/page.do?pageId=8357418 (accessed 9 September 2011).

Lowndes, V. (2001) *Local Partnerships and Public Participation*, Leicester, IPPR Partnerships Commission.

Markwell, S., Watson, J., Speller, V., Platt, J. and Younger, T. (2003) *The Working Partnership, Book 1*, London, Health Development Agency. Available at: www.nice.org.uk/niceMedia/documents/working_partnership_1.pdf (accessed 9 September 2011).

Martens, J. (2007) 'Multisectoral partnerships – future models of multilateralism?' *Dialogue on Globalization Occasional Papers*, no. 29, pp. 1–78.

Milewa, T. (2004) 'Local participatory democracy in Britain's health service: innovation or fragmentation of universal citizenship?', *Social Policy and Administration*, vol. 38, no. 3, pp. 240–52.

Morgan, L.M. (2001) 'Community participation in health: perpetual allure, persistent challenge', *Health Policy and Planning*, vol. 16, no. 3, pp. 121–30.

NHS Health Scotland (2011) 'Food and health alliance' in NHS Health Scotland website. Available at: www.healthscotland.com/food-and-health.aspx (accessed 9 September 2011).

Nishtar, S. (2004) 'Public–private "partnerships" in health – a global call to action', *Health Research Policy and Systems*, vol. 2, p. 5.

Njau, R.J.A., Mosha, F.W. and de Savigny, D. (2009) 'Case studies in public-private-partnership in health with the focus of enhancing the accessibility of health interventions', *Tanzania Journal of Health Research*, vol. 11, no. 4, p. 235.

US Government (2011) 'PPP prevention models' in The United States President's Emergency Plan for Aids Relief website. Available at: www.pepfar.gov/ppp/c23648.htm (accessed 9 September 2011).

Perkins, N., Smith, K., Hunter, D.J., Bambra, C. and Joyce, K. (2010) *'What Counts Is What Works?' New Labour and Partnerships in Public Health*, Bristol, The Policy Press.

Ridolfi, R. (ed.) (2004) *Resource Book on PPP Case Studies*, Brussels, European Commission.

Scottish Government (2011) 'Community Health Partnerships Statutory Guidance' in The Scottish Government website. Available at: www.scotland.gov.uk/Publications/2004/11/20168/45831#6 (accessed 9 September 2011).

Scriven, A. (2011) 'Partnership, collaboration and participation: fundamental principles in a settings approach to health promotion' in Scriven, A. and Hodgins, M. (eds) *Health Promotion Settings: Principles and Practice*, London, Sage, pp. 256-86.

Scriven, A. (2010) 'Partnership, collaboration and participatory approaches in health promotion practice' in Scriven, A., Kouta, C. and Papadopoulos, I. (eds) *Health Promotion for Health Practitioners*, Athens, Paschalides.

Scriven, A. (2007) 'Developing local alliance partnerships through community collaboration and participation' in Handsley, S., Lloyd, C.E., Douglas, J., Earle, S. and Spurr, S.M. (eds) *Policy and Practice in Promoting Public Health*, London, Sage, pp. 256-86.

Shelter (2011) http://england.shelter.org.uk/ (accessed 22 September 2011).

Shelter (2010) *Annual Report and Accounts 2009/2010*, London, Shelter. Available at: http://england.shelter.org.uk/__data/assets/pdf_file/0010/290629/Annual_report_2009-10.pdf (accessed 9 September 2011).

Skidmore, P., Bound, K. and Lownsbrough, H. (2006) *Do Policies to Promote Community Participation in Governance Build Social Capital?*, London, Joseph Rowntree Foundation.

Smith, K., Bambra, C., Perkins, N., Hunter, D., Joyce, K. and Blenkinsopp, E. (2008) *Partnerships in Public Health: A Healthy Outcome? Summary Findings of a Systematic Literature Review. Research Summary No. 1*, Durham, Durham University.

Thanet District Council (2011) 'Partnership framework. Working together for a better Thanet: defining a partnership' in Thanet District Council website. Available at: www.thanet.gov.uk/council__democracy/governance/partnership_working/2_defining_a_partnership.aspx (accessed 9 September 2011).

Watson, J., Speller, V., Markwell, S. and Platt, S. (2000) 'The Verona benchmark – applying evidence to improve the quality of partnership', *Promotion and Education*, vol. VII, no. 2, pp. 16–23.

Welsh Assembly Government (2011) 'Local service boards' in Welsh Assembly Government website. Available at: http://wales.gov.uk/topics/improvingservices/localserviceboards/?lang=en (accessed 9 September 2011).

World Health Organization (WHO) (1998) *Health Promotion Glossary*, Geneva, WHO. Available at: www.who.int/hpr/NPH/docs/hp_glossary_en.pdf (accessed 9 September 2011).

World Health Organization (WHO) (2002) Community Participation in Local Health and Sustainable Development: Approaches and Techniques, European Sustainable Development and Health Series: 4, Geneva, WHO. Available at: www.euro.who.int/__data/assets/pdf_file/0013/101065/E78652.pdf (accessed 9 September 2011).

World Health Organization (WHO) (2006) *Partnerships for Malaria Control: Engaging the Formal and Informal Private Sectors*, Geneva, WHO. Available at: http://apps.who.int/tdr/publications/tdr-research-publications/partnership-malaria-control/pdf/partner_malaria.pdf (accessed 9 September 2011).

World Health Organization (WHO) (2009) *Building a Working Definition of Partnership African Partnerships for Patient Safety (APPS)*, Geneva: WHO. Available at: www.who.int/patientsafety/implementation/apps/resources/defining_partnerships-apps.pdf (accessed 9 September 2011).

Chapter 14: Understanding and influencing policy change

Linda Jones

Introduction

What is public policy and why is it important for public health practitioners to understand it? Public policy is generally seen as the web of decisions made by international, national, regional and local government, and given expression in the form of legislation, regulation and guidance. It is important because it frames and directs much of public health practice. For example, Wales restructured public health through integrated health boards and created Public Health Wales to unify and integrate practice across Wales. Scotland and Northern Ireland have also sought to improve the delivery of public health through greater integration. In England this was attempted later, in 2011, and took the form of relocating public health into local authorities, reversing nearly 40 years of control of public health by the National Health Service (NHS). The precise results of this shift are unlikely to be clear for several years, if then, but the radical intent and implications of this legislation are undeniable (Walshe and Ham, 2011).

Public policy does not need the force of law to be influential and it is helpful to think about policy development in a much broader way. National, regional and local strategies and organisational policies, embodying authoritative guidance rather than legislative force, also help to shape public health practice. At a global level, countries may pledge to work towards agreed goals through processes that are largely based on good will. For example, Health for All targets, set by the World Health Organization (WHO) to achieve better health by the year 2000 (WHO, 1977), kick-started the development of health strategies in many countries: in the UK, England, Wales, Scotland and Northern Ireland each produced a national health strategy with targets for health improvement. The Ottawa Charter (WHO, 1986) had no force of law but influenced public health practice through mainstreaming a vision of empowerment, participation and action on social determinants of health (Porter, 2006).

This chapter explores public policy and the policy-making process, using examples from the public health field and beyond. It discusses how policies are made and why issues get on to the policy agenda. It briefly explores different models of policy making and examines how conflicts of value and interest affect policy change. It suggests that public health practitioners can influence policy decisions directly, for example through lobbying and pressure group membership, and by the important role they play in policy implementation. But in order to do so they need to understand the ideology of policy and the nature of the policy-making process itself.

14.1 Understanding public policy

Public policy making is shaped by competing political philosophies and interests as well as political circumstances and practicalities. Political parties make manifesto commitments but when in office must transform these into policy through parliamentary processes of debate and scrutiny: outcomes may be very different from original intentions. A policy authorises and stamps approval on a particular way forward while marginalising others. For this reason policy has been characterised as 'a web of decisions and actions that allocate values' (Easton, 1965, p. 130). Values are those aspects that people regard as important and they may be reflected in physical or symbolic goods and services such as tax cuts or extra investment in health services. Policy, Easton suggested, is about the authoritative allocation of values; in other words, the ability of those in positions of influence at any level inside or outside formal government to sanction or withhold approval in relation to particular goods and services.

Public policy and ideology

Public health has had its share of philosophical debates and value conflicts, not least about the relative responsibility of the state and the individual in matters of health (see Chapter 5) and the legitimacy or otherwise of state intervention. It is grounded partly in utilitarianism (concerned with maximising benefit or 'utility' for the majority) – a philosophical approach that provided much of the underpinning for nineteenth-century public health measures in the UK, such as sanitary reform and factory legislation. These were driven through in spite of individualist and liberal *laissez-faire* traditions that emphasised personal freedom, self-reliance, market economics and the dangers of state power. At some points in the twentieth century, especially during war and its aftermath, government policies safeguarding health became considerably bolder. Rationing, universal healthcare, family allowances, unemployment benefit, social housing and old age pensions were introduced in various forms by politicians and contributed to better standards of health and rising life expectancy in the UK population. But decisions about health, housing, education, unemployment, disability and so on, have continued to vex and divide politicians and citizens in the twenty-first century.

Debates about the proper role of the state, the balance between freedom and authority and whether state intervention is fundamentally benign or malign, have marked the whole history of public health and remain important today (Jochelson, 2005). These deeper philosophical fissures underlie debates about upstream/downstream work and high-risk/whole population approaches and are captured graphically by Beattie (1991) in his model of health promotion (see Chapter 6). Beattie's matrix model, with its authority-negotiation mode of intervention axis and its collectivist-individual axis, enables us to appreciate different philosophical traditions in public health. Some have espoused collective action – whether legislation or community-based – others have endorsed personal choice and self-reliance. But Beattie also makes the point that collective action can be authoritative and state-sponsored or negotiated, as can individual-focused action. Thus, very different public health traditions are encompassed in this matrix.

By the late 1990s another dialogue had developed claiming that state, market and individuals could complement and support each other in a new contract for social democracy (Giddens, 1998). This so-called 'third way' became linked to 'New Labour' experiments in the 2000s, which moved beyond 'state versus market' conflict towards public-private partnership. While the state had a duty to create an environment that supported health, it had to be done in partnership with voluntary and private sectors, it was argued, and with individual citizens, who themselves were responsible for making healthy choices (Wanless, 2004; Corrigan, 2007). Alongside this emerged a conceptualisation of the state as neither hero nor villain but rather a steward who protected the body politic in the least intrusive way possible (Jochelson, 2005; Nuffield Council on Bioethics, 2007). This stewardship model, set out in the Nuffield Council bioethics report *Public Health: Ethical Issues*, comprised a public health framework and ladder of iterative engagement against which health problems would be tested. This involves weighing 'the benefits to individuals and society against the erosion of individual freedom' and assessing 'economic costs and benefits alongside health and societal benefits' (Nuffield Council on Bioethics, 2007, p. 42).

Coercive measures could be considered if serious threats emerged (e.g. 'mad cow' disease; 'bird' flu; bio-terrorism) but interventions should be proportionate to the risks involved, avoid being intrusive and respect people's preferences. The Nuffield ladder is set out in Figure 14.1.

The ladder of possible policy action is as follows:

Eliminate choice. Regulate in such a way as to entirely eliminate choice, for example through compulsory isolation of patients with infectious disease.

Restrict choice. Regulate in such a way as to restrict the options available to people with the aim of protecting them, for example, removing unhealthy ingredients from foods, or unhealthy foods from shops or restaurants.

Guide choice through disincentives. Fiscal and other disincentives can be put in place to influence people not to pursue certain activities, for example, through taxes on cigarettes, or by discouraging the use of cars in inner cities through charging schemes or limitations of parking spaces.

Guide choices through incentives. Regulations can be offered that guide choices by fiscal and other incentives, for example offering tax-breaks for the purchase of bicycles that are used as a means of travelling to work.

Guide choices through changing the default policy. For example, in a restaurant, instead of providing chips as a standard side dish (with healthier options available) menus could be changed to provide a more healthy option as standard (with chips as an option available).

Enable choice. Enable individuals to change their behaviours, for example by offering participation in an NHS 'stop smoking' programme, building cycle lanes, or providing free fruit in schools.

Provide information. Inform and educate the public, for example as part of campaigns to encourage people to walk more or eat five portions of fruit and vegetables per day.

Do nothing or simply monitor the current situation.

Figure 14.1 The Nuffield Council on Bioethics intervention ladder: the ladder of possible policy action
(Source: Nuffield Council on Bioethics, 2007, p. 42)

While the Nuffield approach seems to replace ideology with common sense, it does not really solve debates about what constitutes a serious public health threat. Questions about how far health inequalities are acceptable, how much focus there should be on vulnerable social groups or what is required in a healthy environment still challenge us because they are, inevitably, not just empirical but ideological. They lead us back to the philosophical debates we noted earlier.

Public health and welfare policy

Such conflict should not surprise us because public health sits squarely within the broader terrain of social welfare policy, a territory that has always been highly contested. Social theorists have continually highlighted the ideological differences that underpin debates about welfare (Hayek, 1976; Lee and Raban, 1983; Giddens, 1998). Despite attempts to reconcile state and market through 'third way' politics, there remain significant philosophical and value conflicts that manifest themselves in politics and policy decisions. An attempt to situate public health within the framework of social welfare is set out in Figure 14.2. The figure captures differences not only about the level of state involvement in welfare but also what type of involvement is appropriate. How far should the state compensate for inequalities in the marketplace? Should it strive to create equality, more equal opportunities or merely provide minimum protection against hardship? The figure plots the following types of state welfare:

- **Conservatism** – characterised by a preference for authoritative persuasion (appeals to the family and the nation) and reluctance to embrace state planning, legislate for health or pursue equality beyond minimum social welfare and security. The focus is on persuading people to change their behaviour largely through health education messages, campaigns or voluntary agreements with producers and retailers.

- **Collectivism** – characterised by a readiness to embrace state planning and support for a comprehensive welfare system, through which better health and greater equality can be delivered. Policies in the early 2000s in the UK – minimum wage legislation, tax credits and the extension of child welfare service such as Sure Start – could all be seen as examples of collectivism at work, underpinned by belief in an active and benign state. Collectivism in public health in the UK has included anti-smoking legislation.

- **Market liberalism** – characterised by distrust of the state, seen as largely malign, a heavy emphasis on the freedom of the individual, a strong trust in market mechanisms to bring about progress and better health and acceptance of inequality. The Thatcher government of the 1980s is usually cited as an example of market liberalism at work: curtailing the power of trade unions, cutting banking regulation, encouraging private healthcare and unfettered individualism. In public health this would mean individual action – personal choices and changes, negotiations about health through counselling, private investment – rather than reliance on state support.

- **Communitarianism** – characterised by a rejection of the state as oppressive but a high commitment to creating equality through community action and shared ownership (e.g. through co-production, cooperatives and social enterprises). Quite a number of voluntary sector and municipal initiatives – community gardens, the SUSTRANS cycle network, jointly-owned and not-for-profit whole food shops – exemplify this approach, although some of them also get state support. Community development is a feature of public health work, characterised by a commitment to empowerment and working in partnership with people to identify and respond to their expressed health needs.

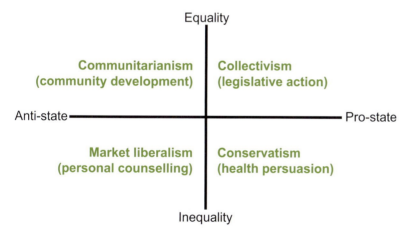

Figure 14.2 Typology of welfare approaches

(Source: adapted from Lee and Raban, 1983; Beattie, 1991).

What are the advantages and drawbacks of this type of diagrammatic representation of debates?

This type of analytical model has value in exposing and enabling reflection on the social and political perspectives underlying public health and other policies, although not all policies will fit neatly into one of these quadrants. Some public health approaches will reflect a more or less ready adoption of state involvement or a stronger or weaker commitment to pursue equality. The 'third way' approach, encapsulated in some 'New Labour' welfare policies in the early 2000s, embodied aspects of collectivism but the England White Paper *Choosing Health: Making Healthy Choices Easier Choices* (Department of Health [DoH], 2004) had a great deal to say about individual responsibility for making healthy choices and working with the private sector and to this extent also embraced market liberalism. We noted that communitarian approaches, for example the work of charities, may rely to some extent on collectivism and state support.

Also positions can shift over time. Consider the rising tide of concern about obesity. If 'responsibility deals' between government and food retailers (DoH, 2011) fail to deliver better labelling, more accurate advertising and support for healthy choices, will the state be tempted to introduce legislative solutions? Will market liberalism be deemed to have failed and will conservatism or a more collectivist approach be adopted, given the costs and seriousness of the health issue?

Policies can also have different meanings, depending on the political tradition espoused. By the beginning of the second decade of the twenty-first century, for example, all UK national governments had signed up to reducing inequalities in health. But this will undoubtedly be interpreted differently in the four nations and by different political parties. Some will be more ready to tolerate state action, as the Scottish National Party (SNP) minority government was in trying to tackle alcohol misuse by introducing minimum pricing for alcohol in Scotland in 2009, and others more likely to endorse a market or *laissez faire* approach (Box 14.1).

Box 14.1 Timeline of alcohol policy development in the UK

- 1987 – Guidelines for alcohol consumption are established by an expert committee at 21 units for men per week and 14 units for women: lower than some other countries (e.g. France).

- 2007 – A Scottish government study identifies the cost of alcohol misuse as £3.56 billion.

- By 2009 – Influential health organisations and chief medical officers in the UK endorse government action on alcohol misuse, including minimum pricing per unit of alcohol. There is public support for some action (e.g. in Scotland), strong opposition from the drinks industry and little political support in England.

- 2009 – SNP minority government introduce the Scotland Alcohol Bill, initially with provision for 45p per unit pricing. MPs pass the bill but with the minimum pricing removed (most Labour MPs vote against and the Liberal Democrats abstain).

- 2010 – A National Institute for Health and Clinical Excellence (NICE) two-year research study report on dealing with alcohol misuse notes that the cost per year for healthcare, crime, disorder and lost productivity is £27 billion. NICE, the British Medical Association (BMA) and Royal College of Physicians call for minimum pricing of alcohol to rise to 50p per unit.

- 2010 – The coalition government proposes a range of 21-28p per unit for England. This is criticised by health organisations as too weak and is not progressed.

- 2010 – Greater Manchester investigates the potential for using a public nuisance by-law to bring in 50p per unit minimum pricing for all pubs and off-licences.

- 2011 – Voluntary 'responsibility deals' are established with producers and retailers in England. They include a responsible drinking deal on labelling, sponsorship code and 'Drinkaware' support. Eight national organisations, including Diabetes UK, Alcohol Concern and the British Heart Foundation refuse to sign, claiming that the drinks industry is dictating terms. The Faculty of Public Health, public health agencies and two royal colleges call for minimum pricing.

- 2011 – The Westminster Commons Science and Technology Committee is asked to examine the evidence behind the existing alcohol unit guidelines, amid a claim from a 1987 working group member that with no decent data they made a sort of intelligent guess. The committee's remit includes examining evidence for guidelines and comparing with other countries.
- 2011 – SNP majority government aims to reintroduce minimum pricing measure.

(Sources: Scottish Government, 2007; Adetunji, 2011; DoH, 2011; NICE, 2010; Parliament UK, 2011)

14.2 Making public policy

Policy making is about the exercise of power. Public policies may be seen as 'authoritative statements of intent about action', with the assumption that 'as government has the ultimate authority to act, it is their policies which become a focus for debate and action' (Allsop, 1995). The role of central government is a key one but it is not a homogeneous body: (fairly) transient politicians, generalist career administrators and professional officers with specialist backgrounds may all have different interests to pursue. Minority and coalition governments need to negotiate and compromise and may rely more on administrative means to enact policy. Focusing too exclusively on government underplays the gulf between policy and implementation.

An alternative view characterises policy as the consequence of the actions taken by individuals in the process of implementation, which might distort or change the original intention (Barrett and Fudge, 1981). The first comment emphasises that policy is deliberate, systematic and government-led; the second highlights the potential for anyone at any level to be involved. It reminds us that policy does not just mean the latest government pronouncement but also how it is put into practice and its intended and unintended consequences.

Who makes policy?

It might be argued that the most important influence on public health policy making has been NHS priorities, since over time public health has been of relatively minor importance compared with the treatment of disease. In all the nations of the UK, and indeed around the world, the overwhelming majority of expenditure, debate and policy time is taken up with discussions about healthcare provision.

Public health is devolved to the UK nations and organisational frameworks for public health differ across the four nations but the trend is for public health functions to be unified in one body, with a greater level of autonomy than in the past (see Chapter 1, Box 1.4). Policies are shaped by robust interaction between national governments, public health and other government bodies and departments and a range of stakeholders and influential interested parties. Government reports from select committees and specialist work groups can be influential in this process. Most policy does not require legislation but is developed through formal processes of management and consultation, with initial research carried out to assess that it will not create an unnecessary burden on healthcare systems. While some policy is radical, much will build on or be limited by previous policy decisions or adapt policies used elsewhere. Policy development is necessarily dynamic: shaped by external and global forces such as multinational corporations, United Nations (UN) institutions (e.g. the World Bank), the WHO and the European Community (EC).

The wider policy community consists of representatives of major producer groups, such as directors of public health and general practitioners (GPs). They may be directly consulted or represented by influential professional associations, such as the Faculty of Public Health, the BMA and the Royal College of Nursing (RCN). Regional and local administrative bodies will be involved: health boards in Scotland and Wales, health and social care boards in Northern Ireland, and local authorities and the new health and wellbeing boards in England. A range of pressure groups – advisory bodies, commissions, charities, patient and consumer groups and business interests – will feature too and policy will be influenced by *ad hoc* bodies, such as public inquiries which explore and report back on particular issues. Some analysts have focused especially on the interplay of pressure groups, noting the ability of 'insider' groups and policy networks to shape agendas (Coxall, 2001) and to capitalise on public concerns (the 'shroud waving' of doctors when faced with possible hospital closures is one example).

Expertise may also be important, especially in public health policy where evidence-based decision making is emphasised. For example, although the 2010 Marmot Review was commissioned by a Labour government, it had a significant influence on the 2011 England White Paper on public health produced by the coalition government because of its promotion as an 'independent' review and its very thorough evidence base. However, investigations and outcomes will inevitably be framed by the types of questions asked and these will be based on assumptions and priorities that may be influenced more by politics and ideology than by a disinterested search for truth (Black, 2001; Kelly et al., 2004; Petticrew et al., 2004).

The role of the media in shaping, pushing and blocking policy change should not be underestimated. The construction of 'risk' in contemporary society owes much to media messages, as the debate about the safety of the measles, mumps and rubella (MMR) vaccination programme demonstrates (see Box 14.2). Established vaccination policy was severely undermined, rates fell and departments of health were forced into campaigning mode to drive rates up again.

Box 14.2 MMR and the media

The MMR vaccine was first developed in the 1960s and NHS policy in the UK has been to vaccinate all children within 24 months of birth. In 1996 vaccination rates were 92 per cent and measles cases were almost unheard of.

A research report by Andrew Wakefield et al. published in *The Lancet* in 1998, and further research reported in 2002, wrongly linked MMR to autism and bowel disease. This was reported widely and inaccurately by much of the media, who allowed Wakefield to conduct 'science by press conference' and helped scare parents into rejecting the MMR vaccine. Epidemiological studies in several countries demonstrated no such links, but sections of the press and social networks in the UK and USA continued to claim MMR was unsafe. The views of celebrities and parents of autistic children were given extensive exposure in the press and politicians were pursued to demand whether or not they had vaccinated their children.

Vaccination rates fell to 85 per cent in 2006 and had not fully recovered by 2011. Measles was declared endemic in 2008 and rates were still rising in mid 2011. In 2005 a mumps epidemic produced 5000 new cases in its first month. In 2008 chief medical officers launched a 'catch-up campaign', urging GPs to improve MMR take-up rates and parents to get their children vaccinated.

In 2010 Wakefield was struck off the General Medical Council (GMC) register and his work declared fraudulent. *Sunday Times* journalist Brian Deer had helped to expose Wakefield using freedom of information law.

Sources: McIntyre and Leask, 2008; Goldacre, 2009; Godlee et al., 2011)

The key dimensions of the policy-making community in public health are set out in Figure 14.3.

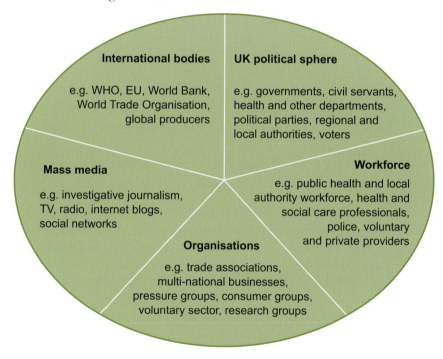

Figure 14.3 Dimensions of the policy-making community

Although governments make plans and state intentions in legislation or regulation, this is only one part of the policy process. It also involves mediation and negotiation between central decision makers and those who implement policies (Barrett, 2004). As they are implemented, policies become adapted and transformed by the actions, inactions and priorities of other people into something rather different. Indeed, Allsop (1995) accepts that 'what policy is can only be seen in terms of

417

outcomes.' In other words, what governments decide to do and what actually gets done are different and both are important to study.

In some ways policy is action: policy does not always come into being through decision making. A particular set of actions may be taken at grassroots level to deal with a crisis, for example excessive pressure on community nursing staff during an influenza epidemic, and these become the accepted way of working. Managers who can see the benefits of the change might then ratify the actions through formal decision or the actions might simply become a part of what new entrants learn from the 'old hands' when coming into the area. So top-down studies of decision making need to be balanced by bottom-up research into actions, which may produce equally potent policy changes.

There are several stages in the making of a policy and many opportunities for policy to change. A decision is not a policy, or even an action, and the subsequent translation of a decision into action shifts the focus to other players. The people who make decisions in an attempt to create a policy are rarely the same as the people who will implement the decisions. Ham (2009, p. 114) has commented that 'a decision network, often of considerable complexity, may therefore be involved in producing action.' Conversely, policy makers rarely operate with a blank sheet. They are influenced and constrained by earlier decisions from other policy sectors as well as their own (Walt, 1995).

Policy analysts have also highlighted the importance of studying non-decision making, inaction and resistance, arguing that a focus on decision making has ignored the importance of policy maintenance and inertia (Ham, 2009). For example, since the 1980s the DoH has tried in various ways to persuade general practitioners to engage in more active health education and promotion. This met with limited success, even after GPs began to be paid on the basis of locally agreed health promotion initiatives, because they did not see health promotion as a priority or were opposed in principle to introducing it into consultations with patients (Astrop and McWilliam, 1996). In spite of more recent contractual and financial incentives, GP advising on smoking, alcohol intake, diet and physical activity – especially the latter two – remains very patchy (Boyce et al., 2010).

You may be able to think of policies, which managers in your own organisation attempted to implement, that were effectively sabotaged when key, but perhaps quite junior, members of the workforce refused to respond. Or perhaps the outward form of the policy was implemented but the intention of the policy was undermined or ignored.

A role for public health practitioners

For many grassroots workers policy might seem to be something imposed on them from above, but in practice there are many possible ways in which their influence might count. Those who seek to influence and change policy so that it puts a higher priority on health, wherever they work, have several alternative strategies they might adopt. They might influence colleagues or managers at work to make changes: for example, pressing for more healthy choices in a staff canteen or persuading their manager to sponsor a health event. They could attempt to influence initial decisions about health made at a national or local level by working through their trade union representatives or other pressure groups, community groups and voluntary agencies. Ewles and Simnett (2005) called this the 'societal change' approach, which is concerned with changing the attitude of society towards a behaviour through policy. They used the example of smoking and identified desirable policy changes that have now partly been realised:

> Aim – make smoking socially unacceptable, so it is easier not to smoke than to smoke.
>
> Activity – no-smoking policy in all public places. Cigarette sales less accessible, especially to children, promotion of non-smoking as a social norm. Limiting and challenging tobacco advertising and sports sponsorship.
>
> (Ewles and Simnett, 2005, p. 43)

Until recently such changes seemed unlikely, yet the ban on smoking in public places now exists and other restrictions have followed. So while influencing societal change might appear unrealistic, prompting the response that policy change is a concern strictly for managers or national policy makers, there is some evidence that health pressure groups and the weight of health evidence can have an impact, despite the power of big tobacco companies. Suppose that we substituted 'car use' for smoking in the example above. This might currently seem absurd but in the future, given energy costs, environmental change and health risks, it is not entirely implausible.

What would be the aim and types of actions needed to accomplish change in car use?

The aim would be to make car use socially unacceptable, so it is easier not to drive than to drive. Activities could embrace promoting no-car-use policy for all urban journeys under five miles; introducing 20 mph zones on all built-up roads; removing car parking facilities, except for 'park and ride'; introducing bike lease and rental schemes; improvement and promotion of public transport, walking and cycling as social norms; and limiting and challenging car advertising and sponsorship.

Changing car culture and use would certainly be much more difficult, not least because of the individual benefits that car ownership bestows and the lack of obvious dis-benefits – disease or death – for most car users. However, the health benefits of lower car use are well established: a more physically active lifestyle, reducing the risks of being overweight and diseases associated with inactivity (Transport and Health Study Group, 2011). Reducing atmospheric pollution from car emissions lowers the risk of respiratory disorders and less and slower traffic means fewer accidents and road deaths, especially involving children. There is evidence from Denmark and the Netherlands of how car culture has been challenged over time and a culture of walking and cycling has been encouraged (Tolley, 2003). As in the case of smoking, an alliance of parents, health professionals, teachers, local authorities, pressure groups and researchers might slowly shift the culture and the public health workforce might be actively involved in this process.

Thinking about policy as a web of decisions, at all levels and not just 'at the top', involving inaction and inertia as well as individual or group action, can be quite an empowering approach. Seemingly small actions can make a difference. Being alert to the potential for making and changing policy in order to promote health is a realistic way to start.

14.3 The policy-making process

There have been many attempts to describe policy making but most analysts use a process approach in which different stages are described (Figure 14.4). This ideal type assumes a flow from identification of the problem to be solved, to assessment of options for action, formation of the policy, delivery and review (which feeds into future action). However, the relationship between policy, evidence and action is complex and there is little agreement on how far such a process is put into operation as a set of deliberate, systematic steps (Walt, 1995; Kelly et al., 2004). The rational view and the incremental view offer distinctive versions of the policy-making process.

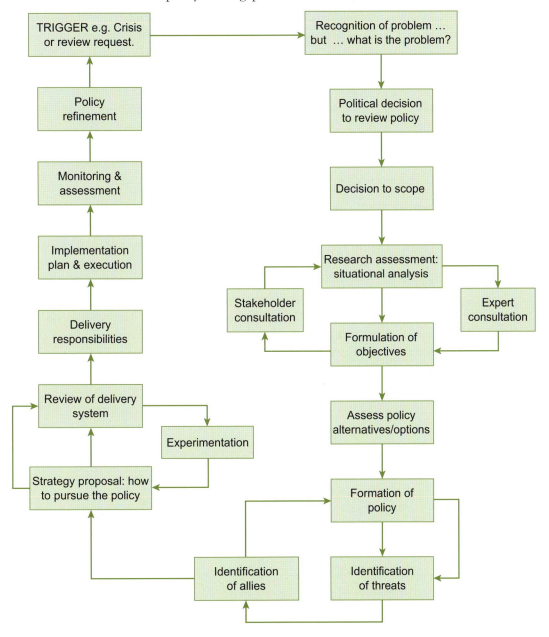

Figure 14.4 An idealised cycle of continual policy-making improvement

(Source: Lang et al., 2009, p. 14)

A rational view

The 'rational' model of policy making set out in Figure 14.4 would suggest that policy makers start by identifying a problem and, using guiding objectives and values, analyse the various alternatives for dealing with it. Having assessed the various options and their relative political and resource costs, policy makers choose the option that maximises their objectives and values. Collins (2005) usefully defines a process for public health policy analysis which incorporates this type of rational and systematic approach. But there is considerable scepticism about whether this approach is feasible. In the first place, problems are not discrete and cannot necessarily be dealt with in isolation. For example, securing better primary-care services or more effective public health services is bound up with resource questions about secondary care.

Second, policy makers may be less concerned about finding a rational solution than a politically acceptable one. They are not likely to be wholly objective in their assessment and, as we have noted, ideological considerations about the superiority of collectivism or market liberalism may mean that some policy options are ignored. Even if a problem is relatively uncontentious, policy makers are unlikely to have the time to gather and weigh up all the evidence. Therefore, evidence may well be partial, conflicting and contested. Some seemingly straightforward public health issues, such as teenage pregnancy, have provoked differences in problem definition and policy response. In relation to complex problems, for example global environmental concerns, conflicting evidence might mean that it may be impossible to be sure about what needs to be done. Finally, past decisions will influence and may well limit the range of policy options available. The major reconfiguration of the benefits system planned by the UK coalition government, for example, will limit and shape the options for reform of any incoming government, even if it strongly opposed the change.

An incremental view

The rational model has been criticised as unrealistic and it has been claimed that most policy change happens in a much more disjointed and piecemeal way. An early observer of policy change, Lindblom (1959; 1975), used the phrases 'incrementalism' (changing outcomes by minor adjustments) and 'muddling through' to describe much of policy analysis and change. He drew attention to incremental change, the inability to make clear decisions and the preference of most players to analyse policy problems one at a time and make minor adjustments rather than explore the whole policy framework. The features of incrementalism can be defined as:

- a blurring of the distinction between objectives and implementation, with objectives not clearly thought through
- appraisal of only a limited range of policy options
- a restricted analysis of these options and their consequences
- policy choice based on consensus rather than systematic cost–benefit analysis
- acceptance of the remedial, incremental and temporary nature of any change.

This draws attention to the practical difficulties involved in any policy change: the weight of vested interests, organisational inertia and the problems of implementation that this raises. At times when more radical policy initiatives have been attempted the outcomes have not always been very lasting or substantial (Harrison et al., 1990), partly because they have fixated on changing structures and neglected policies that would help transform organisational culture (Hunter, 2005). In public health, Dooris and Hunter (2007) have argued that practitioners are poorly equipped in the organisational development and change management skills that are required to grasp opportunities and bring about significant improvements in health.

How convincing do you find 'incrementalism' as an explanation of policy change?

Critics of incrementalism argue that it is at root a conservative analysis – suggesting that it is acceptable to make small adjustments. This may be appropriate in a society where there is a high degree of social stability, but it cannot adequately explain how more dramatic change can happen. To explain policy change fully both models may be necessary; indeed, in his study of economic policy change, Hall (1975) suggested that there are three types of policy change. He delineated:

- first-order change – which is incremental, a process of making minor adjustments over time
- second-order change – which will involve the development of new policy and approaches
- third-order change – which may involve a change in the accepted framework/ideas about a policy (a change of paradigm).

'Paradigm change' means changing the language, framing and whole debate about an issue so that it becomes reconceptualised. An example of this in public health in the UK could be the wrangle over health inequalities. The 'new right' Thatcher government of the 1980s redefined 'inequalities in health' as 'health variations', implying that these were natural, produced by genes or individual decisions about health, and no action was needed. Only in the later 1990s did the term 'inequalities' re-emerge and a programme of action gather pace, to the point where tackling inequalities in health has become a policy orthodoxy for all UK political parties.

14.4 Influences on policy making

Governments have considerable power to set agendas and create policies but incrementalism suggests there are effective boundaries on policy change, created by the implications of past decisions, political pressures and the complexities of policy making itself. In addition, there is the question of how much influence can be exerted by the wider public, as opposed to the more influential members of the 'policy-making community'.

In defining an idealised cycle of policy making, Figure 14.4 draws attention to stakeholder and expert influences on policy formation but how do 'problems' get recognised in the first place? Why are some problems responded to and others ignored? Who decides that a 'crisis' exists and that it must trigger a response? An exploration of two models of policy making – pluralism and conflict – offers some answers to these questions.

A pluralist or consensus view

Pluralism explores political activity as a series of processes which must be kept in balance and it draws on biology to furnish the idea of interaction and interdependence (Easton, 1965). Figure 14.5 is a simple systems model of policy making that begins to identify some of the main processes and stages that pluralism identifies.

This model pays attention to some central aspects of the policy process: the pressures on the political system or 'black box' from the wider environment and the feedback loop from outputs to inputs. At the 'inputs' point, 'demands' refers to pressures exerted by groups and individuals at all levels for some kind of change; for example, more resources for public health, better services for people with mental health

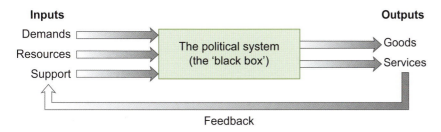

Figure 14.5 A simple systems approach to policy making

(Source: adapted from Easton, 1965)

problems, a ban on alcohol advertising and so on. As noted in Section 14.2, there is a large community of competing internal and external interests ready to make demands on the system. 'Resources' refers to natural, financial or human resources that enable governments to respond to demands. For example, an insufficient budget or a lack of expertise in the policy area may mean that it is not feasible to develop the policy. 'Support' refers to the extent to which the political system counts on wider public support to sustain it. If support for politicians, the political system or policies dwindles because of a failure to meet demands, the system becomes unstable. Instability might also result if demands greatly exceed political capacity.

The key feature of a pluralist view is that the system is adaptive. Instability at the 'input' end will result in rebalancing to create a new equilibrium or 'consensus' and similar adjustment will happen at the 'outputs' end. If 'outputs' in the form of goods and services are not acceptable and this creates greater pressures at the 'inputs' end of the process, the political system will adapt, Easton (1965) argues, and restabilise through policy or personnel changes. In the UK this is ultimately resolved by a general election, but before this happens governments with very slender majorities may change their policies in order to maximise support. Coalition governments in the UK nations try to avoid this through clear statements about their common agenda. In any case, a 'pluralist' view of policy making assumes that a consensus or balance is maintained between inputs and outputs in any political system (Walt, 1995).

The limits of a pluralist analysis

On the other hand, it is clear that policy change is not that simple. Easton's analysis is underpinned by an essentially consensual conception of policy making. In other words, it assumes that all the players in the policy-making process are able to exert some influence and make their needs and demands felt. It assumes that the state is more or less even-handed in the way it manages demands, balancing conflicting values and different interest groups. Others have drawn attention to the deficiencies in this analysis and argued that only some powerful or insider groups may influence policy making. The concept of 'bounded' pluralism was developed, highlighting how some powerful groups, such as major retailers, bankers or professional bodies, may unduly influence decision making, whereas others find their needs continually ignored.

Indeed, the assumption in pluralism that demands will be heard is underpinned by a further assumption that people's needs can be expressed. Yet, as noted in Chapter 9, not every group has the ability to articulate their needs. It is those groups better able to define their needs, express them in forms acceptable to professionals and muster support from influential groups to have those needs met that will be successful in changing policy (Bradshaw, 1980). In a more radical view, Lukes (1974) identified 'a third face of power', claiming that people may be controlled by the policy system to accept prescribed parameters so that they are not even aware that they have legitimate interests or rights to influence policy making.

Can you think of an example of a group that currently finds it difficult to influence policy making?

Marginalised groups in current policy making would include those who are homeless or unemployed. Many are not on electoral rolls and cannot express their needs, so coming together to press for change is very difficult. Governments can argue that there is no evidence of support for policy change and therefore no need to act. Some groups find it very difficult to make their voice heard; for example, those in prison or with mental health problems.

A conflict analysis

A 'conflict' view of the policy process argues that many voices may never be heard. There will always be some more powerful groups who are able to influence policy unduly whereas others can never get their concerns onto the policy agenda. In the UK health sector, for example, powerful professional groups such as the medical royal colleges or the BMA, have at times wielded considerable influence over policy to the exclusion of other producer groups, such as nurses (Dingwall et al., 1988). Public health has also had a very weak voice in policy making, not least because of the focus of the NHS on sickness and treatment. The voice of the service user has until recently gone largely unheard (Branfield and Beresford, 2006).

From being outsiders influencing policy and making demands, some groups become insiders, enmeshed in the policy process. Arguably, doctors formed one of these groups up to the 1990s. Medical influence in the setting up of the NHS ensured that hospital doctors received very generous contracts and that family doctors remained independent practitioners, subcontracted to the NHS. However, the key role of doctors in the provision of services did not protect them against successive reorganisations (Hunter, 2003), and they have not managed to resist restructuring plans for the health sector in England (DoH, 2010). While opposition from hospital doctors and many GPs to aspects of NHS restructuring and increased competition led to a 'pause' in NHS reforms in 2011, the coalition government subsequently moved ahead with changes enabling the entry of more private providers and an extended healthcare market.

New insider groups seem to be emerging in public health, as governments use voluntary agreements (such as responsibility deals – see Box 14.1) to tackle health problems. The coalition government in England has based its policy approach on working with corporate and voluntary-sector networks on food, alcohol, physical activity, health at work and behaviour change. Companies co-chair the networks and 'pledge' action in areas such as labelling and sponsorship. Resignations from these networks by health organisations followed concerns about the undue influence of companies and their use of marketing and datasets to drive policy (Adetunji, 2011).

Conflict theorists also draw attention to the closure that can be effected by powerful insiders. For example, politicians and officials may create their own agenda and not respond to outside demands. What happens within the 'black box' part of the policy process may at times effectively recast or negate external demands.

> Through the manipulation of language and the creation of crises, the authorities may impose their own definition of problems and help to frame the political agenda. Recognition of these processes is an important corrective to the naïve assumptions found in some applications of systems theory.
>
> (Ham, 1999)

In 1990 the creation of an internal market in healthcare was not welcomed by the health-sector workforce or the public. Policy was driven from within the 'black box' by Prime Minister Margaret Thatcher and Kenneth Clarke, the Secretary of State for Health. It could also be argued that this happened with the 2010 health White Paper in England. Having pledged before the election an end to top-down restructuring, the coalition government proposed radical changes and managed to alienate key health professional groups in the process (Gulland, 2011). In support of the changes it cited what turned out to be misleading statistics about poor performance and satisfaction levels (Goldacre, 2011). The Freedom of Information Act, which helped uncover evidence in the MMR case discussed earlier, has also been used to great effect to open up the 'black box' and reveal the inner workings of government.

The limits of a conflict analysis

The argument that only some powerful insider groups can influence policy making has been resisted on the grounds that it is ultimately too rigid and does not explain why policies do change, sometimes in quite radical ways (Walt, 1995). At the same time, it is evident that governments and their allies exercise a high degree of control over what can legitimately be considered to be within the national public policy domain. For example, in 1982 the Central Policy Review Staff, a cross-government think-tank, published a report calling for a comprehensive strategy on alcohol that included higher taxes, restricted sales and advertising, and better enforcement of licensing laws (Baggott, 2011). The UK government refused to publish the report or adopt its recommendations. The political leverage of the drinks industry, its economic importance (employment, tax receipts and exports) and political connections enabled it to block policies.

It was successful in persuading government to approach alcohol misuse as an individual rather than a social issue, focusing on symptoms of alcohol-related illness and disorder rather than preventing problems through population-wide policies to control overall alcohol consumption.

(Baggott, 2011, p. 351)

Attempts since the 1980s to control the drinks industry have met with mixed success (see Box 14.1), although all UK countries have increased resources for prevention – for example through the 'brief interventions' policy – and attempted to integrate alcohol with other misuse services.

It seems probable that the notion of 'bounded pluralism' will best describe this conflict between policy making levels and agendas (Hall, 1975). Insider or elite groups may be able to screen out sensitive issues at national level and use the state to serve their own ideological interests, but this is compatible with accepting more open debate about less politically dangerous issues. Analysts have mainly identified economic issues as the 'high' politics over which the political elite keeps control whereas in particular policy fields there may be quite wide debate (Walt, 1995). This may explain why alcohol was screened out while there was public debate about HIV/AIDS and other less potentially damaging concerns.

14.5 A case study of food policy

Food provides a useful and revealing case study of influences on policy making, highlighting different philosophical approaches and conflicts of value over an increasingly important area of public health. For poorer countries, food production, shortages and effective distribution are major concerns but for affluent nations the production values – quality, food safety, the use of biotechnology, biodiversity and environmental impact – have become key aspects of the contemporary policy debate.

The health dimension of food is obvious enough: insufficient intake leads to malnutrition; overconsumption leads to overweight and obesity. Individuals who are seriously overweight experience significantly greater health risks. Diets that encourage weight gain and are high in fat, processed food, salt and sugar, and low in dietary fibre such as fruit and vegetables, are associated with a higher incidence of type 2 diabetes, coronary heart disease and stroke (Foresight, 2007). Around one-third of cancers in developed countries are related to diet.

The medical profession defines obesity as having a body mass index (BMI) exceeding 30 and underweight as 17 or less (BMI is calculated by dividing body weight in kilograms by height in metres squared and dividing by 1000). Despite controversy about BMI as a measurement tool, particularly when applied to children whose patterns of growth vary considerably and for whom the reliability of the BMI is questionable, there is general agreement that the incidence of overweight and obesity is increasing, especially in richer countries. Levels have increased steadily since the late 1990s except in women in professional classes. The Foresight Report (2007), which reviewed the evidence on overweight and obesity in the UK, predicted that if trends continued unchanged, 40 per cent of the adult population would be seriously overweight by 2030. As with most other health-related problems, risks are not evenly distributed: 'obesity is associated with social and economic deprivation across all age ranges' and prevalence is highest in adult males in skilled, semi-skilled and unskilled manual occupations (Marmot, 2010, p. 59). Trends in overweight and obesity in children are shown in Figure 14.6.

These trends have provoked concern in public health circles. However, unlike smoking, food is not an intrinsically harmful product and, unlike HIV/AIDS, it is not a disease, an epidemic or even a legitimate area of public health intervention for many people. Food is also bound up with culture, profoundly influenced by habits, beliefs and values, and an intrinsic part of how groups and individuals define themselves. In short, it is a policy minefield.

Food policy and ideology

Food policy resembles a battleground in which different interests, values and political priorities compete for power and influence. It has become:

> a constant 'juggle' of competing interests and perspectives. Food policy is made, not given. It is a social construct, not ordained by a pre-programmed, perpetual or externally affirmed human order... Within food policy lies a web of social relations, actors and institutions.
>
> (Lang et al., 2009, p. 9)

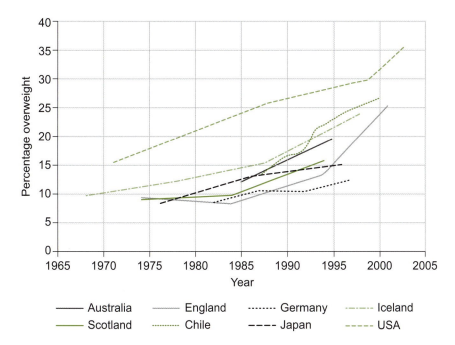

Figure 14.6 Increasing overweight in children around the world
(Source: Foresight, 2007, p. 25)

Food production has long been a matter of concern for governments and until the twentieth-century policy debates focused on output levels, protection of national production and overseas markets. Food quality was regulated to some extent, for example through penalties for food adulteration and in Victorian times through the work of environmental health officers. But the main battles before the twentieth century were between market liberals and conservatives over protection of domestic production, free trade and the opening up of UK markets to cheaper foreign foodstuffs. In the two world wars state planning predominated, and with it came rationing and control of production to maximise output. Even in the 1960s, the Common Agricultural Policy was designed around production: to encourage free trade among European signatories while protecting small national producers. Only in the late twentieth century did debates refocus to food quality, safety and sustainability: on what was being consumed, how was it being produced and who was controlling the process. In public health, trends in overweight and obesity were rising, food safety was in the hands of mass manufacturers or large retailers and experts began to argue that state action was needed to control food quality more effectively

(COMA, 1974, 1984; NACNE, 1983; James, 1997; Donaldson, 2003). Table 14.1 sets out some of the key shifts in food policy in the UK and internationally.

Contemporary debates about food policy reflect the different philosophical positions noted earlier. In the collectivist tradition the state might intervene in several ways: to regulate aspects of final stage production (such as salt and sugar levels or the use of trans-fats in processed food); marketing of food products; parts of the food chain (such as genetically modified seed use); and retailing (through competition laws). However, as you will see, there has been a marked reluctance to go beyond conservatism and more of an emphasis on voluntary agreements with the food industry. The James Report (1997) on nutrition and child health, for example, was criticised as too interventionist and dismissed by the 'third way' Labour government.

For market liberalism, regulation of the food industry is a step too far and even voluntary agreements may be suspect. Tariffs and subsidies encourage inefficiency: a free world market is required, in which the strongest will survive and provide the best deal for the consumer. Beyond minimum safety standards food is approached as a market issue in which consumer choice determines the product range. There was vociferous opposition from the 'new right' to attempts to influence dietary change in the 1980s. The 1983 National Advisory Committee on Nutritional Education (NACNE) guidelines on fat, sugar and salt levels were strongly opposed by the food industry and disliked by government, which then disbanded the committee.

Communitarian approaches are bound up with community action – for example, community shops for hard-to-reach groups, small-scale organic farming and farmers' markets – and reflect distrust of both the government and retailers. A community campaign to try to prevent the Tesco supermarket chain opening a Tesco Metro branch in a Bristol suburb has drawn attention to the social impact of big supermarkets in driving independent food retailers out of business, in the longer term reducing choice and transforming local communities (Williams, 2011).

Table 14.1 Some key shifts in food policy in the UK (1939–2010)

Date	Act/report/event	Focus	Outcomes
1939–1955	Rationing introduced	Food allocation based on nutritional need	Health of babies and children improved overall
1947	Agriculture Act	Rebuilding food production after World War II	Concern is growth and cheap food
1974–1984	Committee on Medical Aspects of Food (COMA) 1st and 2nd Reports	Increasing incidence of heart disease and link to diet	Little government response; focus on production
1980s onwards	Salmonella and BSE large-scale outbreaks	Food safety crisis	Nutrition and safety moving higher up agenda
1990	Food Safety Act	Safety standards and adulteration	Dangers of industrial scale production noted
1994–1997	Nutrition Task Force and James Reports (1997)	Recommendations to improve nutrition and protect child health	Seen by Blair government as too interventionist
2000	Food Standards Act established UK-wide Food Standards Agency (FSA)	Created as independent scientific body not influenced by food industry	Initiatives on labelling, school meals but clashes with food industry and government
2001	Department for Environment, Food and Rural Affairs (DEFRA) created	Integration of production and consumption – 'food policy'	More concern for safety, nutrition, sustainability in food chain
Mid 2000s	Foot-and-mouth outbreak; E.coli in Wales	Lack of effective regulation/ inspection revealed	Renewed concern about food and health
2005	DEFRA's Sustainable food and farming strategy	Improving regulation and sustainability of farming sector but seen as timid by government	Curry Commission set up to rethink British agriculture; Cabinet Office-led review – *Food Matters* (2008)
2010	DEFRA's Food 2030 Strategy	Reduce dependence on global markets; increase sustainable UK production; kids' cooking club network	Links food, health, environment, climate change; backs traffic light food labelling
2010	FSA disbanded in England	Nutrition to DoH; food inspection to DEFRA	Only food safety and hygiene role

The policy-making community

Who is the policy-making community in food policy? Clearly, national government is a major player and devolved governments in Scotland, Wales and Northern Ireland have been more willing to pursue proactive policies than England over recent years. Until the 1970s farmers' interests were more likely to predominate and the Ministry of Agriculture, Fisheries and Food (MAFF), which had responsibility for producers and for food policy, was frequently criticised for its toleration of factory farming and industrial, pesticide and fertiliser-driven agriculture, and its neglect of consumer interests. The setting of risk factor targets in the 1990s brought a clearer health dimension into food policy, with a stronger role for the DoH. In 2000 the UK Food Standards Agency (FSA) was created, separating food policy from agricultural production.

Food manufacturers and retailers, especially the major supermarket chains, have considerable influence and may be seen as 'insiders' in policy making in the sense that voluntary agreements over additives, packaging, advertising, and so on need to be negotiated with these major chains, which together constitute nearly 70 per cent of the UK food retail market. Manufacturing and retail chains are also increasingly global, sourcing from around the world and retailing in several countries. The United Nations, WHO and other global bodies have focused intermittently on food, especially food safety and the supply chain. Their reports have kick-started action in member nations, although until the twenty-first century they were preoccupied with food supply rather than quality.

Food policy and health experts are intermittently influential, with some reports, such as the United Nations report on the *Commission on Nutrition Challenges of the 21st Century* (2000) and the Foresight Report (2007) nudging policy change but others, in spite of a strong evidence base, being sidelined (e.g. James, 1997; NACNE, 1983). Consumer groups such as 'Which?' have become quite powerful and the media has a major role, through news reporting, television programmes and celebrity chefs. Supermarkets themselves have a strong media presence through marketing, sponsorship and customer-targeted literature. Market liberals remind us that consumers also have power, although it is questionable how far the buying habits of individuals can actually shape policy. The food policy-making community is set out in Table 14.2.

Table 14.2 The food policy-making community: key sectors and interests

Local level examples	National level examples	European region examples	International and global examples
State and public sector			
Local authorities (e.g. environmental health, trading standards; public health practitioners, nutritionists, local health services; schools; households)	Agriculture, health, environment ministries, plus economy, trade, consumer, education interests Government bodies and agencies e.g. NICE Legislatures and MPS	EU Commission Regulators Directorates for health, trade, agriculture, environment EU agencies e.g. food safety Legislature and MEPs	World Trade Organisation United Nations and agencies (Food and Agriculture Organization, WHO) Food standards Standing conferences (trade, environment) World Food Programme Framework convention on climate change
Private and corporate sector			
Farms and farmers Allotments associations Agricultural supply chain Local producers and retailers, restaurants and canteens Banks Local press and other media Haulage firms	National farmers' unions, product associations, large landowners, marketing boards, businesses, cooperatives Organic food movement Agricultural suppliers (e.g. pesticide producers, animal feed) and supply chain caterers (e.g. food processors, supermarkets and other retailers) Trade associations National finance Mass media Trade and haulage associations	EU trade associations European landowners association Trade associations, supply chains, manufacturers' associations, national franchises EU regulatory and trade agreement bureaucracies Specialised lobbying companies Airline companies	World Trade Organisation Multinational businesses, largest trade associations, and transnational cooperatives Life science multinational (e.g. Monsanto) and trading and processing companies (e.g. Unilever, Danone, Nestlé) International supermarkets (e.g. Wal-Mart) and restaurant chains (e.g. Pizza Hut, McDonalds) World Bank, IMF Global advertising agencies Airlines

Local level examples	National level examples	European region examples	International and global examples
Civil society			
Food poverty action groups Community food projects Professions Households and the general public	Consumer associations, NGOs (e.g. National Heart Forum) National Consumer Council NHS and health professional bodies	Friends of the Earth, European-level pressure groups European consumers association (BEUC) Scientific organisations	International consumer networks (IAFCO) Greenpeace International, *La Leche* League Global science advisory groups

(Source: adapted from Lang et al., 2009, pp. 88-94)

The policy-making process – rational or incremental?

Is food policy making characterised by rational or incremental development? And is there any evidence of third-order change – the change of paradigm that Hall (1993) discussed in economic policy? The answer may be that at times all three types of change have been significant in UK food policy.

In the late 1980s and early 1990s there was a dramatic shift in relation to food policy, which reoriented it towards food safety and public health. Having assumed since the late nineteenth century that food safety was under control, with public health inspection and monitoring systems in place, the UK government was rocked by two major food safety scandals: salmonella and bovine spongiform encephalopathy (BSE). First, industrial-scale food processing and catering gave rise to increasing levels of food poisoning, mainly through salmonella in poultry and eggs, then cattle infected with BSE (or 'mad cow disease' as it became known) and the contaminated meat entered the human food chain. Lang et al. (1997) draw attention to the level of initial complacency in the UK (and across Europe) about these outbreaks and the slow speed of response that reflected a continuing preoccupation with farmers and output as opposed to public health or consumer protection. However, the shift in policy, when it came, was dramatic:

The result (of complacency and inaction) was international fury, a crisis over food safety that spread worldwide, changes in laws, and even the resignation of the entire Commission of the European Commission. It spawned a wave of food safety institutions – the European Food Safety Authority, the UK's Food Standards Agency, etc. – all set up at arm's length from day-to-day control by politicians. In the UK, it led to the abolition of the Ministry of Agriculture, Fisheries and Food … subsuming its residue into a more environmentally-focused department, the Department for Environment, Food and Rural Affairs (Defra). Food safety can truly be said to have heralded the demise of policy focus on agriculture.

(Lang et al., 2009, p. 40)

Food supply crises in poor countries and the environmental costs of industrialised farming (e.g. high water use, deforestation, land contamination and oil-intensive haulage) also influenced policy but it was the food safety crisis, shaking the developed world out of its complacency, that produced what was arguably a third-order 'paradigm shift' in policy. By 2010 the UK had structures and policies that put health and safety centre stage through DEFRA, tougher food standards legislation through the FSA and the beginning of a more concerted approach to diet-related health problems, in particular obesity (National Audit Office, 2001; Foresight Report, 2007).

Was this a genuine breakthrough in which policy was reconceptualised? Or was it second order: a rational approach to food policy that disrupted existing systems but in which new policies overlaid, rather than replaced, existing policies and philosophies? In a way, the answer to this question can only be given over time but there is some evidence that, having made a major structural reform, piecemeal policy change is now in fashion. Lang et al. (2009, p. 3) argue that:

there are already many signs of policy cacophony – competing powerful voices drowning out equally worthy positions when there is a case for integration and symphony. Actions to ensure decent, health-enhancing food supply and equitable consumption require integration and coherence.

It is clear that food policy in the twenty-first century has remained contentious and piecemeal. It has also exhibited features of an incremental approach in which governments shift this way and that, trying to accommodate competing interests such as retailers, producers, environmentalists, public health professionals, bankers, consumers and so on. Policy decisions about matters such as regulating packaging, labelling, additives and advertising have shifted over time – even when the same government remained in power. However, there are signs of fractures within the food industry, with some companies thinking longer-term about social responsibility, health and community engagement. What has also emerged from recent upheavals is a much stronger consumer lobby, some of which has made common cause with some parts of the food industry. For example, parents, teachers, public health nutritionists and the Local Authority Caterers' Association worked with celebrity chef Jamie Oliver in the 2000s to transform school dinners. They were quick to defend the policy (and Oliver himself) against England Secretary of State for Health Andrew Lansley, who dismissed the scheme as ineffective and to refute his evidence, demonstrating how allegiances are shifting (McSmith, 2010). Such alliances might have a significant impact of the nature and pace of future policy change.

Influences on policy making

We can now reflect on the character of food policy making. Overall, does it best fit with a pluralist or a conflict model? The intriguing answer may be that this has shifted over time. Until the 1990s there were some marked features of a conflict model, with powerful insiders and excluded outsiders. Food supply, as you have seen, was the key goal. Food producers and retailers were therefore predominant in policy making and MAFF was criticised as simply an extension of the food industry. Food safety was assumed to be secure and the DoH had little involvement in diet-related health policy. Existing regulation was assumed to be adequate, with 'sovereign consumers' making free choices in a largely self-regulating market. Some voices – experts concerned about health impacts, environmental critics concerned about pesticides and land degradation (Carson, 1965) and consumer groups – had very little chance to make their voices heard. Others, arguably most citizens, remained unaware of the issues and dangers.

Applying Lukes' concept of a 'third face of power' (1974), we could claim that the general public could not engage in debates about food policy because the policy process and terms of the debate, including the techniques and systems used by the food industry, were never revealed to public scrutiny. The insider relationships between MAFF, the farming lobby, food manufacturers and retailers minimised criticism and debate. In Bradshaw's (1980) terms, the general public did not have 'felt' needs, let alone 'expressed' needs; their 'normative' needs were framed by political and professional judgements that food supply, rather than concerns about how it was produced or what impact production was having on health or the environment, was the critical need to be met.

After the food scandals of the 1980s, the rising tide of concern about environmental damage and the growing pressure on health services arising from obesity-related ill health disrupted this complacency, policy development became more pluralist and open to wider debate. Within government, public health arguments became more influential (Donaldson, 2003) and ministers became more interventionist, although they still relied on health education to shift public attitudes and showed only intermittent determination to regulate food standards, restrict advertising and continue with firm targets for tackling obesity. The Scottish Executive had developed a national diet action plan in the mid 1990s, but by 2000 every UK nation had set targets for reducing obesity and put in place cross-departmental agreements.

New voices and interest groups became prominent and successfully challenged authoritative positions. For example, claims by the food marketing industry that its advertising informs but does not pressure consumers into particular food choices were systematically refuted by evidence from the Hastings Review, which demonstrated that marketing had a measurable impact on children and young people's diets (Hastings et al., 2004). The FSA became a powerful, evidence-based leader in improving diet and food safety (Box 14.3, page 440). The environmental lobby amassed evidence about the health risks of pesticides and factory farming that was difficult to ignore and a political movement (the Green Party) began to win council and then national election seats.

Box 14.3 The Food Standards Agency: a brief history

The Food Standards Agency (FSA) was established in 2000 after the salmonella and BSE crises as an arms-length UK-wide organisation to create 'clear blue water between us and safety difficulties', as one Labour minister was reported to have said.

The remit of all four branches of the FSA was to improve food safety and standards and protect the health of the population in relation to food. It had a nutrition, regulatory and food safety and hygiene role with responsibility for food-labelling policy.

As it settled into its role, the FSA pursued proactive policies, especially in relation to public safety, which brought it into conflict with government. It endorsed the EU-proposed traffic light system of food labelling, welcomed by the BMA, British Heart Foundation and also supermarket chains Sainsbury's and Marks and Spencer, but strongly opposed by the Food and Drink Federation and chains such as Tesco, Nestlé and Danone (which helped defeat the scheme in Europe).

In 2010, Andrew Lansley, Secretary of State for Health in England, announced scaling back of FSA England to focus only on food safety and hygiene. He stated that 'nannying' and lecturing had not worked. Nutrition and labelling was moved into the DoH and inspection into DEFRA. Critics claimed that the food lobby had won and the 'responsibility deal' for food that followed reinforced this view. In Wales, nutrition moved to the Welsh Assembly Government but other functions were retained. Scotland and Northern Ireland have retained all their original functions.

(Ramesh, 2010)

As new interest groups and evidence emerged, the food industry itself began to fragment (Lang and Heasman, 2004). Strains between farmers, manufacturers and retailers had been evident for some time, with large supermarkets and food-processing chains driving down prices paid to farmers (in the UK and overseas), maximising their own profits but also satisfying consumers by keeping food prices low. The farming lobby became more fragmented, with organic farmers in direct opposition to mass producers. We noted earlier that some retailers developed a campaigning and community dimension, championing 'healthy eating' and adopting the language of public health and organic farming to make 'healthy choices easier choices'. Whether this is done because of a new sense of corporate social responsibility or merely to safeguard their position, it has helped to raise public consciousness about diet and health.

How far do you agree that food policy making is more pluralist and what limitations do you think there are to this?

Food policy making in the UK in the twenty-first century is arguably more pluralist and open to wider influence than in the twentieth-century because a much wider range of bodies and interest groups can make their voices heard, including a stronger consumer voice. However, it may be seen as an example of 'bounded' rather than untrammelled pluralism in which the policy-making community is still restricted, even if more diverse. The delivery of cheap food, convenience food and wide choice to the UK consumer means that the public is not heavily engaged in campaigning for less intensive production, fairer pricing or healthier choices. Governments are unable or unwilling to risk alienating retailers and manufacturers by introducing further regulation of fats, additives and food processing. They can also shift the balance of power between producer and consumer (see Section 14.3). Multinational corporations have a great deal of power and food marketing plays a major part in shaping food preferences and choices. Health is one priority among many, and by no means the most important one, although public health expertise is valued more highly than in the past. There is a long way to go before diet becomes viewed, let alone regulated, in a similar way to smoking.

Conclusion

Public health policy is not only about decision-taking and policy creation. It is also about making change and this involves policy implementation. All those involved in public health can play a significant part in the policy process through joining pressure groups and campaigns, through their membership of professional bodies which educate policy makers, by helping to set agendas and lobby for change and through exercising their rights as citizens. In implementation, evaluation and policy review there are particular opportunities for well-informed public health advocates to make their voices heard.

The creation of policy does not mean that it is necessarily translated into action. Quite often this requires the commitment of people in the organisation to push the policy through and make it work. Conversely, without champions, policies for change may not succeed. Looking for opportunities to endorse and support health-promoting policies, and to modify policies that might damage health, can be part of any public health-related role, especially in alliance with like-minded colleagues or agencies.

References

Adetunji, J. (2011) 'Too close? The drink industry's unsteady deal with government', *The Guardian*, 7 April. Available at: www.guardian.co.uk/public-leaders-network/2011/apr/07/close-drinks-industry-unsteady-government (accessed 5 September 2011).

Allsop, J. (1995) *Health Policy and the NHS: Towards 2000*, London, Longman.

Astrop, P. and McWilliam, J. (1996) 'The role of the family health services authorities in promoting health' in Scriven, A. and Orme, J. (eds) *Health Promotion: Professional Perspectives*, London, Macmillan, pp.44-53.

Baggott, R. (2011) *Public Health: Policy and Politics* (2nd edition), Basingstoke, Palgrave Macmillan.

Barrett, S. (2004) 'Implementation studies – time for a revival?', *Public Administration*, vol. 82, no. 2, pp. 249-62.

Barrett, S. and Fudge, C. (1981) *Policy and Action: Essays on the Implementation of Public Policy*, London, Methuen.

Beattie, A. (1991) 'Knowledge and control in health promotion: a test case for social theory' in Gabe, J., Calnan, M. and Bury, M. (eds) *The Sociology of the Health Service*, London, Routledge, pp. 162-202.

Black, N. (2001) 'Evidence based policy: proceed with care', *British Medical Journal*, vol. 323, pp. 275-79.

Boyce, T., Peckham, S., Hann, S. and Trenholm, S. (2010) *A Pro-active Approach: Health Promotion and Ill-health Prevention*, London, Kings Fund.

Bradshaw, J. (1980) 'An end to differentials?', *New Society*, vol. 54, pp. 64-65.

Branfield, F. and Beresford, P. (2006) *Making User Involvement Work: Supporting Service User Networking and Knowledge*, York, Joseph Rowntree Foundation.

Carson, R. (1965) *Silent Spring*, Harmondsworth, Penguin.

Collins, T. (2005) 'Health policy analysis: a simple tool for policy makers', *Public Health,* vol. 119, no. 3, pp. 192-96.

Committee on Medical Aspects of Food (1984) *Diet and Cardiovascular Disease*, London, HMSO.

Committee on Medical Aspects of Food (1974) *Diet and Coronary Heart Disease*, London, DHSS.

Corrigan, P. (2007) 'New social democratic politics of health in England today' in Griffiths, S. and Hunter, D. (eds) *New Perspectives in Public Health* (2nd edition), Oxford, Radcliff, pp. 79-86.

Coxall, W. (2001) *Pressure Groups in British Politics*, London, Longman.

Department of Health (DoH) (2011) *Public Health Responsibility Deal*, London, Department of Health. Available at: www.dh.gov.uk/en/Publichealth/Publichealthresponsibilitydeal/index.htm (accessed 5 September 2011).

Department of Health (DoH) (2010) *Equity and Excellence: Liberating the NHS* (Cmnd 7881), London, Department of Health. Available at: www.dh.gov.uk/en/Publicationsandstatistics/Publications/PublicationsPolicyAndGuidance/DH_117353 (accessed 5 September 2011).

Department of Health (DoH) (2004) *Choosing Health: Making Healthy Choices Easier*, London, Department of Health. Available at: http://webarchive.nationalarchives.gov.uk/+/www.dh.gov.uk/en/Publicationsandstatistics/Publications/PublicationsPolicyAndGuidance/DH_4094550 (accessed 5 September 2011).

Dingwall, R., Rafferty, A.M. and Webster, C. (1988) *An Introduction to the Social History of Nursing*, London, Routledge.

Donaldson, L. (2003) *Annual Report of the Chief Medical Officer of Health for England 2002*, London, Department of Health.

Dooris, M. and Hunter, D. (2007) 'Organisations and settings for promoting public health' in Lloyd, C.E., Handsley, S., Douglas, J., Earle, S. and Spurr, S. (eds) *Policy and Practice in Promoting Public Health*, London, Sage/The Open University, pp. 95-125.

Easton, D. (1965) *A Systems Analysis of Political Life*, New York, Wiley.

Ewles, L. and Simnett, I. (2005) *Promoting Health: A Practical Guide* (5th edition), Edinburgh, Ballière Tindall.

Foresight (2007) *Tackling Obesities: Future Choices*, London, Government Office for Science.

Giddens, A. (1998) *The Third Way: The Renewal of Social Democracy*, Cambridge, Polity Press.

Godlee, F., Smith, J. and Marcovitch, H. (2011) 'Wakefield's article linking MMR vaccine and autism was fraudulent', *British Medical Journal*, vol. 342, p. d1678.

Goldacre, B. (2009) *Bad Science*, London, Harper Perennial.

Goldacre, B. 'NHS leaflet mixes past and present' The Guardian, 16 April 2011.

Gulland, A. (2011) 'Welcome to the century of the patient', *British Medical Journal*, vol. 342, p.d2038.

Hall, P. (ed) (1975) *Change, Choice and Conflict in Social Policy*, London, Methuen.

Hall, P. (1993) 'Policy paradigms, social learning and the state', *Comparative Politics*, vol. 125, pp. 275-296.

Ham, C. (1999) *Health Policy in Britain*, Basingstoke, Macmillan.

Ham, C. (2009) *Health Policy in Britain: Public Policy and Politics* (6th edition), London, Palgrave.

Hastings, G., Stead, M., MacDermott, L., Forsyth, A., Mackintosh, A.M., Rayner, M., Godfrey, C., Caraher, M. and Angus, K. (2004) *Review of Research on the Effects of Food Promotion to Children. Final Report to the Food Standards Agency by the Centre for Social Marketing, University of Strathclyde*, London, Food Standards Agency. Available at: www.food.gov.uk/multimedia/pdfs/foodpromotiontochildren1.pdf (accessed 5 September 2011).

Harrison, S., Hunter, D. and Pollitt, C. (1990) *The Dynamics of British Health Policy*, London, Unwin.

Hayek, F. (1976) *The Constitution of Liberty*, London, Routledge.

Hunter, D. (ed) (2005) *Managing for Health*, London, Routledge.

Hunter, D. (2003) *Public Health Policy*, London, Routledge.

James, P. (1997) *An Interim Proposal for Nutritional Education*, London, Ministry of Agriculture, Forestry and Fisheries.

Jochelson, K. (2005) 'Nanny or steward: the role of government in public health', *Public Health*, vol. 120, pp. 1149-55.

Kelly, M.P., Speller, V. and Meyrick, J. (2004) *Getting Evidence into Practice in Public Health*, London, Health Development Agency.

Lang, T., Barling, D. and Caraher, M. (2009) *Food Policy: Integrating Health, Society and the Environment*, Oxford, Oxford University Press.

Lang, T. and Heasman, M. (2004) *Food Wars: The Global Battle for Mouths, Minds and Markets*, London, Earthscan.

Lang, T., Millstone, E. and Rayner, M. (1997) *Food Standards and the State: A Fresh Start*, London, Thames Valley University Centre for Food Policy.

Lee, P. and Raban, C. (1983) 'Welfare and ideology' in Loney, M., Boswell, D. and Clarke, J. (eds) *Social Policy and Social Welfare*, Milton Keynes, Open University Press.

Lindblom, C.E. (1959) 'The science of muddling through', *Public Administration Review*, vol. 19, no. 2, pp. 79-88.

Lindblom, C.E. (1975) 'Still muddling, not yet through', *Public Administration Review*, vol. 39, no. 6, pp. 517-26.

Lukes, S. (1974) *Power: A Radical View*, London, Macmillan.

Marmot, M. (chair) (2010) *Fair Society, Healthy Lives. Strategic Review of Health Inequalities in England Post-2010*, London, The Marmot Review. Available at: www.marmotreview.org/AssetLibrary/pdfs/Reports/FairSocietyHealthyLives.pdf (accessed 5 September 2011).

McIntyre, P. and Leask, J. (2008) 'Improving uptake of MMR', *British Medical Journal*, vol. 336, no. 7647, pp. 729-30.

McSmith, A. (2010) 'Jamie Oliver health approach "doesn't work" says Health Secretary', *The Independent*, 30 June. Available at: www.independent.co.uk/news/uk/politics/jamie-oliver-health-approach-doesnt-work-says-health-secretary-2014780.html (accessed 5 September 2011).

National Advisory Committee on Nutrition Education (NACNE) (1983) *A Discussion Paper on Proposals for Nutrition Guidance for Health Education in Britain*, London, Health Education Council.

National Audit Office (2001) *Tackling Obesity in England*, London, HMSO. Available at: www.nao.org.uk/publications/0001/tackling_obesity_in_england.aspx (accessed 5 September 2011).

National Institute for Health and Clinical Excellence (NICE) (2010) *Alcohol-use Disorders – Preventing Harmful Drinking. Public Health Guidance Note (PH24)*, London, NICE. Available at: http://guidance.nice.org.uk/PH24/EducationResource/trainingslideset/ppt/English (accessed 5 September 2011).

Nuffield Council on Bioethics (2007) *Public Health Ethical Issues*, London, Nuffield Council on Bioethics.

Parliament UK (2011) 'Committees' in Parliament UK website. Available at: www.parliament.uk/business/committees/ (accessed on 5 September 2011).

Petticrew, M., Whitehead, M., Macintyre, S., Graham, H. and Egan, M. (2004) 'Evidence for public health policy on inequalities: 1: The reality according to policymakers' in *Journal of Epidemiology and Community Health*, vol. 58, pp. 811-16.

Porter, C. (2006) 'Ottawa to Bangkok: changing health promotion discourse', *Health Promotion International*, vol. 22, no. 1, pp. 72-79.

Ramesh, R. (2010) 'Food Standards Agency to be abolished by health secretary', *The Guardian*, 12 July. Available at: www.guardian.co.uk/politics/2010/jul/11/food-standards-agency-abolished-health-secretary (accessed 5 September 2011).

Scottish Government (2007) *The Societal Cost of Alcohol Misuse in Scotland*, Edinburgh, Scottish Government.

Tolley, R. (ed) (2003) *Sustainable Transport*, Sawston, Woodhead Publishing Ltd.

Transport and Health Study Group (2011) *Health on the Move 2*, Stockport, Transport and Health Study Group.

United Nations (2000) *Commission on Nutrition Challenges of the 21st Century*, New York, United Nations.

Walshe, K. and Ham, C. (2011) 'Can the government's proposals for NHS reform be made to work?', *British Medical Journal*, vol. 342, p. d2038.

Walt, G. (1995) *Health Policy: An Introduction to Process and Power*, London, Zed.

Wanless, D. (2004) *Securing Good Health for the Whole Population: Population Health Trends*, London, HM Treasury.

Williams, Z. (2011) 'The Tesco riot is no surprise given people's powerlessness', *The Guardian*, 28 April. Available at: www.guardian.co.uk/commentisfree/2011/apr/28/tesco-riot-planning-law-bristol (accessed 5 September 2011).

World Health Organization (WHO) (1986) *Ottawa Charter for Health Promotion*, Geneva, WHO.

World Health Organization (WHO) (1977) *Health for All by the Year 2000*, Geneva, WHO.

Chapter 15: Building healthier futures: barriers and enablers

Linda Jones

Introduction

Public health faces an uncertain future. It has become bolder, more ambitious and more overtly political. It has signed up to World Health Organization (WHO) goals to reduce inequalities in health within countries and between countries. It has paraded its intentions to build a healthier future: developing new initiatives, forging stronger alliances and seeking greater influence in policy making.

The potency of 'health' – the general public's desire for it and politicians' preoccupation to protect it while controlling its rising costs – has assisted public health to gain some ground. Claims about the advantages of ill-health prevention (and, more radically, of promoting wellbeing) are now more widely understood and sometimes accepted, as in the case of smoking. Other policy sectors, such as transport and food, have appreciated that linking their plans to a health message could enable them to carry more weight.

Across the UK there have been decisive moves towards creating more integrated public health services, amidst recognition that much health and ill health is generated outside the health sector (Marmot, 2010). But how effective are these services likely to be? What factors will influence progress? Internationally, there have been some successes in refocusing health development and developing stronger regulatory frameworks (Lee, 2010). But how feasible is further progress within structures and systems so heavily influenced by economic considerations and multinational corporate power?

This chapter investigates opportunities and challenges for public health practice in the twenty-first century. It places public health within a global, regional and national context and assesses how far key dimensions of 'healthier futures' – vision and values, leadership, resources and structures – are in place or in development to deliver those futures. It reflects on the 'toolbox' of contemporary public health practice and considers whether the skill-set used today will need to be supplemented by new approaches in the future. In doing so, it draws on evidence set out in earlier chapters and seeks to assemble an agenda for further action.

15.1 Facing the future: challenges and opportunities

So where does public health stand in the early twenty-first century? Table 1.4 in Chapter 1 suggests that public health in the UK may be entering a phase of development, characterised by 'integration' and marked by a growing concern to tackle health inequalities and environmental change alongside its health protection and preventive work. Could it be that by combining its nineteenth-century population focus on environmental improvement and its twentieth-century preoccupation with individual behaviour, public health will rebalance itself to create a twenty-first-century integrated, multi-professional service? Will this mean that public health repositions itself alongside other welfare services in intellectual and operational terms? Can downstream lifestyle approaches and upstream social determinants approaches begin to work more constructively together to tackle the complexity of dealing with the wider determinants of ill health?

In some ways, lifestyle approaches seem well entrenched. For example, Chapter 10 notes how 'nudge theory', in spite of its critics, has become the latest potential 'magic bullet' in the battle to change health behaviours, at least in England. Behaviour change is seen as less complex and challenging than community engagement and empowerment, which can often be marginalised as practitioners work to hit targets and secure funding (see Chapter 11). But there are signs of new thinking in response to emerging and renewed health challenges, including efforts to link together public health and other welfare services. Moreover, ever more sophisticated individual-level treatment and prevention may not in the longer term provide a feasible or sustainable way forward to health.

What factors do you think might encourage a shift towards more population-level public health?

Several factors at global level have strengthened the case for regulatory frameworks, including the resurgence of infectious diseases and environmental threats from pollution and climate change. In addition, drug resistance, hospital-acquired infection and the resurgence of infectious diseases are highlighting some of the limitations of modern medicine, while its costs continue to rise. The success of individual-focused disease prevention has been limited and some new public health concerns, such as obesity and excessive drinking, are proving very difficult to tackle without increased interagency working and stronger regulation. We explore these challenges below. It is doubtful whether any of them can be controlled through interventions at the level of the individual.

The challenge of globalisation

Much has been written about globalisation but there is a lack of systematic research evidence of its impact on population health (Beaglehole and Bonita, 2009). International trade has burgeoned, production has become globalised, technological innovation has speeded up and population movements are more pronounced. But is this beneficial or detrimental to health? It is clear that some health-related work becomes more challenging; for example, enforcing food and other safety standards when a much greater percentage of products are shifted around countries for processing (Lang et al., 2009). Other work may become easier, such as health development with remote communities. Improvements in communications are facilitating the coordination of global responses to pandemics, but on the other hand economic migration and leisure and business travel offer new possibilities of exposure to infections for which people may have not developed resistance, and allow new strains of infections to develop. In the face of such challenges, advice on safe travel, healthy eating and individual protection, while important, is unlikely to substitute adequately for concerted national and international action. Table 15.1 sets out some risks and benefits directly and indirectly associated with globalisation.

Table 15.1 Globalisation and health: some risks and benefits

Dimension	Direct and indirect benefits for health	Direct and indirect risks to health
Accelerated economic growth	Rising living standards Longer life expectancy (although may be unequally distributed) Investment in education, health and welfare infrastructure can grow	Recession likely to impact globally, threatening living standards Increasing gap between rich and poor nations (and within nations) Values of rich (e.g. economic liberalism) constrain poor countries' development
Rapid technological innovation	Production costs fall – cheaper food, medicines, etc. ICT communications can support education and economic development Improved management of global health risks	Poor countries geared to export (e.g. food, raw materials) versus domestic development Digital divide – poor lose out More effective marketing of health-damaging products (e.g. tobacco, processed foods)
Increased mobility	Economic migration boosts poor countries' income Travel promotes cultural exchange, innovation, etc.	Transnational companies press to reduce labour costs, threatening health and safety Skilled labour migrates, undermining development Easier spread of infectious diseases; pandemics and new disease strains
Environmental impact	Better housing, amenities and transport are developed and can be afforded as national incomes rise	Energy-intensive production and consumption (e.g. car, air travel) increases pollution, greenhouse gases, climate change Depletion of natural resources: land take, deforestation, decline in open spaces and biodiversity

Economic growth and health

Table 15.1 makes the point that it is not globalisation as such that is a threat to health but the way that its impact is managed. Increased interconnectedness through population mobility and open borders can be liberating, but not if it creates a global free-market economy that undermines health. Public health researchers have drawn attention to the tensions between neoliberalism and social justice, in particular the dangers of a deepening gulf between rich and poor countries. Criticism has been levelled at the World Bank (WB) and the World Trade Organization (WTO) for the negative side effects of their liberalisation policies on the economies of poor countries (WHO, 2008; McMichael and Beaglehole, 2009; Marmot, 2010). Multinational corporations, with their huge purchasing power, influence production priorities and economic development in poorer countries, sometimes detrimentally.

At the root of debates about globalisation, it may be argued, lies a rather different concern: one about unlimited economic growth (Jones, 2000). While there is considerable evidence that economic growth can bring health benefits through improved living standards (McKeown, 1976; Wilkinson, R.G., 2005), unrestrained economic growth that entails the rapid consumption of finite resources, pollution and global instability is likely to damage population health, at least in the longer term (Schumacher, 1974; Popay et al., 1993; McMichael and Beaglehole, 2009). WHO has shifted position on this issue. In 2001 it published the *Report of the National Commission on Macroeconomics and Health* which emphasised the importance of investing in population health to support economic growth. But more recently, for example, in the WHO Commission Report on Social Determinants of Health, *Closing the Gap in a Generation* (2008), it has acknowledged that economic growth should be linked to the fair distribution of health, wellbeing and sustainability. In other words, economic growth should not be seen as an end in itself but as a means to an end; it should be used to enhance health and wellbeing and to tackle inequalities in health. This was stated forcefully in the 2010 Marmot Report *Fair Society, Healthy Lives*, which commented:

> It is time to move beyond economic growth as the sole measure of social success ... Wellbeing should be a more important societal goal than simply more economic growth. Prominent among the measures of wellbeing should be levels of inequalities in health. Environmental sustainability, too, should be a more important societal goal than simply more economic growth.
>
> (Marmot, 2010, p. 18)

There are two related issues to consider here. First, it is not economic growth as such that is key, but economic distribution of the growth that does occur. R.G. Wilkinson (2005; 2008) has argued that societies with a more equal distribution of income thrive and are better off in health terms. In contrast, countries with much larger income differentials, he claims, also have larger differences between the health status of different social groups. Beyond a certain point the health of high-income groups does not improve, so they benefit little in health terms from their extra income, but below a certain point a lack of income correlates very strongly with poor health, disability and premature mortality (see Chapter 2).

Second, the preoccupation with economic growth leads to a bizarre situation in which any wealth creation is considered valuable. Back in the 1990s, Popay et al. pointed out that including costs for cleaning up oil spillages, dealing with traffic accidents and long-distance road haulage in a country's Gross National Product (GNP – the sum of all economic output each year) distorted the figures. Preventing pollution and accidents and having local or home-grown food would make more environmental sense; however, they would make a far less significant contribution to GNP. They commented that 'similarly, cigarettes and alcohol production are "wealth producing" from an economic perspective, but from a health perspective they are "ill health producing" ...' (Popay et al., 1993, p. 275). So measures of economic growth include some inappropriate activities and overlook others, including all those that are informal or unpaid. Neither income distribution nor the composition of GNP can be ignored if public health really wants to tackle health inequalities.

Public health and environmental impacts

Issues about productivity provoke consideration of environmental change, which presents new challenges to public health (Haines et al., 2006). Climate change, which is generally acknowledged to be driven by industrial growth and related human activities, brings new risks for human health. Global warming, with associated droughts, heat waves, floods, ozone depletion and air pollution, are all calculated as being likely to increase in the future (Wilkinson, P., 2005). Rising average temperatures may increase the incidence of some infectious diseases, such as malaria, as well as some chronic conditions, such as respiratory diseases. Bentham and Langford (reported in Baggott, 2011) noted that a 1 per cent rise in temperature was associated with a 5 per cent increase in reported cases of food poisoning.

By 2011, 192 governments (but not the USA) had ratified the Kyoto Protocol (agreed in 1997 and in force from 2005) which focused on tackling climate change by cutting greenhouse gases and other emissions, but progress remained patchy (Victor, 2011a). The first commitment period of Kyoto was until 2012, with increasingly fractious attempts to gain further agreement. Critics of the UN-led cumbersome, global-negotiation process have claimed that it should be replaced by smaller regional forums focused on driving major emitters (such as the European Union [EU], USA and China) and major corporations to make substantial change happen (Victor, 2011b; Harvey, 2011). Such a shift would enable regional or national governments to drive work forward. However, environmental groups such as Greenpeace have claimed that it would 'send a destructive signal to business and undermine the green economy' (Victor, 2011a).

The Health Protection Agency (HPA) in the UK produced a report in 2008 entitled *The Health Effects of Climate Change in the UK*. It offered a useful account of health impact, indicating that the rise in heat-related deaths over the next decade (estimated as in excess of 3000) would probably be offset by the fall in winter deaths due to higher average temperatures. It noted other health risks, for example the potential of floods to contaminate water supplies and food crops. It emphasised preparedness and public health guidance.

What responses do you think people involved in public health should make to concerns about environmental health risks?

Responsible choices about food, travel and other types of consumption are needed at individual and organisational levels, but they must be matched by systematic and sustained action at national and global level. This may seem too remote to influence, but environmental campaigns and concepts such as 'Think Global, Act Local', or its more recent conceptualisation as 'Glocalism', highlight the way in which global and local issues are linked and individual action is possible. Table 15.2 suggests some ways in which individuals and agencies might contribute to sustainability in their private and professional lives.

Table 15.2 Action for sustainability at different levels: some examples

Consumer action – walk or cycle, buy green products and local produce
Household action – insulate, store rainwater, avoid food waste, recycle
Citizen action – join a pressure group, start a local campaign, lobby your councillor and MP
Community action – establish a skills exchange scheme, start a community garden, organise a 'walking bus' of children to school
Professional action – prioritise sustainability at work, support community initiatives, harness external resources for green action
Local authority action – use health impact assessment tools, energy-saving advice, set and enforce targets, involve local people in environmental priority setting
Organisational action – save energy in transport, cleaning, heating and lighting, restrict car parking, lobby for public transport links
National and international action – set policy frameworks and targets, get political commitment, monitor targets, enforce regulations and inspection, provide resource to encourage change at lower levels

(Source: adapted from Jones, 2000, p. 214)

The concept of sustainability widens the debate about environmental impact and offers an ecological account of the interconnections of humans and the environment. It moves our social relationships, patterns of production and consumption, use of finite natural resources and concern for the ecosystem centre stage, and raises issues about our responsibilities to current and future generations. Within public health there has been growing acceptance of the conclusion of the United Nations (UN) *Report of the World Commission on Environment and Development: Our Common Future* (1987) that 'even the narrow notion of physical sustainability implies a concern for social equity between generations that must logically be extended to equity within each generation' (UN, 1987, p. 166). Among other strategies, Agenda 21 (UNCED, 1992), Health 21 (WHO, 1998a) and the UN Millennium Development Goals (MDG) (UN, 2000) have all included a commitment to generational and intergenerational environmental sustainability. But the challenges remain substantial and public health can only work in partnership.

The MDG include targets to:

- 'integrate the principles of sustainable development into country policies and programme; reverse loss of environmental resources' (although this lacked a target date)

- make a 'significant reduction' in biodiversity loss by 2010

- 'reduce by half the proportion of people without sustainable access to drinking water by 2015'.

The 2010 target was missed and MDG monitoring indicates that the 2015 target will not be met (UN, 2000).

New challenges for health protection

Some of the old challenges facing society in the past are returning in different guises as new challenges today. The industrial scale of modern medicine and explosion in use of drug therapies has brought new types of systemic health concerns. More drug-resistant strains of infectious diseases, such as tuberculosis, have developed through widespread and sometimes indiscriminate use of antibiotics in humans (Baggott, 2011) and via animals through the food chain. Ivan Illich (1977) termed this 'iatrogenesis' (damage done by the provider) and argued that modern health systems were increasingly the enemy rather than the champion of good health.

Poor hygiene and antibiotic resistance have been factors in the growth of hospital-acquired infections of which the best-known are Clostridium difficile (C. difficile) and methicillin-resistant Staphylococcus aureus (MRSA). In England for example, the Department of Health (DoH) (2004) reported that around 9000 deaths each year could be attributed to hospital-acquired infections and calculated the costs of treating them as around £1 billion. This resulted in strategies, targets and monitoring of MRSA and C. difficile, although other infections were overlooked (National Audit Office, 2009). Health-persuasion messages were slow to work in the context of MRSA and C. difficile, which were brought under control through systems-level strategies driven through by the Health Protection Agency and managers at all levels of the health service. In both cases remedial programmes have been effective; in mid 2011 MRSA cases stood at a record low with fewer than 100 infections per month across National Health Service (NHS) trusts in England. C. difficile cases in June 2011 were 16 per cent lower than in June 2010 (Press Association, 2011).

Risks – and costs – are evident in other areas of health protection too. In Chapter 14 we noted how complacency about food safety standards in the UK and Europe as a whole was challenged by salmonella outbreaks and 'mad cow' disease (BSE), which had a human impact through the degenerative brain disease Creutzfeldt-Jakob disease (CJD). The estimated cost of the BSE outbreak was £20 billion (Jones, 2007), a figure no doubt recorded as contributing positively to GNP. While CJD sufferers are so far few in number, outbreaks of salmonella in eggs, listeria in cheese and E.coli from undercooked meat products have resulted in thousands of casualties across the UK (Pennington, 2003). Around 80,000 cases of food poisoning are reported each year and around 500 deaths occur. Box 15.1 examines the outbreak and response to E.coli in Wales.

Box 15.1 The E.coli outbreak in South Wales (2005)

The first cases of E.coli 1057 in children were reported to the National Public Health Service for Wales on 16 June 2005 and within two days the food source had been identified and control measures put in place. The outbreak was traced to cross-contamination from raw to cooked meat products caused by faulty equipment and flagrant disregard of safety procedures by a local butcher who supplied meat to schools in the Bridgend area. An emergency prohibition notice was issued under section 12 of the 1990 Food Safety Act and, after a second notice, the premises (shop and abattoir) were closed. The Food Standards Agency (FSA) issued a Food Alert for Action (FARA notice) to all local authorities in Wales to remove all cooked meat products from schools. One hundred and fifty-seven children were affected across 44 schools, 65 per cent of cases infected from the original source. Thirty-one were treated in hospital and one child died.

The subsequent public inquiry report praised the coordination across the public health services and concluded that 'but for the quality of the analysis and control measures, the outbreak would have been considerably more severe and prolonged' (para. 48). In contrast, it severely criticised council environmental health officers for failing 'to assess the business management of food safety as well as they could, or should, have done' (para. 27) and for not picking up flaws in the company's plans. Meat Hygiene Service regulations were not followed and the abattoir was allowed to stay open in spite of breaching regulations. Bridgend Council was criticised for a 'seriously flawed' schools meals contract process (para. 37), which also was poorly monitored.

(FSA, 2009)

What improvements does the E.coli outbreak (Box 15.1) suggest might be needed to protect the public's health?

There is strong evidence that public health services coped well with the E.coli crisis, but some indication that cooperation between different agencies and organisations was not adequate and that enforcement was lax. Stronger enforcement of regulations and better coordinated systems-level responses are required to counter such hazards to health in the future, including integration of national, local authority and public health services.

Healthcare services have not delivered health for all despite their rising costs and, as noted earlier, marked health inequalities persist despite upward trends in wealth and average incomes (Wilkinson, R.G., 2005). As the cost of healthcare services continues to rise – fuelled by rising public expectations, longer life spans and new treatments – further growth may become unsustainable. At present, politicians largely value individual treatment and behaviour-change work but for economic reasons they may in future be prepared to invest more in prevention and health protection at a population level.

Counting in social welfare?

If public health is to succeed in delivering better physical and mental health for populations and individuals, it must count in social welfare. Health has always been about much more than healthcare provision. The challenges identified above are just another indication that health is unlikely to be delivered in isolation, but rather through working in a more integrated way with other policy sectors, in particular with other areas of social welfare.

Most countries have developed some type of welfare system and in wealthier countries this is often comprehensive. In the UK, for example, welfare policies evolved piecemeal but were brought together in the 1940s through the creation of the 'welfare state'. This provided social security for the workforce against sickness and unemployment, public housing, free access to education and a universal, free national health service. Underpinning all this was economic growth, bringing 'full employment' to deliver the jobs and taxation receipts that would pay for social security (Beveridge, 1942).

Such policies for social welfare, while they have varied considerably in terms of how they are financed and delivered, have been essential building blocks of the public's health. They have supported the most vulnerable groups in the population, provided health-sustaining services and played a modest part in some countries in redistributing resources. Indeed, we might claim in the UK that there is considerably more understanding of the social determinants of health in social services, housing and education than there is in most of the NHS. The language and cultures are very different but social workers, community and youth workers, housing officers and teachers are often at the 'sharp end' of managing social problems and have insight into the wider determinants of ill health in direct ways that NHS staff – and even some public health staff – do not. If the integration phase of public health development is to be realised, closer cooperation and joint planning between public health, health and other welfare services is essential. In some parts of the UK, notably Northern Ireland, the planning of care through health and social care boards delivers part of this agenda but there is still much joining up to do there (Appleby, 2005) and in the rest of the UK.

15.2 Responses: health policy to 'health in all policies'

Until the late twentieth century healthcare systems, governments and even the public health workforce demonstrated little enthusiasm for more integrated working or much recognition of the longstanding contribution of other social policy sectors in creating or sustaining health. Conversely, the health sector did not feature strongly in the development of other social policies. Rather, sectors developed policies with relatively little regard for other sectors and in many countries this is still widespread.

Within public health, WHO pioneered 'healthy public policy', calling for strategic action by national governments to create greater integration across policy sectors in the cause of health (see Box 15.2, page 460). It distinguished between 'traditional public health policy [which] is mainly geared towards securing and improving medical care and prevention ...

uni-sectoral and short-term in nature' and healthy public policy which 'is basically multi-sectoral in nature, moving beyond healthcare with a long-term view to create a healthy society' (WHO, 1990).

Box 15.2 Healthy public policy in the Adelaide Charter

Healthy public policy is characterized by an explicit concern for health and equity in all areas of policy and by an accountability for health impact. The main aim of healthy public policy is to create a supportive environment to enable people to lead healthy lives. Such a policy makes healthy choices possible or easier for citizens. It makes social and physical environments health enhancing. In the pursuit of healthy public policy, government sectors concerned with agriculture, trade, education, industry and communications need to take into account health as an essential factor when formulating policy. These sectors should be accountable for the health consequences of their policy decisions. They should pay as much attention to health as to economic considerations.

(WHO, 1988, p. 1)

Changing language, changing priorities?

The development of thinking about public policy integration was reflected in the 'WHO health promotion glossary', published in 1986 in a new journal, *Health Promotion International*. The glossary began to track the use of new terms, drawing its material from position papers, research work and statements from WHO conferences (see Box 15.3 for a list of key WHO conferences on health). Early entries were 'intersectoral policy' and 'new public health', defined as 'concern for the effect of the total environment on health' and referring back to the old public health movement of the nineteenth century (Nutbeam, 1986). When the glossary was updated in 1998 'healthy public policy' and 'settings for health' were added (Nutbeam, 1998) and in its next update (Smith et al., 2006) 'global health' was added to the glossary, representing a further stage in a developing dialogue about health and illness. Global health is defined as the 'transnational impact of globalisation on health determinants and problems which are beyond the control of individual nations.' Alongside this is a parallel dialogue about how public health and health-promotion practice should be framed and developed: 'capacity building', 'health impact assessment' and 'evidence-based health promotion' have all become familiar terms.

Box 15.3 The politics of health: some major WHO landmarks in health policy development

1977 – *Health for All by the Year 2000* set health targets mainly for reduction of disease, with emphasis on health as a human right and equity.

1978 – *Declaration of Alma Ata on Primary Health Care* calls for shift of resources towards primary-care and community settings.

1986 – *Ottawa Charter for Health Promotion* focused on building healthy public policy through creating supportive environments, strengthening personal and professional skills, community action and reorienting health services.

1988 – *Adelaide Recommendations on Healthy Public Policy* focus on wider determinants of health and steps towards building healthy public policies.

1998 – *Health for All for the 21st Century* revised the 1977 targets with greater emphasis on partnership, sustainable development and social determinants of health.

2002 – *Global Strategy for Food Safety*

2005 – *Framework Convention on Tobacco Control* (2003); binding convention, in effect from 2005.

2005 – *The Bangkok Charter for Health Promotion in a Globalized World* emphasised settings, intersectoral work and integration.

2010 – *Global Strategy to Reduce the Harmful Use of Alcohol*

2010 – *Adelaide Statement on Health in All Policies*

The glossary not only signals how language is changing but, linked to that, the vision that lies behind language and the priorities and approaches that are uppermost at particular times. Thus 'intersectoral policy' of the mid 1980s had become 'intersectoral collaboration' by the late 1990s, emphasising that partnership not just policy-making, was important. By 1998, 'healthy public policy' had entered the glossary alongside 'sustainable development' and 'determinants of health' (Nutbeam, 1998). Critics and policy makers alike began to couch their strategies in this language and to shift terminology to reflect its evolution. Campaigners in the UK, for example, combined 'new public health' and 'healthy public policy' as part of their reformist crusade:

> Many contemporary health problems are ... social rather than solely individual problems; underlying them are concrete issues of local and national public policy, and what are needed to address these problems are 'Healthy Public Policies' – policies in many fields which support the promotion of health. In the New Public Health the environment is social and psychological as well as physical.
>
> (Ashton and Seymour, 1988, p. 21)

Many countries adopted the language of healthy public policy and attempted to create it through 'intersectoral' and 'joined-up government' at national level and stimulate partnerships and alliances at regional and local levels. In the UK, Wales was in the forefront of this work, with a focus on national coordination and the 'duty to collaborate' and other countries set up 'interdepartmental' groups and committees. After 2000, public health policies significantly strengthened arrangements, with 'duties' and 'responsibilities' placed on other sectors to assess policies for their health impact.

Vision and values: health in all policies?

In the early twenty-first century, the language and the vision changed again: 'healthy public policy' evolved into 'health in all policies' (Kickbusch, 2008). 'Health in all policies' was defined as:

> an innovative strategy that reflects the critical role that health plays in the economies and social life of 21st century societies. It introduces better health – improved population health outcomes – and closing the health gap as shared goals across all parts of government. It aims to address complex health challenges through an integrated policy response across portfolio boundaries. By incorporating a concern with health impacts into the policy development process of all sectors and agencies, it allows government to address the key determinants of health in a more

systematic manner. It also takes into account the benefit of improved population health for the goals of other sectors.

(Kickbusch, 2008, p. 1)

What do you think are the key differences between a 'healthy public policy' and a 'health in all policies' approach?

Several key elements from 'healthy public policy' remained in 'health in all policies', such as integration, intersectoralism and systemic rather than piecemeal approaches. Healthy public policy focused mainly on the total environment at a population level rather than individual level, thereby aiming to distinguish itself from healthcare, whereas 'health in all policies' included a greater focus on better health in the round, including healthcare quality. The 'social determinants of health', a phrase very widely used especially after the publication of the WHO Commission Report on the Social Determinants of Health (2008), signalled a concern to address the social, economic, political and cultural causes of ill health at all levels and across all sectors.

Kickbusch et al. (2008) have documented the way in which the targets from the Adelaide Charter (WHO, 1988) were used to review South Australia's strategic plans, resulting in significant revision of policies in several sectors. The work culminated in a statement from a panel of WHO and South Australian health promotion experts on goals, stakeholders and techniques for creating 'health in all policies'. Box 15.4 sets out what the panel saw as being the key drivers for 'health in all policies'.

Box 15.4 Key drivers for 'health in all policies'

- Create strong alliances and partnerships that recognise mutual interests, and share targets.
- Build whole-government commitment by engaging the head of government, cabinet and/or parliament, as well as the administrative leadership.
- Develop strong high-level policy processes.
- Embed responsibilities into governments' overall strategies, goals and targets.
- Ensure joint decision making and accountability for outcomes.

- Enable openness and full consultative approaches to encourage stakeholder endorsement and advocacy.
- Encourage experimentation and innovation to find new models that integrate social, economic and environmental goals.
- Pool intellectual resources, integrating research and sharing wisdom from the field.
- Provide feedback mechanisms so that progress is evaluated and monitored at the highest level.

(WHO and the Government of South Australia, 2010)

What is the significance of the shift to 'health in all policies' and does the change of language denote a breakthrough moment? Kickbusch (2010) and others argue that steady progress has been made, with health rising up international and national agendas and even influencing national election outcomes. Health has become vital as a measure of overall government performance and the opportunity to deploy the health workforce to influence policies at all levels should be seized. This involves pressing for joined-up government and creating partnerships with civil society and the private sector. Krech and Buckett (2010, p. 258) have written about 'windows of opportunity' to 'change mind sets and decision-making cultures' at all levels and in all sectors.

On the other hand, in health promotion in particular, there is some sense of a 'lost generation'. After the breakthrough signalled by the Ottawa Charter (WHO, 1986) and the plethora of subsequent statements, strategies and policy frameworks that followed it (see Box 15.3), the dreams of healthy public policy – of intersectoral collaboration, population-level initiatives to reduce inequalities in health and support to transform communities – have faded. Progress has been slower and more difficult than anticipated; opposition has been stronger. Hopes have not been realised. In a challenging critique, Porter (2006) goes further, arguing that Ottawa principles have been subverted and more recent statements by WHO have replaced people-focused principles of equity and participation with technocratic and consumerist approaches.

Public health analysts have highlighted the difficulties encountered in driving through and implementing change, even where there is strong evidence that it is needed; inequalities in health persist in richer countries with comprehensive healthcare services.

In the UK, where healthcare is (almost entirely) free and accessible for all at the point of use, successive research reports since the 1960s have highlighted a continuing social class gradient in health. As noted in Chapter 2, semi-skilled and unskilled manual workers have shorter lives, experience more ill health and are much more likely to suffer debilitating long-term conditions than their non-manual and professional counterparts. Intermittently, governments have developed strategies and targets to tackle such inequalities. At other times, governments have explained that such variations are inevitable, that equality is an undesirable goal or that solutions can be delivered by individuals modifying their own behaviour. Whatever the approach, there is fairly little evidence that public health or the health sector in general has been capable of significantly reducing health inequalities (Marmot, 2010).

In Sweden, the conceptualisation of health as relating largely to social welfare meant that intersectoral policy did not engage other high-priority areas such as transport, planning and economic development. In addition, there was too much focus on making policy and too little on implementation of what was enacted to deliver the change agenda of the Ottawa Charter (Mannheimer et al., 2007). In the USA, concerns about individual freedom and responsibility severely constricted the ability of reformers to harness the power of state governments or federal government in the cause of health (Winkelstein, 2009).

In Canada, despite evidence that socioeconomic changes had most impact on health, the chosen approach focused on access to healthcare and persuasion to reduce unhealthy living (Collins and Hayes, 2007). Ottawa did not get implemented in Canada, partly because there was no consensus on the evidence and research findings were not translated into clear policy positions. Policy making was compartmentalised, with health care, not public health, the dominant voice for health. Politicians had short-term goals focusing on the next election and other policy sectors resented what they saw as health imperialism. The politicians in power, and the media, were resistant to structural interventions.

What barriers to change exist in your own organisation and how might they be overcome?

Some of these barriers are all too familiar, at whatever level change is sought: information challenges about the evidence, rigid institutional structures, powerful interest groups and political beliefs may all work against change (Low and Theriault, 2008; Raphael, 2009). Persistence and determination will inevitably be needed and progress will be slow. Groups and organisations, especially powerful ones, are unlikely to accept the pre-eminence of health as a goal as opposed to their existing ambitions and goals, established priorities, desire for profits or accepted cultural norms. Kickbusch has commented of the 'health in all policies' approach that:

> It is not unusual that such a process can create tensions within government as conflicts over values and diverging interests can emerge. Resolution can be achieved through persistent and systematic engagement with political processes and key decision-makers.

(Kickbusch, 2010, p. 263)

Implications for public health practitioners

Value conflicts and diverging interests exist not only in governments but also at all levels and across a range of sectors and organisations. A key part of the public health role, whether engaged in developing a small-scale initiative at local level or negotiating a policy change in a complex organisation, is to understand, engage with and move beyond competing interests to create healthier outcomes. In addition, resolution through negotiation means compromise and part of the debate about progress in building healthier futures relates to ethical dilemmas about what constitutes an ethical compromise as opposed to a betrayal of principles. Box 15.5 offers a global-level example of such a dilemma, posed by an organisation that now has a major role in global health: the Gates Foundation.

Box 15.5 'Money clashes with mission'?: *The Los Angeles Times* and the Gates Foundation

Since 1994 the Gates Foundation, set up by Bill Gates, CEO of Microsoft, and his wife Melinda, has funded health and development projects around the world. Nearly $US25 billion has been invested, of which around $US14.5 billion has been spent on global health and $US3.5 billion on development. It ranks alongside the WHO as a major investor and decision maker about priorities for health action. It funds public health projects, focusing on infectious diseases (such as malaria), HIV/AIDS and 'neglected' diseases. Through the Global Alliance for Vaccination and Immunisation (GAVI) it makes vaccines available for the poorest countries. Its development work includes projects to improve nutrition; maternal, neonatal and child health; and tobacco control.

In January 2007 *The Los Angeles Times* ran a story about the vast profits made from investments by the Gates Foundation that damage people's health. Their reporter highlighted how the Gates Foundation had invested heavily in subprime lenders and other businesses that did not support, and could be actively undermining, people's health and wellbeing. He claimed that in the case of the Gates Foundation, 'money clashes with mission' and 'undercut its good works', citing examples of damage and ill health directly linked to their investments. The Gates Foundation responded in the following terms:

> The stories you told of people who are suffering touched us all. But it is naive to suggest that an individual stockholder can stop that suffering. Changes in our investment practices would have little or no impact on these issues. While shareholder activism has worthwhile goals, we believe a much more direct way to help people is by making grants and working with other donors to improve health, reduce poverty and strengthen education.

(Piller, 2007)

What stance would you take in such a case? From the viewpoint of the Gates Foundation, it was drawing a clear distinction between business ethics and charitable giving. Grants and partnerships were direct ways of improving health, whereas structural change through shareholder pressure to change investment practices would have negligible effect. However, a 'health in all policies' approach might well involve systematic assessment of the degree to which these investment practices sustained and promoted health as opposed to undermining it. The risk in such a review is that it might 'turn off the tap' of charitable giving by the Gates Foundation. The dilemma is a real one for practitioners at many levels: public health alliances and interventions increasingly include commercial and corporate sponsors. What ethical stance is appropriate? If *The Los Angeles Times* criticism is justified, does $US25 billion invested in health outweigh 'vast profits' from likely health-damaging investments? Is the evidence of beneficence or non-maleficence (see Chapter 5) robust enough to justify the Gates Foundation's position?

15.3 Supporting public health development

Some of the main threats to health today, as noted earlier, do not respect national borders and arise from complex interactions associated with globalisation (Lee and Collin, 2005). Conversely, some of the resources to support health are sustained by global action and facilitated by globalisation. To what extent are capabilities for public health development being strengthened at global, regional and national levels?

Structures, frameworks and governance: working for health?

Global institutions have joined with wealthy G8 nations to create partnerships for public health, for example the Global Fund to combat AIDS, tuberculosis and malaria (GFTAM). Some of the global profits of Microsoft have found their way, via the Gates Foundation, into major health and development projects in the poorest countries (see Box 15.5). A host of other non-governmental organisations (NGOs), such as Oxfam and Médecins Sans Frontières, attract worldwide donations to invest in health projects in poor countries. The WHO itself, with an annual budget in 2006–2007 of $US3.3 billion, draws 70 per cent of its income from international agencies, foundations, countries and other partners and only 25 per cent from regular membership dues. There are signs that a sense of corporate social responsibility is leading some multinationals into greater involvement in health-policy development and even regulation. Opinion is divided about whether this reflects a genuine concern for the poor and sick or whether it is a means to gain influence and greater respectability: very likely it is both (Bakan, 2005).

One important effect of global threats to health, which we noted earlier, has been increasing acknowledgement of the need for global responses. Potentially pandemic influenza outbreaks have led to much greater coordination by national health agencies at global level, led by the WHO. Global regulation of greenhouse gases and other emissions, although under attack as a way forward, has made an impact in some countries as noted in Section 15.1 and evidence of health impact has been a major way of moving it forward. On some issues, even against powerful opposing interests, the WHO has worked successfully to bring about reforms, although other areas such as diet and nutrition have proved more intractable (Lee, 2010). In the case of tobacco, a recognised carcinogen and still the main cause of premature death globally, a global regulatory framework was drawn up that is providing a model for other industries and sectors. The framework and an outline of its development are set out in Box 15.6.

Box 15.6 Global regulation of tobacco

It is predicted that tobacco will cause 10 million deaths annually by 2030, concentrated in poorer and developing countries. Tobacco is a highly addictive substance and its production, marketing and consumption serves the powerful interests of multinational corporations. Smoking has declined in wealthier countries since the 1980s, assisted in the EU by tougher safeguards on advertising and tar levels and high taxes in some states. But it has grown rapidly in low- and middle-income states in Africa and south-east Asia, with 70 per cent of tobacco-related deaths predicted in future to be in these 'emerging markets'.

Until 1998 the WHO developed tobacco control strategies, which relied on persuading member states to conform and urging global agencies (such as the World Bank) to take tobacco control seriously. The Framework Convention on Tobacco Control was devised to address the transnational aspects, such as illicit trade and cross-border marketing. The Framework Convention Alliance established by the WHO played a key role in mobilising and harnessing NGOs and organisations from many different countries and at all levels. They became partners with strong involvement in lobbying, developing reports and leading campaigning. The Framework Convention on Tobacco Control came into effect in 2005 and nearly 200 countries have signed it and 60 have ratified it. Strong leadership, clearly defined goals, the involvement of civil society, the requirement for national signatories (rather than a voluntary code) and very strong health evidence of harm (which tobacco companies could not avoid acknowledging) were some of the reasons for its success.

(Chapman, 2007; Lee, 2010)

Regulation and leadership for health does not just happen at global level. Regional players such as the EU also intervene and influence health across national borders. The European Region Office of the WHO (1998a) produced *Health 21, the Health for All Framework for the European Region*, which laid out a set of targets for achievement in stages by 2020. This strategy includes targets related to health improvement, systems enhancement and reduction of health inequalities, although only the last of these has specific target figures included. These require a reduction of one-third in the health-status gap between member states of the European region by 2020, and a reduction by one quarter in the gap between socioeconomic groups within each member state by 2020. It has prompted action in many countries, including continuing commitment to action across all UK nations, but seems very unlikely to be achieved in the light of widespread economic recession. Job cuts, rising living costs and a growth in unemployment across the EU have resulted in rising levels of poverty and insecurity: conditions in which people's health is at much greater risk.

Since 2002 the EU has been implementing its public health strategy, with an emphasis on public protection that has been reinforced through the Lisbon Treaty (EU, 2009). Monitoring and coordination against cross-border health threats and of safety standards was supplemented in 2009 by an explicit reference to wellbeing as well as to physical health, suggesting that in the future health might move higher up the agenda (Baggott, 2011). However, the EU health budget is tiny and its Directorate of Health and Consumers is relatively weak: other sectors such as economic policy and agriculture are much more powerful and can exert influence on health policy (Greer, 2009).

At national level, governments and health systems play a key role in public health, not only in secondary and tertiary prevention but also in health protection measures such as infection control and emergency relief. There is some encouraging evidence of integration in public health services. The Public Health Agency of Canada, for example, was established in 2005 to integrate national public health functions and enable a more systematic approach to problems such as health inequalities (Stachenko et al., 2009). In several other countries, including the UK at national level, similar structural integration has taken place so that health protection and health improvement work can be coordinated.

Why do you think national-level coordination is so important for global public health in the future?

It has been argued that 'progress in global health is first and foremost dependent on the performance of health systems at the national and local level' (Kickbusch and Seck, 2010, p. 154). Global surveillance, management and response systems are only as strong as their weakest link when a pandemic or natural disaster threatens. In the UK there are strong systems in place but new threats to health, such as those from terrorism, have highlighted a lack of coordination between different services (e.g. the coordination of health, fire and transport services in the case of the 7 July 2005 bombing in London and see Box 15.2 for the issues arising from the 2005 E.coli outbreak in Wales). In poor or war-torn countries, lack of investment in public health measures such as water and sanitation, and an inadequate or poorly trained public health workforce, pose not just a national but also a global danger.

At national level there is also emerging evidence that systematic and sustained scrutiny of policies to identify their health-threatening features, and then to amend them to protect people's health or create better health outcomes, can be made to work. Guidelines that have emerged from the experience of the South Australian government reviewing its strategic plans identify some of the techniques and approaches that can enable 'health in all policies' to begin to be delivered (Kickbusch et al., 2008). These are set out in Box 15.7 (page 472) and include already well-known tools, such as impact assessment and some more novel approaches. 'Health lens analysis', for example, involves a process of systematic scrutiny against set criteria by an expert panel. While the focus of the tools in Box 15.7 is regional government level, many are equally applicable at local and organisational level.

> **Box 15.7 Enabling 'health in all policies'**
>
> Tools and instruments that have shown to be useful at different stages of the policy cycle include:
>
> - inter-ministerial and inter-departmental committees
> - community consultations and citizens' juries
> - cross-sector action teams
> - partnership platforms
> - integrated budgets and accounting
> - health lens analysis
> - cross-cutting information and evaluation systems
> - impact assessments
> - joined-up workforce development
> - legislative frameworks.
>
> (WHO and the Government of South Australia, 2010)

At global level, however, many public health experts remain gloomy about making further progress, unless better global governance of health can be secured. As the authority of the WHO has been weakened, an array of trade and business groupings, public–private alliances, NGOs and regional organisations has become involved in directing, financing and managing aspects of public health. The resultant 'unstructured plurality' (Beck and Lau, 2005) is destabilising – not least because of a lack of accountability. The voice of the WHO has often been ignored and its leadership criticised (Horton, 2006). The World Bank and the WTO have gained ground, but doubts remain about their commitment to health. Lee et al. (2009) highlight the actions of the WTO in breaching the health protection regulations agreed by its members when it suits richer countries to do so. Considerations of trade and profit, not health, are the major drivers of multinational enterprise (Bakan, 2005; Ollila, 2005).

But other observers have argued that increasing complexity and fragmentation in health politics has resulted in a more shifting and pluralist climate in which even powerful players can be held to account in some areas. Sustained criticism of the health consequences of market liberal World Bank policies on lending to poor countries, for example, did persuade it to adopt a revised approach, which included capability building and poverty-reduction programmes, together with adoption of tobacco control policies (McMichael and Beaglehole, 2009). In 2006 the World Health Assembly called for greater linkage to health across different sectors and was successful in prompting the World Bank and the WTO to develop a framework on trade and health policies.

Kickbusch and Seck (2010) have argued that effective global health governance is an essential element in ensuring that resources are used effectively and ethically, that organisations and agencies are held to account for what they do in the name of health and that initiatives are coordinated. Projects should not be duplicated or nations left unable to cope with initiatives because they lack adequate infrastructure or workforce. This requires organisation and leadership, from the WHO or an equivalent agency, 'to ensure transparency and accountability in global health governance and play a brokering role in relation to the health impacts of other agencies' (Kickbusch and Seck, 2010, p. 157).

What about the workforce?

If cross-border leadership and organisational coherence is still lacking, how far is the public health workforce ready to 'fill the gap' in dealing with new threats and by working in new ways? To what extent can an approach that seeks to include 'health in all policies' be made to work at grassroots level?

In wealthier countries, where healthcare systems are sophisticated and comprehensive, a dedicated public health workforce usually exists, largely focused on surveillance, primary prevention and health protection but increasingly trying to engage in tackling health inequalities. Secondary and tertiary prevention may be dealt with by professionals who are mainly engaged in providing primary, acute and social care. Beyond this is what is termed in the UK the 'wider public health workforce' (Griffiths et al., 2005), which includes not only the health and social care workforce but also a very wide range of people at all levels in public, private and voluntary sectors who have, or need to have, the understanding and skills to participate in public health-related work. To achieve 'health in all policies' requires engagement from this very wide community, which is partly why public health workforce training and professional development in the UK, as noted in Chapter 4, is now moving up the political agenda.

In contrast, many poorer countries are struggling with an under-strength, sometimes poorly trained and poorly paid health workforce.

Some health professionals, such as nurses who might have had a public health dimension to their work, are migrating to more secure and better paid jobs in Europe and the USA (Dovlo, 2009), although there have been systematic attempts, not least in the UK, to prevent health services recruiting in this way. Some African nations have developed 'task shifting' and created extended roles for community-health workers with a combined public health and primary healthcare remit (WHO, 2007; McPake and Mensah, 2008). Box 15.8 describes task shifting in Uganda to deal with the HIV/AIDS crisis. HIV/AIDS has been particularly destructive because of its impact on the healthcare workforce and on other professional groups, such as teachers.

Box 15.8 Tackling the HIV/AIDS epidemic: task shifting in Uganda

In Uganda, task shifting is the basis for providing antiretroviral therapy. Uganda's nurses are now undertaking a range of tasks that were formerly the responsibility of doctors, such as: managing people living with HIV who have opportunistic infections; diagnosing tuberculosis sputum positive; prescribing medicine to prevent other infections; and deciding on medical eligibility for antiretroviral therapy.

In turn, tasks that were formerly the responsibility of nurses have been shifted to community health workers, who have training in a range of theoretical and practical clinical skills but not professional qualifications. These tasks include: HIV testing; counselling and education; monitoring and supporting adherence to therapy; clinical follow-up; and taking weight and vital signs.

In addition, a range of non-professional types of healthcare workers receive specific task-related training. These include community members who focus on education on HIV prevention, adherence to medication and ongoing support and monitoring, and people living with HIV give support in triage, education and counselling.

(WHO, 2007, p. 4)

Task shifting is designed to safeguard healthcare quality, an important dimension of public health but largely aimed at 'fire-fighting' a huge health crisis. It inevitably focuses on medical treatment and on tertiary prevention. In general in poor countries, the public health workforce is under-resourced, relying on the efforts of NGOs in the poorest countries to provide a sometimes haphazard array of sanitation, nutrition, maternal and child-health interventions that may or may not reach those in greatest need. Having reviewed evidence from around the world, including Europe, Beaglehole and Bonita (2009) reached the gloomy conclusion that:

> The public health workforce is not in a position to respond appropriately to the old, let alone the new challenges … With very few exceptions, governments have neglected public health workforce development and the public health infrastructure in general …. In all countries the proportion of the health budget allocated to public health activities is less than 5 per cent, and usually of the order of 1–2 per cent … Building the public health workforce is a long-term undertaking and will require a substantial commitment of new resources ….
>
> (Beaglehole and Bonita, 2009, p. 286)

Graham (2010) has echoed some of these concerns, arguing in particular that public health is preoccupied with current problems and is failing to identify and prepare for the ecological and systems challenges of the future.

The 'health in all policies' approach acknowledges these difficulties. The South Australia government experiment (Kickbusch et al., 2008) identifies a key role for all health services – not just public health – in challenging policies, developing the evidence base and leading change. Public health needs to mobilise groups across the health sector and other sectors, indicating that analysing, negotiating and influencing skills will be key to its future role. The skill-set required was set out in the Adelaide statement (WHO and the Government of South Australia, 2010) and is highly relevant to public health practice at organisational and local level. It includes:

- understanding the political agendas and administrative imperatives of other sectors
- building the knowledge and evidence base of policy options and strategies

- assessing comparative health consequences of options within the policy development process
- creating regular platforms for dialogue and problem solving with other sectors
- evaluating the effectiveness of intersectoral work and integrated policy making
- building capacity through better mechanisms, resources, agency support and skilled and dedicated staff
- working with other arms of government to achieve their goals and in so doing advance health and wellbeing.

In what ways could this skill-set be useful for public health work in organisations or at local level?

Those already engaged in public health practice might be familiar with these techniques already. Capacity building, partnership, intersectoral work, research and option appraisal are all well documented, not least by the authors in this book, as important techniques to deploy. What is striking is that by bringing these together into a type of 'toolkit' the strategic importance of public health practice is immediately highlighted. At whatever level it is deployed, this toolkit focuses on enabling, advocacy, horizon-scanning and capacity building rather than just on 'doing' interventions, guidance work, activity or advice sessions, screening, and so on. This does not mean that such 'doing' work is not important; for most practitioners in local authorities, the health sector, education, social services, and so on it is, and will continue to be, the core of their work. But if 'health in all policies' is to be achieved it will require more than just pronouncements by governments, scrutiny of plans or even new regulations, difficult though they will be to develop. It will require champions of public health at all levels who can ensure that the policies for health are enacted in organisations and local institutions, implementation is rigorous and transparent, and consultation and participation is fair and effective. It will also require new alliances, not least with powerful voices within clinical medicine.

The potential rewards are great. If health is systematically considered and protected through policy making and implementation, 'health in all policies' could deliver significant reductions in health inequalities. It could mean a greater concern for health, for example as new housing is built, transport is planned, cities are reshaped, or facilities and amenities are developed.

15.4 Alternative futures?

What is the likely future for public health across the UK and at international level? To what extent does public health possess the vision, values, structures, workforce and resources to extend its role? Much depends on the extent to which health and wellbeing continue to be seen as important objectives for politicians, businesses and the general public. Table 15.3 (page 478) sketches alternative futures for public health. This is a risky activity and in doing it, acknowledgement is made of the limitations of models and 'ideal types'. These scenarios are altogether more modest in their intentions – a heuristic device to get anyone interested in public health to reflect on future directions and on what part they themselves might play in realising desired goals.

Amid the judgements and predictions, it should be noted that a further scenario – the deterioration of public health over the next decade – has not been included. There is evidence in this chapter to indicate a risk that, amid climate change, global recession and restructuring, health might get squeezed off international and national agendas. The negative implications of globalisation (see Table 15.1) might drive to the margins its potential for assisting in health development. However, many indicators are pointing in the other direction: towards a healthier future for public health.

In what ways do you think the 'fully engaged' scenario in Table 15.3 presents a likely future for public health?

There is some reason for cautious optimism. As noted at the start of this chapter, other sectors are viewing health, at the least, as a convenient banner under which to press for policy change. The WHO Framework Convention on Tobacco Control (WHO, 2003) has demonstrated that such an approach is practical, at least on an issue which can gather strong international support. In some countries, including the UK, public health services are becoming more integrated and some greater concern for workforce development is visible. The leadership of WHO has been revived, in particular in leading global thinking about intersectoralism and the strengthening of vulnerable health systems through workforce and governance development. However, challenges remain, not least the tendency for governments and practitioners to focus downstream on behaviour change and miss opportunities to engage in more fundamental and potentially transformative action on the social determinants of health.

Table 15.3 Alternative futures for public health

Dimensions	'Business as usual'*	'Fully engaged'*
Vision and values	Focus on lifestyle changes with variable commitment to reducing health inequalities	Population health, health equity and wellbeing as national and global priorities
	Public health partially or not integrated; different sectors continue with own priorities	Public health integrated across social, economic and health policies
	Values base of voluntarism; much reactive engagement	Values base of social justice and empowerment
Scope and focus	Scope unclear; some joining-up of public health functions and intersectoral initiatives but focus largely on healthcare	Encompasses action at all levels and across all sectors to improve population health
	Global strategy partially or not implemented at national level	Connects national strategies to global strategies, feeding both ways
Leadership and workforce development	Continued lack of investment in public health workforce development at all levels (public health stays at 2–5 per cent of total health budget)	Investment in public health strategic leadership development to tackle broader agenda (e.g. inequalities, climate change, mental health)
	Ad hoc, temporary workforce recruitment to address new concerns (e.g. obesity)	Development work with other sectors to embed public health priorities
	Lack of cohesion and shared vision	Wider public health workforce development prioritised to ensure skill-set and values enshrined
Structures and resourcing	Some global frameworks adopted but reluctance to use regulation/legislation	Frameworks at global, regional, national and local level, as appropriate
	Search for 'magic bullet' solution to problems	National health systems strengthened; research supported
	Much work/funding remains initiative based and short term	Two-way partnership at all levels
		Decisive shift of funding to preventive, social determinants and health inequalities work

* The terms 'business as usual' and 'fully engaged' are those used by Wanless (2004) to describe the different extent to which England might choose to drive forward the public health agenda.

Conclusion

This chapter has highlighted a wide range of issues that present new challenges for public health, including globalisation and climate change. In doing so it has also focused on investigating how public health is responding to these challenges at national, regional and, in particular, global levels. The evolution of Health for All principles into 'healthy public policy' and 'health in all policies' has been accompanied by a growing confidence that public health has something unique to contribute to debates about health and wellbeing.

While it is important for public health to contribute to a robust and efficient national health system, it should also be influencing policy makers, agencies and organisations in sectors other than health to give greater priority to population health and wellbeing and to focus upstream on tackling the structural causes of ill health. In a 'fully engaged' future, public health and the public health workforce should be striving not just for efficiency and effectiveness but for social justice.

References

Appleby, J. (2005) *Independent Review of Health and Social Services Care in Northern Ireland*, Belfast, Department of Health, Social Services and Public Safety, Northern Ireland.

Ashton, J. and Seymour, H. (1988) *The New Public Health*, Milton Keynes, Open University Press.

Baggott, R. (2011) *Public Health: Policy and Politics* (2nd edition), Basingstoke, Palgrave Macmillan.

Bakan, S. (2005) *The Corporation: The Pathological Pursuit of Profit and Power*, London, Constable.

Beaglehole, R. and Bonita, R. (2009) 'Strengthening public health for the new era' in *Global Public Health: A New Era*, Oxford, Oxford University Press, pp. 283–98.

Beck, U. and Lau, C. (2005) 'Second modernity as a research agenda: theoretical and empirical explorations in the "meta-change" of modern society', *The British Journal of Sociology*, vol. 56, pp. 525–57.

Beveridge, W. (1942) *Full Employment in a Free Society*, London, George Allen and Unwin.

Chapman, S. (2007) *Public Health Advocacy and Tobacco Control: Making Smoking History*, Oxford, Blackwell.

Collins, P.A. and Hayes, M.V. (2007) 'Twenty years since Ottawa and Epp: researchers' reflections on challenges, gains and future prospects for reducing health inequalities in Canada', *Health Promotion International*, vol. 22, no. 4, pp. 337–45.

Department of Health (DoH) (2003) *Winning Ways: Working Together to Reduce Healthcare Associated Infection in England: Report From the Chief Medical Officer*, London, Department of Health. Available at: www.dh.gov.uk/en/Publicationsandstatistics/Publications/PublicationsPolicyAndGuidance/DH_4064682 (accessed 10 September 2011).

Department of Health (DoH) (2004) *Towards Cleaner Hospitals and Lower Rates of Infection*, London, Department of Health. Available at: www.dh.gov.uk/en/Publicationsandstatistics/Publications/PublicationsPolicyAndGuidance/DH_4085649 (accessed 10 September 2011).

Dovlo, D. (2009) *Health Sector Reform and Deployment, Training and Motivation of Human Resources towards Equity in Health Care: Issues and Concerns in Ghana*, Bellville, HRH (Human Resource for Health) for Africa, University of the Western Cape. Available at: http://hrhforafrica.org.za/index.php?option=com_library&task=book_detail&book_name=Health+Sector+Reform+and+Deployment,+Training+and+Motivation+of+Human+Resources+towards+Equity+in+Health+Care+:+Issues+and+Concerns+in+Ghana&id=62&Itemid=71 (accessed 26 September 2011).

European Union (EU) (2009) *The Lisbon Treaty*, Brussels, European Union.

Food Standards Authority (FSA) (2009) *The Public Inquiry into the September 2005 Outbreak of E coli 0157 in South Wales*, Cardiff, National Assembly for Wales. Available at: http://wales.gov.uk/ecolidocs/3008707/reporten.pdf?skip=1&lang=en (accessed 10 September 2011).

Graham, H. (2010) 'Where is the future in public health?', *The Milbank Quarterly*, vol. 88, no. 2, pp. 149–168.

Greer, S. (2009) *The Politics of European Union Health Policies*, Maidenhead, Open University Press.

Griffiths, J., Jewell, T. and Donnelly, P. (2005) 'The three domains of public health', *Public Health*, vol. 119, pp. 907–13.

Haines, A., Kovats, R., Campbell-Lendrum, D. and Corvalan, C. (2006) 'Climate change and human health: impacts, vulnerability and mitigation', *The Lancet*, vol. 367, pp. 2109–11.

Harvey, F. (2011) 'Sir David King: we should abandon Kyoto Protocol on climate change', *The Guardian*, 15 July. Available at: www.guardian.co.uk/environment/2011/jul/15/david-king-abandon-kyoto-protocol?INTCMP=SRCH (accessed 10 September 2011).

Health Protection Agency (2008) *The Health Effects of Climate Change in the UK*, London, Health Protection Agency/Department of Health. Available at: www.dh.gov.uk/en/Publicationsandstatistics/Publications/PublicationsPolicyAndGuidance/DH_4007935 (accessed 10 September 2011).

Horton, R. (2006) 'WHO: strengthening the road to renewal', *The Lancet*, vol. 367, pp. 1793–95.

Illich, I. (1977) *Limits to Medicine: The Expropriation of Health*, Harmondsworth, Penguin.

Jones, L. (2000) 'Health promotion and environmental politics' in Jones, L. and Sidell, M. (eds) *The Challenge of Promoting Health: Exploration and Action*, Basingstoke, Macmillan, pp. 183–206.

Jones, T. (2007) 'Are we winning the battle?', *Health Protection Matters*, vol. 8, pp. 5–7.

Kickbusch, I. (2010) 'Health in all policies: where to from here?', *Health Promotion International*, vol. 25, no. 3, pp. 261–4.

Kickbusch, I. (2008) *Policy Innovation for Health*, New York, Springer.

Kickbusch, I. and Seck, B. (2010) 'Global public health' in Douglas, J., Earle, S., Handsley, S., Jones, L., Lloyd, C.E. and Spurr, S. (eds) *A Reader in Promoting Public Health* (2nd edition), London, Sage, pp. 151–59.

Kickbusch, I., McCann, W. and Sherbon, T. (2008) 'Adelaide revisited: from healthy public policy to health in all policies', *Health Promotion International*, vol. 23, no. 1, p. 104.

Krech, R. and Buckett, K. (2010) 'The Adelaide statement on health in all policies: moving towards shared governance for health and wellbeing', *Health Promotion International*, vol. 25, no. 2, pp. 258–60.

Lang, T., Barling, D. and Caraher, M. (2009) *Food Policy: Integrating Health, Environment and Society*, Oxford, Oxford University Press.

Lee, K. (2010) 'Global health promotion: how can we strengthen governance and build effective strategies?' in Douglas, J., Earle, S., Handsley, S., Jones, L., Lloyd, C.E. and Spurr, S. (eds) *A Reader in Promoting Public Health*, London, Sage, pp. 171–6.

Lee, K. and Collin, J. (eds) (2005) *Global Change and Health*, Maidenhead, McGraw-Hill/Open University Press.

Lee, K., Sridhar, D. and Patel, M. (2009) 'Bridging the divide: global governance of trade and health', *The Lancet*, vol. 373, pp. 416–22.

Low, J. and Theriault, L. (2008) 'Health promotion policy in Canada: lessons forgotten, lessons still to learn', *Health Promotion International*, vol. 23, no. 2, pp.200–6.

Mannheimer, L.N., Lehto, J. and Ostlin, P. (2007) 'Window of opportunity for intersectoral health policy in Sweden – open, half-open or half-shut?', *Health Promotion International*, vol. 22, no. 4, pp. 307–15.

Marmot, M. (chair) (2010) *Fair Society, Healthy Lives: Strategic Review of Health Inequalities in England Post-2010*, London, The Marmot Review. Available at: www.marmotreview.org/AssetLibrary/pdfs/Reports/FairSocietyHealthyLives. pdf (accessed 10 September 2011).

McKeown, T. (1976) *The Role of Medicine: Dream, Mirage or Nemesis*, London, Nuffield Provincial Hospitals Trust.

McMichael, A. and Beaglehole, R. (2009) 'The global context for public health' in *Global Public Health: A New Era*, Oxford, Oxford University Press, pp. 1–22.

McPake, B. and Mensah, K. (2008) 'Task shifting in health care in resource-poor countries', *The Lancet*, vol. 372, no. 9642, pp. 870–71.

National Audit Office (2009) *Reducing Healthcare Associated Infections in Hospitals in England*, London, The Stationery Office. Available at: www.nao.org.uk/ whats_new/0809/0809560.aspx (accessed 10 September 2011).

Nutbeam, D. (1998) 'Health promotion glossary: new terms', *Health Promotion International*, vol. 13, no. 4, pp. 349–59.

Nutbeam, D. (1986) 'Health promotion glossary', *Health Promotion International*, vol. 1, no. 1, pp. 113–27.

Ollila, E. (2005) 'Global health priorities: priorities of the wealthy?', *Globalisation and Health*, vol. 1, no. 6, p. 106.

Pennington, H. (2003) *When Food Kills: BSE, E Coli and Disaster Science*, Oxford, Oxford University Press.

Piller, C. (2007) 'Gates Foundation to keep its investment approach', *Los Angeles Times*, 14 January. Available at: http://latimes.com.business/la-na-gates14jan14.1.1844117.story (accessed 10 September 2011).

Popay, J., Griffiths, J., Draper, P. and Dennis, J. (1993) 'The impact of industrialisation on world health' in Beattie, A., Gott, M., Jones, L. and Sidell, M. *Health and Wellbeing: A Reader*, Basingstoke, Macmillan, pp. 272–80.

Porter, C. (2006) 'Ottawa to Bangkok: changing health promotion discourse', *Health Promotion International*, vol. 22, no. 1, pp. 72–79.

Press Association (2011) 'MRSA rates in England at record low, figures show', *The Guardian*, 4 August. Available at: www.guardian.co.uk/society/2011/aug/03/mrsa-rates-england-record-low (accessed 10 September 2011).

Raphael, D. (2009) 'Mainstream media coverage and the social determinants of health in Canada: is it time to call it a day?', *Health Promotion International*, vol. 26, no. 2, pp. 220–29.

Schumacher, E.F. (1974) *Small Is Beautiful*, London, Abacus.

Smith, B.J., Tang, K.C. and Nutbeam, D. (2006) 'WHO health promotion glossary: new terms', *Health Promotion International*, vol. 21, no. 4, p. 342.

Stachenko, S., Legowski, B. and Geneau, R. (2009) 'Improving Canada's response to public health challenges: the creation of a new public health agency' in *Global Public Health: A New Era*, Oxford, Oxford University Press, pp. 123–38.

United Nations (UN) (2000) *Millennium Development Goals*, New York, United Nations. Available at: www.un.org/millenniumgoals/poverty.shtml (accessed 10 September 2011).

United Nations (UN) (1997) *Kyoto Protocol*, New York, United Nations. Available at: http://unfccc.int/resource/docs/convkp/kpeng.pdf (accessed 10 September 2011).

United Nations (UN) (1987) *Report of the World Commission on Environment and Development: Our Common Future*, New York, United Nations. Available at: www.un-documents.net/wced-ocf.htm (accessed 10 September 2011).

UNCED (1992) United Nations Conference on Environment and Development, Brazil.

Victor, D.G. (2011a) 'Why the UN can never stop climate change', *The Guardian*, 4 April. Available at: www.guardian.co.uk/environment/2011/apr/04/un-climate-change?intcmp=239 (accessed 10 September 2011).

Victor, D.G. (2011b) *Global Warming Gridlock*, Cambridge, Cambridge University Press.

Wanless, D. (2004) *Securing Good Health for the Whole Population*, London, HM Treasury.

Wilkinson, P. (2005) 'Global environmental change and health' in Scriven, A. and Garman, S. (eds) *Promoting Health, Global Perspectives*, Basingstoke, Palgrave Macmillan, pp. 129–42.

Wilkinson, R.G. (2008) *The Spirit Level*, London, Routledge.

Wilkinson, R.G. (2005) *The Impact of Inequality*, London, Routledge.

Winkelstein, D. (2009) 'The development of American public health policy', *Journal of Public Health Policy*, vol. 30, no. 1, pp. 40–48.

World Health Organization (WHO) (2010) *Global Strategy to Reduce the Harmful Use of Alcohol*, Geneva, World Health Organization. Available at: www.searo. who.int/LinkFiles/Meeting_reports_GSRH-Alcohol.pdf (accessed 2 October 2011).

World Health Organization (WHO) (2008) *Closing the Gap in a Generation. Report of the WHO Commission on the Social Determinants of Health*, Geneva, World Health Organization. Available at: http://whqlibdoc.who.int/publications/2008/ 9789241563703_eng.pdf (accessed 10 September 2011).

World Health Organization (WHO) (2007) *Report on Task-shifting*, Geneva, World Health Organization.

World Health Organization (WHO) (2005) *The Bangkok Charter for Health Promotion in a Globalized World*, Geneva, World Health Organization. Available at: .www.who.int/healthpromotion/conferences/6gchp/hpr_050829_ BCHP.pdf (accessed 2 October 2011).

World Health Organization (WHO) (2003) *Framework Convention on Tobacco Control*, Geneva, World Health Organization.

World Health Organization (WHO) (2002) *Global Strategy for Food Safety: Safer Food for Better Health*, Geneva, World Health Organization. Available at: www. who.int/foodsafety/publications/general/en/strategy_en.pdf (accessed 2 October 2011).

World Health Organization (WHO) (2001) *Report of the Commission on Macroeconomics and Health: Macroeconomics and Health: Investing in Health for Economic Development*, Geneva, World Health Organization. Available at: www. who.int/macrohealth/action/Report of the National Commission.pdf (accessed 10 September 2011).

World Health Organization (WHO) (1998a) *Health 21, the Health for All Framework for the European Region*, Copenhagen, European Regional Office. Available at: www.euro.who.int/__data/assets/pdf_file/0010/98398/ wa540ga199heeng.pdf (accessed 10 September 2011).

World Health Organization (WHO) (1998b) *Health Promotion Glossary*, Geneva, World Health Organization. Available at: www.who.int/hpr/NPH/docs/ hp_glossary_en.pdf (accessed 10 September 2011).

World Health Organization (WHO) (1990) *Investment in Health*, Geneva, World Health Organization.

World Health Organization (WHO) (1988) *Adelaide Recommendations on Healthy Public Policy*, Geneva, World Health Organization. Available at: www.who.int/healthpromotion/conferences/previous/adelaide/en/index.html (accessed 10 September 2011).

World Health Organization (WHO) (1986) *The Ottawa Charter for Health Promotion*, Geneva, World Health Organization. Available at: www.who.int/hpr/NPH/docs/ottawa_charter_hp.pdf (accessed 10 September 2011).

World Health Organization (WHO) (1978) *Alma Ata Declaration*, World Health Organization. Available at: www.who.int/hpr/NPH/docs/declaration_almaata.pdf (accessed 2 October 2011).

World Health Organization (WHO) (1977) *Health for All by the Year 2000*, World Health Organization.

World Health Organization and the Government of South Australia (2010) *Adelaide Statement on Health in All Policies*, WHO and the Government of South Australia. Available at: www.who.int/social_determinants/hiap_statement_who_sa_final.pdf (accessed 10 September 2011).

Acknowledgements

Grateful acknowledgement is made to the following sources:

Figures

Figure 1.1 Office for National Statistics; **Figures 2.1a and 2.1b** Courtesy of Gapminder; **Figure 2.2** Data taken from WHO Health for All database, http://data.euro.who.int; **Figure 2.4** Adapted from Norman, P., Gregory, I., Dorling, D. and Baker, A. (2008) 'Geographical trends in infant mortality: England and Wales, 1970– 2006', *Health Statistics Quarterly*, Office for National Statistics; **Figure 2.5** Dahlgren, G. and Whitehead, M. (1991) *Policies and Strategies to Promote Social Equity in Health*, Stockholm, Institute for Futures Studies; **Figure 2.6** Adapted from Organization for Economic Co-operation and Development, 'Income distribution – poverty', *OECD.StatExtracts*, www.oecd.org, OECD; **Figure 3.1** Schein, E.H. (2004) 'The levels of culture', *Organizational Culture and Leadership*, Jossey-Bass; **Figure 3.2** Vangen, S. and Huxham, C. (2003) 'Nurturing collaborative relations: building trust in interorganizational collaboration', *The Journal of Applied Behavioural Science*, vol. 39, no. 1, pp. 5–31; **Figure 3.3** Oakland, J.S. and Turner, S.J. (2006) 'Quality management in the 21st century: implementing successful change', *International Journal of Productivity and Quality Management*, vol. 1, no. 1/2, pp. 69–87; **Figure 4.1** Kolb, D.A. (1984) *Experiential Learning: Experience as the Source of Learning and Development*, Prentice-Hall, Inc., A Division of Pearson Education; **Figure 4.4** Gibbs, G. (1988) *Learning by Doing: a guide to teaching and learning methods*, Oxford Further Education Unit; **Figure 6.1** Adapted from Gabe, J., Calnan, M. and Bury, M. (1991) *The Sociology of the Health Service*, Routledge; **Figure 6.2** Transtheoretical Theory of Change Model, Prochaska, J.O and DiClemente, C.C. (1984) *The Transtheoretical Approach: Crossing Traditional Boundaries of Therapy*, Dow Jones Irwin; **Figure 6.3** Rogers, E.M. and Scott, K.L. (1997) *The Diffusion of Innovations Model and Outreach for the National Network of Libraries of Medicine to Native American Communities*, http://nnlm.gov/archive/pnr/eval/rogers.html, Department of Communication and Journalism, University of New Mexico, National Network of Libraries of Medicine; **Figure 6.4** Caplan, R. and Holland, R. (1990) 'Rethinking health education theory', *Health Education Journal*, vol. 49, pp. 10–12; **Figure 7.2** OECD iLibrary (2010): *Quality of Life*, OECD Fact Book (2010): *Economical, Environmental and Social Statistics*, OECD; **Figure 7.3** Office for National Statistics (2009) 'Infant, neonatal and perinatal mortality rates 2008'. Reproduced under the terms of OGL for PSI, www.nationalarchives.gov.uk/doc/open-government-license; **Figure 7.4** Williams, H., Dodge, M., Higgs, G., et al. (1997) *Mortality and Deprivation in Wales*, Cardiff, University of Wales. Reproduced with permission; **Figure 7.5** Health protection Agency (2010) 'New diagnoses of syphilis and gonorrhoea at GUM clinics by gender, 2000–2009 United Kingdom', *Health Protection Report*, vol. 4, no. 34; **Figure 7.6** Health Education Authority (1995) *A Survey of the UK Population Part 1: Health and Lifestyles*, HEA; **Figure 7.7** Joint United Nations Programme on HIV/AIDS (2008) *AIDS epidemic update*, www.unaids.org, World Health Organization, United Nations; **Figure 7.8** Office for National Statistics (2009) *Smoking and Drinking among Adults (2009) – General Household Survey: A Report on the 2009 General Lifestyle Survey*; **Figure 7.9** The King's Fund; **Figure 10.1** Green, J. and Tones, K. (2010) *Health Promotion Planning and Strategies* (2nd edn), Sage Publications Ltd, fig. 3.3, p. 117; **Figure 10.2** National Healthy Schools Programme (2009) *Whole School Approach to the National Healthy Schools Programme*, Department of Health and Department for Children, Schools and Families; **Figure 11.1** NHS Health Scotland (2003) *LEAP for Health: Learning, Evaluating And Planning*, Glasgow, M&M Press; **Figure 12.2** National Healthy Schools Programme (2009) *Whole School Approach to the National Healthy Schools Programme*, Department of Health and Department for Children, Schools and Families; **Figure 13.2** World Health Organization (WHO) (2002) *Community Participation in Local Health and Sustainable Development: Approaches and Techniques*, European Sustainable Development and Health Series: 4, Geneva, WHO; **Figure 14.1** Based on The Nuffield Council on Bioethics Intervention Ladder; **Figure 14.2** Adapted from Beattie, A. (1991) 'Knowledge and control in health promotion: A test case for social policy and social theory', in Gabe, J., Calnan, M. and Bury, M. (eds) *The Sociology of the Health Service*, Routledge; **Figure 14.4** Adapted from Beattie, A. (1991) 'Knowledge and control in health promotion: a test case for social theory', in Gabe, J., Calnan, M. and Bury, M. (eds) *The Sociology of the Health Service*, London, Routledge and Lee, P. and Raban, C. (1983) 'Welfare and ideology' in Loney, M., Boswell, D. and Clarke, J. (eds) *Social Policy and Social Welfare*, Milton Keynes, Open University Press; **Figure 14.5** Lang, T., Barling, D. and Caraher, M. (2009) *Food Policy: Integrating Health, Society and the Environment*, Oxford, Oxford University Press.

Tables

Table 2.1 World Health Organization (WHO) (2008) *Global Burden of Disease 2004 Update*, WHO. Copyright © 2008 World Health Organization; **Table 9.2** Adapted from Hawe, P., Degeling, D. and Hall, J. (1990) *Evaluating Health Promotion: A Health Worker's Guide*, MacLennan & Petty; **Table 10.1** Behavioural Insights Team (2010) *Applying Behavioural Insight to Health*, Cabinet Office and Institute for Government. Reproduced under the terms of OGL for PSI, www.nationalarchives.gov.uk/doc/open-government-license; **Table 12.1** Adapted from Whitelaw, S., Baxendale, A., Bryce, C., Machardy, L., Young, I. and Witney, E. (2001) 'Settings based health promotion: a review', *Health Promotion International*, vol. 16, no. 4, pp. 339–53, Oxford University Press; **Table 14.2** Adapted from Lang, T., Barling, D. and Caraher, M. (2009) *Food Policy: Integrating Health, Society and the Environment*, Oxford, Oxford University Press.

Text

Box 3.2 Belbin's Team Roles, www.belbin.com, Belbin Associates 2007–2010.

Every effort has been made to contact copyright holders. If any have been inadvertently overlooked the publishers will be pleased to make the necessary arrangements at the first opportunity.

Index